Clinical Studies in

Infant Mental Health

CLINICAL STUDIES

IN INFANT

MENTAL HEALTH

The First Year of Life

EDITOR

SELMA FRAIBERG

In collaboration with Louis Fraiberg

Basic Books, Inc., Publishers

NEW YORK

An earlier version of chapter 7 appeared in the *Journal of the American Academy of Child Psychiatry*, vol. 14, no. 3, Summer 1975, pp. 387–422. An earlier version of chapter 8 appeared as "Infant-Parent Psychoanalysis on Behalf of a Child in a Critical Nutritional State," in *Psychoanalytic Study of the Child*, vol. 31, 1976, pp. 461–491. An earlier version of chapter 12 appeared as "A Model for the Introduction of Infant Mental Health Services to Community Mental Health Agencies," in the *Journal of the American Academy of Child Psychiatry*, vol. 14, no. 3, 1975.

Library of Congress Cataloging in Publication Data

Fraiberg, Selma H
   Clinical studies in infant mental health.

   Includes bibliographies and index.
   1. Infant psychiatry. I. Title. [DNLM: 1. Mental
health—In infancy and childhood.   WS105.5.M3 C641]
RJ502.5.F7   618.9289   79–3078
ISBN 0–495–01170–5

CONTENTS

Contents

Contents

CONTRIBUTORS

EDNA ADELSON is an Assistant Research Scientist in the Department of Psychiatry at the University of Michigan Medical School. She has been a Staff Psychologist at the Child Development Project since 1967.

CAROLYN R. ARADINE is an Associate Professor of Parent–Child Nursing at the University of Michigan School of Nursing and a senior staff member in the Child Development Project of the Department of Psychiatry at the University of Michigan with which she has been associated since 1974.

JOHN W. BENNETT JR., is a Senior Social Worker in the Child Development Project of the Department of Psychiatry at the University of Michigan Medical Center. During the 1975–1976 academic year he was a Grant Foundation Post-Graduate Fellow in Infant Mental Health.

VICKI ANN BENNETT is a Psychotherapist and Infant Mental Health Specialist. During the 1974–1975 academic year she was a Grant Foundation Post-Graduate Fellow in Infant Mental Health.

PETER BLOS, JR., is Acting Director of the Child Development Project and Lecturer in the Department of Psychiatry at the University of Michigan. He is also Lecturer in the Michigan Psychoanalytic Institute.

DEBORAH SPITZ CHERNISS is currently the general editor of the series on child development and social policy published by the Bush Program in Child Development and Social Policy at the University of Michigan, where she has been a Fellow. She worked for three years at the Child Development Project of the Department of Psychiatry at the University of Michigan.

SELMA FRAIBERG is Professor of Child Psychoanalysis in the Departments of Psychiatry and Pediatrics of the University of California San Francisco. She is Director of the Infant-Parent Program at San Francisco General Hospital.

ALICIA F. LIEBERMAN is a Senior Psychologist in the Infant-Parent Program at San Francisco General Hospital (University of California San Francisco).

JEREE PAWL is Associate Director of the Infant-Parent Program at San Francisco General Hospital (University of California San Francisco).

Contributors

VIVIAN SHAPIRO is a Lecturer in the Department of Psychiatry of the University of Michigan Medical School and has been a Senior Social Worker at the Child Development Project since 1972. She is Assistant Professor of Social Work in the School of Social Work of the University of Michigan.

BETTY TABLEMAN is Director of the Michigan Department of Mental Health's prevention programming. She is responsible for implementing infant mental health services through community mental health.

HOWARD UMAN is Chief, Pediatrics Division, U.S. Public Health Service Hospital, Seattle, Washington; Clinical Assistant Professor, Department of Pediatrics, University of Washington, School of Medicine; formerly Behavioral Pediatrics Fellow, University of Washington, 1977–1978, and Pediatrics Trainee at the Child Development Project, University of Michigan, 1976–1977.

PREFACE AND ACKNOWLEDGMENTS

THIS COLLECTION of papers describes major aspects of the clinical methods which we developed at the Child Development Project, University of Michigan, for assessment and treatment of developmental disturbances in infancy. This volume is one of our promised outcomes to two sponsors, the Grant Foundation and the National Institute of Mental Health.

We are indebted to the Grant Foundation for its support of this program during the period 1972 to 1979. Philip Sapir, director of the Grant Foundation during these years, fairly merits the title "godfather" to this program—he was present at the christening and he was present to provide good counsel during the early development of this baby. On behalf of the babies, their families, and ourselves we wish to say "thank you" by exchanging gifts.

From 1974 to 1980 the National Institute of Mental Health supported our program through Grant #MH 24746. This grant was for a research and demonstration project on the effects of intervention in infancy. We proposed to develop clinical methods in the treatment of babies and parents who showed the early signs of attachment disorders and to assess developmental outcomes. Our report of the "outcome" study will appear in later publications. The study of clinical methods can be followed in this volume through illustrative cases. During the years of our NIMH support Dr. Michael Fishman, then our program officer, followed our work with close attention and became our valued advisor at many points in program development and research design. We are deeply grateful to him.

My own work at the Child Development Project ended in July 1979 when the University of California Medical School, San Francisco, invited me and a group of colleagues at the Project to begin a new program in infant mental health at San Francisco General Hospital. The work at the Child Development Project, University of Michigan, continues with Dr. Peter Blos, Jr., as acting director.

Our thanks to Adele Wilson, Beverly Knickerbocker, and Jeri Hixon for preparation of manuscripts and for devoted attention to detail at every step in the process of writing this book.

Clinical Studies in Infant Mental Health

I

Introduction

SELMA FRAIBERG

DURING the past two decades, clinical and developmental research in infancy have given us answers to a multitude of questions that had once seemed unanswerable. Today, we are in possession of a vast scientific treasure acquired through the study of normal and deviant infants, a treasure that should be returned to babies and their families as a gift from science.

We now know that a very large number of the most severe and intractable emotional disorders of children and adults can be traced to developmental disorders and conflicts in the first two years of life, the embryonic period of personality development. Impoverishment in early sense experience, impediments to the formation of human bonds, and conflicts between the baby and his human partners appear as recurrent themes in the developmental histories of many children and adults who suffer severe personality disorders. By the time we meet these patients in child or psychiatric clinics, it may take the whole of our colossal apparatus of psychotherapy and remedial education, as well as years of professional work, to undo or repair the damage to personality. Yet the morbid signs were present in infancy.

As for the developmental side of the story, we now have a consensus among scientists from a wide range of disciplines that the human capacities for love and for learning are rooted in the sensorimotor period of development, the first eighteen months of life. The developmental significance of emotional impoverishment in infancy and the disruption of human bonds in the early years of life is documented in a literature on maternal and sensory deprivation that has sobered a generation of scientists. In the cognitive realm we have amassed a library of studies which have led to the consensus that sensorimotor learning provides the building blocks for all later cognitive development. And from both clinic and laboratory there is strong evidence to support the commonsense view that affective and cognitive development are inextricably interwoven in the development of the infant and child.

In briefest summary:

We know what babies need for the fullest development of their innate capacities.

We know the danger signs in early development.

We know what parents need for their own fulfillment as parents.

The scientific treasure of which we speak is largely stored in our libraries, but the babies themselves have not been its full beneficiaries. Between the library and the baby in need there is a great gulf: We are missing the scientist-intermediary who can bridge this gulf. We need psychiatrists, pediatricians, nurses, psychologists, and social workers who can identify the psychologically imperiled infant, and bring the resources of psychiatry and the community to the baby and his parents in programs of clinical intervention. We need infant mental health specialists in each of these disciplines, and we need a very large measure of training in normal and deviant infant development to enable the mental health professions to engage in a vast collaborative work on behalf of infants. In the United States there are only a small number of mental health specialists who have been equipped through their professional training to engage in preventive work on behalf of infants.

In this volume we will describe our experiences as a psychiatric team in the development of an infant mental health program within a department of psychiatry. It is our hope that this report of clinical problems in the identification and treatment of infants at risk will be useful to colleagues in the mental health professions at a time when we see unprecedented concern for infants and a proliferation of new programs in mental health settings.

The program we will describe here is in no sense to be regarded as a "model." Our own conception of infant mental health would embrace a large number of models, each reflecting the unique problems of a particular infant population, each adapted to the setting in which the work is performed and the professional expertise represented in its staff. We also conceive of infant mental health as a province of community mental health which extends beyond the borders of any clinic or social agency. We are concerned with the implications for social policy, for law, and for social welfare practice.

The Child Development Project: An Infant Program in a Department of Psychiatry

Our current program at the Child Development Project unites clinical services for infants 0 to 3 years of age, a clinical research program, and a training program for mental health specialists in the diagnosis and treatment of infants with a wide range of developmental disorders.

Our clinical program has served approximately 140 families per year in Washtenaw County, Michigan (population approximately 300,000). A network of clinics and social agencies within our own hospital and the larger community constitutes our referral sources. The majority of our infants are referred to us because of very severe disturbances—failure to thrive, neglect, and abuse—often reflecting severe parental psychopathology and family disorder. Most of our families are in the low income range. We do not charge fees.

At the time of this writing (August 1977), our senior staff is composed of two psychoanalytic consultants, a pediatric consultant, a pediatric nurse, three clinical psychologists, and two social workers. All but one of the staff members are part-time. The eight senior staff members represent the full-time equivalent of 4.5 staff members (this includes myself). Six trainees in child psychiatry, pediatrics, pediatric nursing, and clinical psychology (pre- and post-doctoral) carry a limited number of cases in our program.

HISTORY OF THE CHILD DEVELOPMENT PROJECT

Our history as an infant research program should be briefly described since it has undoubtedly influenced the direction of our current infant mental health program and our methods.

The Child Development Project was established in 1965 as a research unit in the Department of Psychiatry, University of Michigan Medical School. Between 1965 and 1972 we were engaged in longitudinal developmental studies of infants blind from birth, an investigation which was supported by the National Institute of Child Health and Development. In the course of our work, we were able to identify the unique adaptive problems for the blind infant during the sensorimotor period, which in many instances led to an impasse in development for the child. We also saw the extraordinary problems for the parents of a blind infant, who not only needed to overcome their grief and despondency to become adequate parents but were cut off from their baby by his sightless eyes and his incomprehensible patterns of development.

As a research team composed of well-trained clinicians in the field of psychiatry, psychology, and social work, we responded to both the pain of these parents and its dangers for the baby; we felt it imperative that we offer our own understanding to the parents and employ our research findings in ways that might facilitate the development of each child and promote the relationship between parents and child. We presented a proposal to the Office of Education Bureau of the Handicapped for a guidance program on behalf of blind infants and received support for this program between 1969 and 1972. We believe this may have been the first infant mental health program of its kind.

It had very significant consequences. First, we developed methods of intervention for this unique population which were later applicable to other infant populations (Fraiberg et al. 1969; Fraiberg 1971). Second, and most important, intervention in infancy for our blind group demonstrably facilitated the development of these children. At the conclusion of this program in 1972 we were able to report that the blind children who had received guidance during the first two years of life demonstrated human attachment, language, and motor capabilities that brought them closer to sighted child ranges than to blind child ranges (Fraiberg 1977). The evidence of significant gains gave us confidence that intervention in infancy was intervention at the most favorable stage of the growth cycle.

We saw the implications for other disadvantaged infants and their parents. As clinicians we knew that emotionally impoverished infants, even though biologically intact, constituted a vast imperiled population within every community. And we also knew, as clinicians, that for the emotionally empty child psychiatric intervention later in childhood could rarely bring him the human qualities which are normally given every baby in the first two years of life.

Accordingly, we submitted a proposal to the Grant Foundation of New York requesting support for a program that would reflect these ideas. In 1972 we received a generous award from the Grant Foundation for a program which we called "An Infant Mental Health Program." The new work began in October 1972 with a small, experienced staff. Edna Adelson, Evelyn Atreya, and I represented the "old" staff, and Vivian Shapiro, an experienced child therapist, joined us at the start of the new program.

During the first two years of this program, we set ourselves the task of developing diagnostic and treatment methods for a new population of infants and their families. We had envisioned dealing with a wide range of developmental disorders in infancy ranging from "moderate to severe." We saw ourselves as serving many families with "everyday" problems in infant rearing: babies, for example, with mild feeding or sleep disturbances. We also expected that a small number of our cases would fall into the "severe" range.

Our projections were wrong. The baby with "the little feeding disturbance" never appeared. From the start we began to get referrals of babies who could be classified in the "severe" range, and today the largest number of our cases are gravely imperiled babies and their families. Our program was defined by community needs and, most certainly, by the fact that we were a clinic in a psychiatric department. Judging from our referrals, we were seen as a clinic for the assessment and treatment of severe disorders in infancy.

When we began this new program, we had no models for program development or for assessment and treatment methods beyond those which we had developed in our earlier program for blind infants. Much that we had learned in our earlier program was to be of great value to us in designing the new program for a broad spectrum of infant disorders. (I will illustrate this very shortly.) But the severity of the infant and family pathology which we saw in our new population required the development of new methods.

Our families in the blind infant program had represented the full spectrum of a normal population, and the incidence of gross parental psychopathology was probably not larger than that in the general population. Guidance methods for a family in crisis because of the birth of a blind child can assume a fair degree of adequacy and adaptive capacity in most parents, and the infant himself, even though biologically imperiled by his blindness, need not be neglected, abused, or the center of parental psychopathology. With the parents as our allies, our methods were primarily those of "developmental guidance" on behalf of the blind infant. It was the baby who was our patient, not his parents. In the rare cases where parental psychopathology impeded our work on behalf of the infant, we sought psychiatric help for the parents.

In our new program we could see developmental guidance as central to the work, but it was clear that we would need to find methods which could reach parents incapacitated by their psychological conflicts. The baby *and* his parents were now our patients.

Yet as we reflect upon the evolution of our infant mental health program from its origins in a research and clinical program for blind infants, we can identify many elements of the new program that originated in the old. The new work, like the old, is largely carried on through home visits, with the baby very much present and the focus of our work with his parents. The range of observations provided by the home visit cannot be duplicated in any way in an office-centered program for infants. And since infants are frequently constrained in a strange situation (as are their parents very often), we are more likely to get the optimal range of the infant's and his parents' capabilities and the quality of their interactions through the familiar setting of the home and its climate.

Our concept of the multidisciplinary approach to infant guidance work had already been well established in the earlier program. Our staff, as I described it, includes representatives from nearly all of the professions that contribute to the mental health of infants. But there is no arbitrary assignment of function. As therapists we all do the same work and employ methods which do not distinguish a clinical psychologist from a social worker. We use each other's expertise in consultation and supervision, in program development, and in teaching.

Our research base has carried over into the new work. Outcome studies of treatment were designed in the early stages of our new work. We also anticipated clinical studies of subgroups in our population. This means that from the start we employed observational procedures and recording methods that would insure objectivity and provide clinical detail and a narrative of process—the data base for all projected studies. One difference in procedure was indicated. In our research program for blind infants we were privileged to make on-the-spot notations in data collection. (The parents were not our patients; the blind baby was the subject of our study; our educational guidance was an outgrowth of that study. The baby, whether as subject or as patient, did not object to our note taking; neither did his parents.) In the new program the parents were our patients, too, and note taking, we felt, would be an impediment to free discourse, to candor, to the expression of intimate feelings. We chose, then, to record after each session and to record, as faithfully as memory permitted, the detailed narrative of each session.

We had learned to use videotape for periodic documentation of development in our work with the blind infants. In our new program we again chose to use video in a natural, unobtrusive way at intervals of approximately three months. In our earlier program the video had also served as a means of helping our parents observe their child's development, and we had developed tactful ways in which the parent could use tape observation for self-observation. This too carried over into our new program.

And finally, certain principles of intervention in infancy which had served us well in our earlier blind program were transferred to the new work. We already knew that nearly all parents of endangered babies could find it within themselves to "bring the best" to their children when a trusted professional ally stood with and by them in periods of stress. We saw ourselves as allies, not as "teachers" or "models." We saw each baby and his family as uniquely constituted, and the pathways which led to successful resolution of developmental problems, we believed, must be uniquely constituted as guidance methods for this baby, this family.

With these experiences from the program for blind infants we entered our new work for an as yet unknown population of imperiled infants and their families.

THE INFANT MENTAL HEALTH PROGRAM

We devoted a four-month period between June 1972 and October 1972 to the development of a referral network within our hospital and within the larger community of Washtenaw County. At the invitation of many clinic and social agency chiefs, we visited, described the objectives of our new program, and invited questions and referral inquiries. We described the projected range of problems and services we were prepared to offer. We emphasized, I remember, at each visit our interest in babies with developmental problems in the moderate range and said we would be prepared to take on "a small number of babies with problems in the severe range." On October 15 we formally opened our program. The phone rang and our first referral came to us from one of the university clinics. "Jane, age 5½ months. Mother in a severe depression. Mother wants to surrender baby for adoption. Baby appears to be neglected. . . ."

201 EAST CATHERINE

The setting for a program such as ours is of considerable importance, we believe. The building that we occupy is an ancient and venerable Ann Arbor monument, a granary in the 1870s, a laundry between 1935 and 1960. For the decade of the 1960s it housed the university's radiation lab. In 1970, when space at the University Hospital became tight, we moved from the medical center to the then vacant building on Catherine Street.

The building is situated in the oldest part of the city, approximately one mile from the medical center and one mile from the University of Michigan's central campus. The neighborhood is regarded as a slum by many people and an area of "urban renewal" by others. Our close neighbors are mainly impoverished families. Junkies and prostitutes have settled into the landscape of decaying buildings, porno shops, massage parlors, and sleazy bars.

Our closest neighbor is the block-long Farmer's Market, which is the town meeting place three days a week from April to November. During these months it is alive with colorful Ann Arbor natives, flower stalls, and the produce of the countryside. Native crafts, mainly pots and macramé, are strung up in booths. At the end of the block, urban renewal has appeared in the form of a remodelled ancient building which now houses a Chinese delicatessen, a fish store, a pickle shop, and various boutiques.

At our end of the street urban renewal has stopped, as though the imagination of the City Plan Commission failed before the task. From my window on the second floor of our building I can take in the view of urban decay which spreads out for a mile or two either side of Fourth Street. We are established residents of the neighborhood. Occasionally one of our neighbors wanders into our building to complain about his relief check (Social Service is across the street) or plots against his life (the Crisis Center is down the street one block), to threaten the City Fathers (City Hall is two blocks away), or to tell his life story to our intake worker, who will steer him to a source of help. All this takes place within a building which is clearly labeled "The Child Development Project."

The old granary which is our house is a splendid building for our work. Within, it is furnished like a home, with white walls, bright carpets, comfortable seating, green plants, and wall hangings which the staff has chosen to delight small children and their parents. On the entrance level we have a brightly furnished reception room (not a "waiting" room, since nobody must wait for an appointment with us), staff offices, each reflecting the taste of its occupant, a large library with an excellent collection of books and periodicals, and a conference room.

On the lower level, away from street noises, are playrooms, one for infants, one for toddlers, furnished with sturdy furniture for the children, comfortable chairs and sofas for parents and therapists. Between appointments the toy shelves look bare. This is because the rooms are "furnished" for each child before an appointment. The therapist chooses appropriate toys and equipment for a baby or toddler of a particular age with particular needs. A toy storage room with catalogued and labeled toys provides all the necessary materials from which the therapist can select. The rationale for this plan is very simple. If each of the playrooms were equipped for all ages and needs, a small child would be overwhelmed and we would see a restless moving from toy to toy, many of which would be inappropriate for his age. Further, our selection of toys becomes a tacit form of education for our parents. Our toys and books are sturdy, well made, often very beautiful objects. We also try to choose some toys which parents of limited income can find in dime stores. In watching their babies and toddlers at play in our rooms, parents make fascinating discoveries regarding the educational function of toys. Soon we find these discoveries reflected in the toys they select for their children. Picture books, carefully chosen for the toddlers, introduce many parents to the discovery that learning to love books can begin in a parent's lap with a picture story. We also have a lending library of toys and books and a gift collection of toys and books for the many babies whose families cannot afford to buy toys. We have found tactful ways of giving these toys to needy families without hurting pride. (Actually, these toys come from a gift fund which is replenished like the Purse of Fortunatus by friends of the Project or parents who wish to show appreciation for our help and from whom we will not accept fees. It is easy then to say to needy parents that the toys are gifts from many friends of the Child Development Project.)

Also on the lower level of the building is one room set aside for psychological testing. In an earlier space plan we had used one of the playrooms, but we soon discovered that our toddlers were puzzled, if not outraged, when they came into "their" playroom to find the room "remodeled" to accommodate testing and to find that something strange and different was required of them today. The tester, even when he had been properly introduced one visit earlier, was now taking the initiative that ordinarily "belonged to" the therapist. In fairness to the children and to facilitate testing, we decided to give testing its own space with its own "rules." The plan has worked well.

Our audiovisual department is also on the lower level, protected from street noises and other interferences with videotaping. One large room serves as a lab housing videotape and editing equipment. All tapes and films are filed and stored for easy retrieval, and an index to each tape leads us quickly into its contents. Taping is done by our audiovisual coordinator or by student assistants trained for this work. We must have psychologically educated eyes behind the camera. Our photographers sit in on our seminars, which brings them close to our work and our objectives, and their beautiful tapes reflect their own understanding of "what is important" in observing a baby and his parents. (As a bonus—and not coincidentally—our student assistants receive their introduction to clinical infant work through their work with us and many, over the years, have chosen careers in related fields.)

The second floor of our building is reached through a broad staircase. At the first landing, children are greeted by a mural of Winnie the Pooh ascending with a cluster of bright balloons. On the second floor are staff offices, graduate students' offices, secretarial offices, the main file room, and the office of Lily Ladin, administrative assistant, who is really several people under the same name. She is assistant director, business manager, chief of protocol, director of public relations, ombudsman, editorial consultant, and official translator in four foreign languages.

On the third floor are more staff offices, graduate student and secretarial offices, a lounge, a small kitchen, and an antique shower stall which is, as yet, unused.

Our housing plan reflects our staff plan. We do not have a social work division, a clinical psychology division, a medical division, a student group, a secretarial group. We are distributed throughout the building in such a way that on the third floor, for example, Peter Blos (our psychiatrist) is across the hall from Bill Schafer (clinical psychologist), and graduate students occupy the offices down the hall. Vivian Shapiro (chief social worker) and Carolyn Aradine (pediatric nurse) are neighbors on the first floor with graduate students whose offices cluster around the perimeter of the building. Edna Adelson (clinical psychologist) and John Bennett (social worker) are my neighbors on the second floor. Jeree Pawl (clinical psychologist) has a commanding view of the stairway traffic on the second floor and offers hospitality to members of all disciplines, without prejudice.

There is normally a heavy flow of traffic between floors since each staff member serves as consultant to all others in his field of expertness, a process which we will see illustrated in our description of the work.

PEDIATRIC HEALTH CARE

During the first two years of our infant mental health program, we discovered that the largest number of babies referred to us (and the most imperiled in every aspect of development) were not receiving well-baby care and had no regular connection with the Washtenaw County medical network. In a community rich in medical resources, the families of these babies rarely met a physician outside of the emergency room. The families in poverty were eligible for Medicaid, of course, but rarely, if ever, had they exercised their privilege of using the clinics or private physicians for sustained family health care and, specifically, pediatric care.

There were three major problems in bringing pediatric care to our families. First, we needed a network of collaborating pediatricians. Second, we needed to educate our families to use the medical services available to them. Third, we needed to educate the pediatricians about our work to help the families on behalf of their babies' health.

When Dr. Ruben Meyer joined our staff as a consulting pediatrician, he developed a pediatric network which brought the highest quality of medical care to our patients. A number of private pediatricians became our collaborators in this program. Both Dr. Meyer and Carolyn Aradine, our pediatric nurse, served as liaison between the project and the pediatric network and maternity health services. Systematic medical recordkeeping was instituted in our program. In 1977, Dr. Stephen Blackman became our pediatric consultant and a member of the health research team.

The therapists assigned to each case took responsibility for educating the family in the basic health care of the infant and, equally important, in understanding the physician's concern with maintenance of health and prevention of illness. The therapists themselves often initiated our families into this new world and its new concepts by driving mothers and babies to the clinic or physician's office, and by sitting with them in the waiting room and offering emotional support in every way they could. They helped parents articulate their questions to professionals, discussed again what physicians had told them, and translated medical terminology into language more readily understood by the families. If children or parents were hospitalized, the therapists also went to visit them.

We discovered one of the reasons that many families in poverty do not ordinarily use the medical resources available to them. For it was not only ignorance we saw, but fear—an irrational fear of doctors and hospitals which was highly complex in origin. Often as we sat with parents and a baby, we saw something close to panic in these grown men and women, a panic that belonged to their own childhood experience of pain and illness. The doctor was a symbol of danger before the patient had ever set eyes upon him. This anxiety diminished when the doctor and his staff became known as persons to our patients (and we could quietly bow out of the role of initiator and symbolic handholder in the waiting room).

In this way our parents (with rare exceptions) became users of medical services like most others, who brought their babies to the doctor for regular checkups, who felt free to ask questions and advice, who recognized early symptoms of illness in their baby and called the doctor promptly. They had learned to trust *their* children's doctors.

In addition, some of these parents had been unable to obtain needed medical care for themselves and were now enabled by the therapists' support, intervention, and education to be less fearful and to seek health care for themselves as well. They learned that doctors, nurses, and hospitals could help them as well as their children.

INTAKE AND THE DECISION PROCESS

Every member of the senior staff serves as "intake worker" on a rotation basis. John Bennett serves as intake coordinator and consultant.

During the years of our NIMH-Grant Foundation program we have averaged 140 referrals and inquiries per year. We regard every referral of a baby as a sign of crisis and respond immediately to the request for service. There is no "waiting list." No baby, in our view, should wait for help; no parents in need should wait for help.

Not every baby among the 140 referred to us will require treatment through our clinic. However, we are prepared to take on the most difficult cases up to the limit of our staff resources. At the first intake conference we explore as fully as possible the special conditions of the baby and family which have led to the request for service. In certain of the cases referred to us, we may judge that another clinic or social agency can serve the families' needs as well as or better than we and suggest alternatives to our referral source. Also, given the size of our staff, we cannot serve all families. In the largest number of cases we offer an extended assessment of the baby and his family (typically five sessions, which includes developmental testing) and consult with the referring clinic or agency at the close of the assessment period for further planning. At the close of the assessment we may conclude together that: (1) the problems identified can be handled within the framework of the referring agency or another agency (we will offer periodic consultation if the clinic wishes); or (2) that the problems identified require the specialized treatment alternatives which we can provide, and we move toward a treatment plan at the Child Development Project.

The following table will provide a picture of the distribution of our cases in these categories in a typical year.

Assessment only or brief treatment	32%
Intensive treatment	40%
Consultation with or referral to other agencies	28%

Thus in any one month, our active caseload is comprised of these categories: (1) assessment in progress; (2) consultation with other agencies; (3) brief treatment; (4) intensive treatment. Every new case begins, of course, in assessment. The treatment of choice may lead to (2), (3), or (4). In later chapters we will describe and illustrate with clinical examples the methods of assessment and the methods employed in each of the categories of service which we provide. It will be useful, however, if we provide a brief description of these services in this preliminary overview.

ASSESSMENT

Each case accepted for service is assigned at intake to a therapist and a supporting team. From the start, the therapist is identified to the family and the referring agency, and will carry through, both in the assessment period and the treatment program. (We place great importance upon this form of intake. Parents in need, parents in crisis, must have *a person*, not an agency, to represent help and promise. The initial transference to this person, who represents a responder to need, may be the crucial determinant in outcome of the work.)

A supporting team (some members of which may, in practice, be invisible to the patient) is assigned at the same time. A supervisor-consultant is appointed to the team. Every staff member, regardless of years of experience or expertness in this work, consults with a senior staff member on a regular weekly or twice-monthly basis. Work with imperiled infants is emotionally draining. The decision-making process is, in a certain sense, life-giving or even life-saving for the child. To share the emotional burden, to achieve the highest degree of objectivity, and to bring our best judgment to the case, we have chosen this method of staffing.

Developmental testing is assigned to another member of the team. In our program, every senior staff member is trained to administer the Bayley Scales of Infant Development. This means that the tester may be a social worker or a clinical psychologist. Clinical psychologists on our staff may consult with members of other disciplines on problems of scoring or interpretation or, in the event that other tests are administered, may take over the testing program. We have found this an effective and economical use of our staff. This means that we have a pool of qualified testers, instead of one or two staff members who would certainly be inundated with testing assignments. It also means that every staff member is as knowledgeable as he needs to be in the area of infant testing.

Our pediatrician becomes a member of the team at the start. Our pediatric nurse may also be assigned to the team at this point. Medical records are gathered, reviewed, and summarized for our records. Consultation on medical issues will take place in the course of the assessment. Liaison with physicians and medical services is established.

On the same basis, our psychiatrist becomes available for consultation on the most difficult diagnostic issues and to participate in the decision process.

A social worker, who is involved in every new case, is automatically part of the assessment team as consultant or coordinator, and as liaison with social agencies and intake sources.

This team may be augmented *ad hoc* with any other member of the staff who has expertise in a particular area bearing upon the assessment of a case.

The assessment itself may cover five to seven sessions, in which the baby and his family are visited at home; one visit is scheduled at the clinic for developmental testing.

At the close of the assessment period, either a staff team or the full staff, in review, will consider all the information which has been gathered, and a decision will be made regarding the best treatment alternatives for the baby and his family. The referring agency is asked to participate with us in the decision process. Thus the treatment of choice may lead in several directions.

CONSULTATION WITH OTHER AGENCIES

Following assessment we may conclude that the baby's needs and the family's needs can be served by the referring agency or another clinic in our community. Our assessment should have identified the central issues in the family which have affected the baby's development. We may conclude that good supportive treatment and education of the parents in certain areas of infant care can be provided by the public health nurse or the family agency. If the agency wishes regular or periodic consultation and review with us, we are prepared to offer such consultation and a developmental reassessment at intervals.

BRIEF TREATMENT

This category of services actually covers a range of treatment options within our own clinic, and is defined arbitrarily as less than six months of service. It includes "crisis intervention" (sometimes as few as three sessions to help parents deal with a critical situation which has arisen in the baby's health or development). It includes "developmental guidance" for a limited period to help parents deal with reactive disturbances in a baby who has suffered trauma (separation, hospitalization, surgery, etc.), or, in some cases, to help parents understand and deal with a perplexing—though not morbid—developmental problem in their infant.

INTENSIVE TREATMENT

This category typically includes cases in the "very severe" range of disturbance, or babies who are judged "at risk" because of physiological or environmental factors. In any one month, these babies constitute the largest part of our caseload. In this group we have our failure to thrive infants, neglected and abused infants, infants and toddlers who already are showing pathological forms of behavior, and babies affected by extreme psychopathology in one or both parents.

In this volume we will include clinical examples of each of these aspects of our work.

The Training Program

Our intramural training program serves both staff education and the education of graduate students and residents in our program.

STAFF EDUCATION

In a new field of mental health such as ours there is no pool of "infant mental health specialists" from which a clinical infant program can draw its personnel at the start of the program. We were fortunate, of course, in that three of the original staff in the blind infant program became the nucleus of the professional staff which served the new infant mental health program. We brought with us our backgrounds in infant research and early childhood development, our clinical experience with infants and their families, and teaching.

In selecting staff for the new program we sought men and women who possessed the highest *clinical* qualifications in child and adult psychotherapy. We were prepared to build into the experiences of these clinicians a thorough knowledge of infant development and clinical methods for work with infants and their parents.

Every new staff member receives a full year of training in seminars and supervised casework, and is assigned a small caseload which will permit a range of experiences and a large amount of time for study. In these respects, the training of a new staff member is nearly identical with that of graduate students and residents, but his prior experience makes an important difference: If he brings to this work large experience in psychotherapy and a strong theoretical base, he finds the transfer of knowledge to this new field a task which is not formidable. If one possesses clinical methods and a strong theoretical foundation, new applications become another exercise of this knowledge and not entirely "a brand-new experience."

Typically our new staff members have felt they needed to saturate themselves both in experiences of infant-parent observation and in wide reading of the literature on infancy that has burgeoned in the past ten years. Observations of normal infant-parent relationships are provided through "study cases"—volunteer families with healthy babies who permit us to visit on a once-a-month basis. Observations of infants with deviant development and parents in conflict with their baby are, of course, everyday experiences provided by our program. Both direct observation and video study are available to the new staff member. Typically, a supervisor or consultant serves as a member of the team, and shared observation sharpens the eyes of the new staff member to subtleties in behavior.

Our library, which is excellent and comprehensive in all areas bearing upon childhood and family relations, provides a resource for independent study and for discussions of the literature in small seminars or conferences with a senior staff member. Our video and film library is a resource which every member of the staff has learned to use with mechanical ease, as freely as one pulls a book from a library shelf. "Would you like to look at a tape with me?" is an invitation offered as frequently as "Are you busy? Can I tell you about something wonderful that just happened?" Our video tapedecks and monitors are in use every hour of the day. The saturation of oneself with observed experience, the storing of thousands of pictures in one's head, becomes indispensable both to new staff members and old in sharpening one's eyes and one's judgments.

Seminars augment the program for all new and old staff members. Our traditional case review seminar on Tuesday afternoon includes all staff members and trainees. A seminar focusing on assessment is scheduled for three months at the beginning of each new academic year. A seminar dealing with technical problems is scheduled for the second part of the academic year.

Each year our program includes distinguished lecturers who bring to us their own work in progress in infant research and applied research. Twice a year we plan two-day work sessions with colleagues in related fields in which we and they present current research interests and problems for intensive study and discussion.

Training and experience in developmental testing of infants is built into the program through supervision and study of taped testings.

This has proven to be a workable plan. Our new staff members as well as our old ones are agreed that the one-year intensive training program for experienced clinicians results in a high level of competence in the new subspecialty of infant mental health.

Staff education goes beyond the intensive training period, of course. The seminars which form the background for training of new staff members and students include senior staff members at all levels of experience. This mix of senior and junior staff in all seminars results in excellent theoretical and practical discussions and debates and makes its own explicit statement to the new staff members and trainees: "No one ever completes his education."

The presentation of cases for staff review should also be added to this description of our educational program. Following a tradition in our program that we have come to value, each presentation by a staff member or trainee is a report which aims at the highest level of clinical observation and inference. The report is the presentation of clinical evidence to one's colleagues in which the central issues are fully documented and the treatment methods are derived from these findings. The discussion that follows such a presentation ideally does not admit "speculation" but only well-formulated clinical hypotheses. Many of the presentations to our Tuesday seminar have in fact been the first drafts of papers later presented at scientific meetings elsewhere. Some have since been published. A selection of these papers appears in this volume; others will appear in future volumes.

GRADUATE TRAINING

In a typical year, our graduate student and resident program includes representatives from a number of professional training programs. We provide a clinical practicum, a research internship, and intramural seminars in which all trainees participate.

Thus in a peak year for the training program (1976–77), we had a senior resident in child psychiatry (who is also a board-certified pediatrician), a senior resident in pediatrics, a pediatric nurse who was at that time a doctoral student in nursing, a post-doctoral student in clinical psychology, a post-degree fellow in social work, three doctoral students in developmental psychology in our research assistants' program, and one research assistant seeking her degree in social work.

The practicum in the clinical program includes a range of cases which are carried under the supervision of senior staff members. Each trainee is assigned a primary supervisor in his own professional field and, in the course of training, may have as many as four other supervisors as other cases are assigned to him. Case conferences with the supervisor are based upon detailed clinical notes of patient sessions (following the recording model previously described) and study of videotape sessions.

The educational program for each fellow and graduate student is tailored to the specific needs of the student. Each student or resident comes to us with a fund of knowledge in his own specialty. Thus the resident in pediatrics or psychiatry or the student in developmental psychology may already have acquired through course work a good background in normal infant development. What he needs from us is not another course in infant development but comparative study of normal and deviant development in infants. The clinical psychology student and the social work student may or may not have had advanced course work in infant development, and we may need to build into their training, through reading and tutorials, a fund of knowledge which is scattered throughout a vast literature in pediatrics and developmental psychology. The developmental psychology student may already have learned to administer infant tests. The resident in psychiatry or pediatrics may not have infant testing in his background. Testing experience and supervision in testing can be provided in our program. Research experience in infancy may not have been available to some of our graduate students and residents, but every student participates in our outcome research and is trained in observation, recording, and the methods of data reduction which we employ in our research design. A student or resident with a research interest of his own is encouraged to pursue it if our own resources can be useful to him.

Our intramural seminars are not designed as "courses." If, indeed, any student or resident is in need of a course to acquire basic information, there are excellent programs in clinical and developmental psychology on our campus, and the department of psychology has been generous in making its own resources available to us.

The seminars are forums. The focus of each seminar is clinical study. We bring to this study of a particular infant and his family everything that is available to us, in psychiatry, pediatrics, developmental and clinical psychology, social work, nursing, and anthropology, that can illuminate this case. Only one seminar, an introductory seminar on clinical assessment, is designed "for students only." All other seminars bring our faculty, professional staff, and students together. The presentations may be made by the students or senior staff members. The seminars are *not* pitched to "the level of experience of the students," which we would consider an injustice to highly intelligent graduate and postgraduate students. The "level" of exposition and discussion is that of the professional staff. Student questions and student participation in discussion are simply part of the dialogue. (And there is no bashfulness on the part of our students.)

When senior staff members present their own clinical material, the student has the opportunity to examine the work of his own faculty, to see not only the highest level of our clinical work but to observe his teachers struggling with difficult and often painful clinical experiences. He will see success with most difficult cases, but he will also see failure, or a less than optimal outcome, and witness the soul searching and honest anguish that the clinician experiences at such times. He will sense the climate in which our work is done and is discussed, one in which every therapist feels the support and understanding of his colleagues, one in which scientific debate and argument can be conducted without pettiness or rancor. We want, and get, lively questions and discussions from our students, but we also impose an unspoken rule upon ourselves: that the questions should be well-formulated and attentive to the data presented, that inferences drawn from these data are fairly derived. No guessing.

When the student presents his work, he follows the model of our professional staff. We ask for a well-organized presentation, preferably written, and documentation from the case record and video. The student's presentation is subjected to the same standards of clinical performance as that of the senior staff. But this does not mean that the student with his still-limited experience is expected to do clinical work on the level of the senior staff (though some, in fact, do). Rather, we should explain, we ask the same questions of the student that we ask ourselves as senior staff. We raise alternative hypotheses if we feel that the case dynamics do not support the student clinician's views. We make suggestions regarding technique which come from our larger experience.

This mix of faculty and graduate students has undoubtedly accelerated the learning of all of our trainees. Our own graduates have repeatedly praised this aspect of their learning.

At the conclusion of one year of training in our program we expect of our graduates "beginning competence" in clinical work with infants and their families. We expect that they will be able to work with a fair degree of independence in the new professional subspecialty of infant mental health. A small number of students have chosen to continue their training with us for a second year. With the second year of training we believe that the level of competence attained by certain trainees qualifies them as specialists in infant mental health, capable of training others in clinical settings or universities. This assessment must include the exceptional gifts of the students and the excellence of their primary graduate school education.

The Research Program

The research objectives of our infant mental health program originated in the two-year pilot program under the Grant Foundation sponsorship and became the basis for our proposal to the National Institute of Mental Health in 1973 for a program which would combine clinical services for infants and a study of the effects of intervention methods for infants and their families with demonstrable impairment in the areas of human attachment.

In the proposal to NIMH, which was later funded for a period of six years, we outlined a plan for data collection and assessment of treatment outcome which would involve the development of rating scales to measure the developmental status of the infant pre-treatment and post-treatment, as well as ratings of parental competence pre-treatment and post-treatment. At the same time, we proposed to examine treatment *methods* through detailed clinical studies.

We were, then, asking two kinds of questions in this study: What are the *results* of treatment measured through the pre-treatment and post-treatment psychological status of the infant and his parents, and what are the *problems and therapeutic methods* that can be identified as contributing to "change" or "no change" in psychological status in the infants and families under study? The two central questions had to be addressed, of course, through different methods of study.

Introduction

At the time of this writing, we are midway through the outcome study of 55 infants and their families in our intensive treatment group. Criteria for assessment have evolved which will give us the stage-specific expectations for optimal development during the first year of life, and these will be expanded to cover the second and third years. Degrees of impairment (moderate to severe) in children and families in the intensive treatment group are rated and will yield, in final analysis, an inventory of items and clinical judgments, which should eventually lead to the development of rating scales which can be employed by infant clinicians. A provisional rating scale has been developed for the children under one year of age. It is being tested for reliability both through senior staff consensus and the outside agreement of independent raters who are themselves specialists in the area of infant development and infant mental health.

In the last phase of our study, we have chosen to add another major area. The entire population of our study since 1972 will be examined for its characteristics at the point of intake. The central question of this inquiry is: "Who are the babies and families and what are their presenting problems?" In short, if a new program for infant mental health emerges in a community and the doors are open to a full range of infant-parent problems, who is referred, what are the problems brought to us, what services are required, what can the infant mental health program offer, and what can the community itself offer in response to the problems which are brought to us?

The second question in our original proposal, "problems and therapeutic methods," can only be examined through a case-by-case analysis of our detailed clinical methods. In this volume we have selected a group of cases which illustrate our methods of clinical assessment, the derivation of the treatment plan from the assessment, and the range of clinical methods employed to bring positive change in cases where babies and parents were severely imperiled in their relationships.

BIBLIOGRAPHY

Fraiberg, S. (1971) "Intervention in Infancy: A Program for Blind Infants," *Journal of the American Academy of Child Psychiatry* 10, No. 3, pp. 381–405.
———. 1977 *Insights from the Blind.* New York: Basic Books.
Fraiberg, S., Smith, M., and Adelson, E. 1969 "An Educational Program for Blind Infants," *Journal of Special Education* 3, No. 2, pp. 121–139.

II

Clinical Assessment of the Infant and His Family

SELMA FRAIBERG

AS IS TYPICAL of a psychiatric facility for infants and their families, our patients are referred to us by a clinic or social service agency or by the parents themselves when the baby shows signs of a developmental disturbance or when his parents are experiencing difficulty in providing for the baby's physical and emotional needs. This first step in "identifying a problem" will not yet tell us whether the problem, as perceived by another interested party, carries the right label, whether the problem as seen by the parents is the problem as seen by trained clinicians, or, in the event that the problem has been fairly identified, whether the baby and his family will be best served by our clinic or by another agency in the community.

The telephone referral will reflect the impressions of the referral source: "Margie, 5 months old. 'Looks neglected' to public health nurse." "Peter, 8 months. Hospital suspects abuse." "Danny, 4 months. Premature baby; mother can't cope." "Cindy, 2 months. Mother 15 years old; mother seems helpless in caring for her." "Mother about to be discharged from mental hospital. Afraid can't care for 18-month-old girl." Self-referrals by parents will include such telegraphic messages as: "My 18-month-old baby is hyperactive; he's driving us crazy." Or, "My 15-month-old baby bangs her head day and night. Do you think we should be concerned about it?"

On the face of it, each of these problems requires careful clinical study. If the family lives in Washtenaw County and if our own staff resources permit us to take on the baby and family for study, we will provide clinical assessment of the baby and his family. Our methods will be described in this chapter.

The Referral Process

INVITATION TO THE FAMILY

The first steps in the referral of a family to our program may be critical for the outcome. Whether or not a baby identified by a referring agency as "having a problem" will get to us depends upon the way in which the problem is interpreted to the family and the way we are introduced. If the public health nurse thinks Margie "looks neglected," how can she communicate to the parents her concern for the baby without appearing to indict them? Neither the nurse nor we want parents to come to us under professional indictment. When parents feel "accused" and frightened, grim fantasies about the Child Development Project may crowd out the benevolent picture of a clinic for babies and their families which the referring agency has offered. Fear and shame may cause many of these needy families to take flight from the proffered help.

In the early days of our program, we were sobered to find that many of the most imperiled babies in our community were not getting to us after referral. If we exerted ourselves to reach these families and succeeded in getting a first interview, we might be greeted by a grim couple who let us know directly or indirectly that we were not welcome. If at this point we managed to get some grudging consent from the parents to talk with us, we would receive a litany of grievances against "people who say they want to help us." And, gradually, as we listened and put the stories together at our regular intake conferences, we began to track the referral process and its perils back to sources which were actually invisible to us.

The referral process had already proceeded a long way by the time, for example, that a pleasant and tactful social worker or nurse talked with the family about coming to see us. It had begun with a procession of doctors, nurses, and social workers who had crisscrossed each other in a frantic emergency room or a busy ward in a large hospital. (There are three large hospitals in our county.) The anonymous health professionals had already begun the process of identifying the baby's problem weeks before the social worker or nurse came on the scene and suggested that the case be referred to us. And, we suspect, by then she didn't have much of a chance.

I will compose a story which is really a composite sketch from many stories that emerged in the early years of our work.

The baby, at 6 months of age, is brought into the emergency room with an upper respiratory infection. He is hospitalized and found to be suffering from severe malnutrition. From the parents' point of view, the baby is sick and the baby has a feeding problem. "He always had trouble keeping his food down." The parents are expecting that "the doctors will find out what is wrong," that "the tests will show something, and then we'll know what to do."

When the medical tests show that there are no primary physiological causes for growth failure in the baby, there is understandable alarm on the part of the physicians and nurses. The baby is in great danger, and the parents seem not to understand this. As the staff's alarm is expressed in the report to the parents, the parents begin to understand that the doctors believe their baby is suffering from neglect. (Rage toward the doctors now.) They will learn that the baby has gained two pounds since he has been in the hospital with a special nurse assigned to him. (Rage toward the nurse, now, who is a better mother than the baby's own mother. And all their self-doubts about their parenting seem confirmed by the implicit accusations from without.) Someone else on the staff may appear to warn the parents that a complaint to Protective Services may need to be filed. (Fear and panic now.) And finally, at the end of this series of interviews, someone appears with a recommendation. The parents will now hear that there is a baby program at the Child Development Project, and they will be referred there for "help." (What help?) Rage, fear, and dreadful suspicion now find their next target—the Child Development Project. (What's that? Probably another court agency with a nice-sounding name to disguise its malevolent purpose.)

This is not a climate for "help." In the early days of our program we sat on many doorsteps hoping for entry into a house with an endangered baby, the door closed against us and a curtain moving in the window. If we succeeded in getting into that house, there might then be a chance to present ourselves as humane and decent people concerned about the baby and his troubled parents. There would then be a chance to listen to parental suspicions and anger against us and the hospital and to turn the negative transference into a positive alliance with the parents on behalf of their baby. (There will be many clinical illustrations of this problem in this volume.)

There is an easier and more effective way open to us and our referral sources. In the course of our collaborative work with hospitals and social agencies, we have worked out together step-by-step methods in which the referring physicians and social workers play an important role in helping frightened parents to use our help.

In a paradigm, the method looks like this: The physician or social worker shares his grave concern with the parents. No scolding. The parents' *own* concerns and anxieties are elicited. "I know how worried you are too. . . . No, the tests have not shown 'physical causes' and we don't understand the picture fully right now. But we are going to do everything possible to help you. We don't know yet why Johnny isn't eating well and growing. We work very closely with the Child Development Project. They have baby specialists in many fields. They visit the baby and his family at home. They are good people. They care about parents and their feelings—just as much as they care about the baby. Would you like to meet somebody from the Child Development Project while the baby is still in the hospital? They can tell you more about their work and answer your questions."

In this form of referral we have a fair chance that the parents will be willing to meet us. We arrange to have a staff member meet the parents at the hospital during the next parental visit that day or the next day. It is now up to us to listen to the parents' concerns, to listen to their grievances against the doctors, the nurses, and all those people who can't find out what's wrong with the baby (and we know that includes us too), to sympathize with them in their terrible plight, and to offer our help. "Together, you and we and the doctors will try to find the answers. We have helped many families. We know how you feel. We hope we will not disappoint you. But if you should find that we are not helping, we hope that you will tell us frankly. We will not be angry." (We are, of course, anticipating distrust and anger and opening the pathways for expression of feelings, now or later.)

We visit the baby on the ward with the parents. We look for any positive signs in the baby's response to his parents—a smile, a gesture—and comment upon it. We make friends with the baby, if he'll let us.

Meantime, as we watch the baby and his parents together, we may pick up some vital clues in the relationship between them. To ourselves we note: "There *are* preferential responses to the mother in this 6-month-old baby. Good." Or: "There are *no* signs of discrimination of mother and stranger. Not so good. But this is the hospital. Will it be different at home?" Or: "No vocalizations from the baby. Also, parents do not speak *to* the baby. Seems stiff in mother's arms. More relaxed in father's." Or: "Hand-eye coordination poor for his age. Lack of experience in reaching for persons, toys? Or is it regression in the hospital? Also, doesn't support himself well in sit. Lack of experience? A secondary effect of malnutrition? CNS damage? No, that was checked out in the hospital."

None of these concerns needs to be shared with the parents at this point. We ourselves don't know the answers.

We watch a feeding in which the mother gives the baby his bottle. A joyless feeding, perhaps. But this is the hospital. Can we judge a feeding on the basis of behavior in this strange situation, the mother herself anxious and being observed?

With this initial picture of the baby and his parents, we sit down for a long talk with the parents. We invite their questions. About the baby. About ourselves. We allow the parents to interview *us*, to find out everything they need to know in order to give us their initial trust. We describe our work. We ask, finally, if the parents would like us to begin visiting and to see together how we can all help Johnny with his feeding problems.

In this approach we have avoided the unhappy situation in which parents feel threatened or punished, and we now have a fair chance that the parents can form an alliance with us on behalf of their endangered baby and will be able to make a commitment to treatment. The winning (and earning) of this initial trust is the first step in treatment and will be closely related to outcome.

But what about clear-cut neglect and abuse cases in which a complaint has already been filed at Protective Services, or where our own moral and legal obligations require us to inform parents that if they cannot work with us, or if they refuse our treatment, charges will be brought against them and the baby may be taken into protective custody? Isn't that punitive? No, to our mind it is a statement of reality and such a statement need not be delivered either as an accusation or a hostile threat. It can be presented as a sad fact.

To construct another paradigm: We say, "Yes, this is a very serious charge. Yes, if things do not improve there is the danger of losing the baby. But we are the people who care about keeping babies and their families together and the court wants to give you every chance to become the kind of parents you would like to be. We will give you all the help we can so that you can give your baby what he needs. If we cannot help you, it's true that placement of the baby may be the only solution. But we have helped many parents with problems such as yours and we are willing to do everything possible to help you."

Except in rare cases such as those where there is severe parental psychosis, this method has brought a very large number of "hard-to-reach" parents, charged with neglect or abuse, into a therapeutic alliance with us. (One clinical example, "Greg," is presented in Chapter VII.)

27

THE TRANSFERENCE TO "THE BABY SPECIALIST"

We are guided in our work by psychoanalytic principles. To establish an alliance during the assessment period, to establish a relationship which may lead to treatment following assessment, we need to draw upon everything we know about the nature of transference. We need trust in order to do our work, but the largest number of our parents have not known trust in their own childhood experiences with parents and parent figures. The "helping person" is a figure contaminated from the beginning by the betrayal which many of our parents experienced in their own families at the hands of the first "helping persons," mothers or fathers. We need a strong desire from our families to be "good parents," but many of them have no models of good parenting on which to build. We need from them a wish to change, to become another kind of person, another kind of parent. However, the majority of our parents, when they first come to us, do not see change as a product of self-observation and personal growth, or of learning. They see it as something that *happens* to you. It is the result of "good luck" or "bad luck." For successful therapeutic work, we need something called, in our jargon, "motivation." Most of our patients do not come to us with the "self-motivation" that is so highly valued in psychotherapy. They have been "motivated" by someone else. Usually, it was someone who was reading "danger" while the parents were waiting for the baby to outgrow the problem or for their luck to change.

On the face of it, such patients would be regarded in all conventional psychotherapies as unpromising patients. Since we can demonstrate and will illustrate in this volume that these patients, the parents, can become "highly motivated," and that their imperiled babies have been brought to adequacy in a very large number of instances, where does the motivation come from?

From the baby, of course. If there is one theme that runs throughout the pages of our case records it is "I want something better for my baby than what I had myself." It comes from parents who have been neglecting, or abusing, their babies. It comes from a mother with a postpartum depression who seems not to hear her baby's cries. It is the baby then, who provides the "motivation," and if we understand this and become the allies of his parents, on his behalf, we have the essential conditions for a therapeutic relationship.

The hope of "something better for my baby" becomes available for the positive transference to the therapist. And we need this positive transference for our guidance on behalf of the child. But the negative transference to the therapist may exist side by side with the positive transference, and much of the success of our work will depend upon therapeutic skills in understanding and modifying the negative transference in treatment.

The work on behalf of the baby arouses many buried or unsettled childhood conflicts in the parents. The therapist is simultaneously both "good parent" or "idealized parent" and "bad parent," who cannot be fully trusted, toward whom anger, rage, disappointment, or fear will be reexperienced even when the therapist is manifestly a benevolent figure. Thus an understanding of the psychoanalytic principles of transference and transference resistance become indispensable to the therapist in this work, as in all other therapeutic work.

In some of our cases we may not get to even the first stage of help, the assessment itself, without finding a path through formidable resistance. The negative transference is manifest at the first meeting.

Beth (Chapter IX) is 17½, an unwed mother. Her baby, Trudy, 4 months old, is starving. Trudy has dropped far below the third percentile on her growth chart and all evidence shows that Beth is unable to feed her baby. The baby is dirty, neglected, developmentally retarded. Beth has refused all help at our hospital and has refused to accept a referral to the Child Development Project. The situation is critical. After two months of futile attempts to make an appointment with Beth, Edna Adelson of our staff arranges to see Beth and Trudy at the hospital, following an out-patient visit. Beth knows that Mrs. Adelson is coming to talk with her and also knows that the hospital is on the verge of making a report to Protective Services. She knows that Mrs. Adelson is not a representative of Protective Services, but Beth's stored up rage against "people who are trying to take my baby from me" is ready for another target. Mrs. Adelson enters the consulting room where the physician has just finished her examination and the hospital social worker is present to introduce Mrs. Adelson.

Beth greets Mrs. Adelson with a tirade. Everyone is blaming Beth for not feeding her baby. Everyone is blaming her because the baby throws up all the time. She "keeps coming to this damn clinic every week for checkups and the doctors haven't found out yet why Trudy throws up all the time." Mrs. Adelson listens patiently to this torrent. Out of the corner of her eye she sees Trudy in a bundle of rags, a limp little bundle herself, with pipestem arms and legs, a solemn face, staring eyes. We should not ask Mrs. Adelson what is going on in her mind. If the impulse to pick up the baby and take her home has entered her mind we would all forgive her (for the impulse, that is). If the doctors and nurses and social workers at the hospital are frightened for Trudy and angry with this sullen, contemptuous child-mother, we can forgive them too.

The torrent goes on. A recital of grievances against the hospital, the daycare center, and the welfare program (AFDC). She, Beth, has been telling the doctors and telling the doctors that the baby throws up, and they won't do anything. "They won't listen to me. Nobody listens to me. Nobody understands." (Not true, Mrs. Adelson thinks to herself, knowing that the whole staff in that clinic had devoted itself to Beth and Trudy for weeks, and that it is Beth who doesn't listen.) But Mrs. Adelson is hearing a message in this litany of complaints: *"Nobody listens to me. Nobody understands."* Finally, Mrs. Adelson finds a moment to speak. "Well, then," she says, "if you have been trying to get answers and you feel that nobody is listening to you, you have a right to feel angry at everyone who is trying to help you. I am listening very hard. I want to understand everything you are saying. If I do not understand you, you will have the right to be angry at me too. And you can tell me that."

With these words, there is a change in the atmosphere. Beth looks incredulous. Her voice softens. The flood of complaints begins to dry up. She begins to look like the frightened child she is, and Mrs. Adelson, the witch-mother, undergoes a transformation (as I interpret this session) and becomes, very simply, Mrs. Adelson, a woman and a psychologist who knows a great deal about parents and babies.

In technical language, we would say that Mrs. Adelson "handled the negative transference" and "cleared the path to a positive therapeutic alliance." In fact, this first session became the critical session for establishing a relationship with Beth. It also led to excellent therapeutic work and guidance on behalf of Trudy which brought her to nutritional adequacy in a few months! It was by no means the only period in treatment in which the negative transference renewed itself and was interpreted, but clearly, if the negative transference had not been dealt with in this first session there would probably not have been any further sessions. The outcome for Trudy would have been placement in a foster home. (More terrible was the chance that Trudy might not survive.) The outcome for Beth would have been a tragedy beyond repair.

But it was not only "handling the negative transference" which was crucial in the first session. Mrs. Adelson had picked up a thread in this litany of complaints: the repetition of the phrase "Nobody listens to me. Nobody understands." True, this is a common enough complaint among patients, but there was something in this refrain that called for a selective therapeutic response. When Mrs. Adelson responded, it was to these words, and she used these words selectively in her statement to Beth. Nobody can know in a first session what such phrases mean on the most profound level. But in a few weeks, when we had come to know Beth and Trudy better, these words took on a special poignancy.

Beth had been a war orphan, found abandoned at an unknown age on the streets of a war-torn country. She was starving when she was ad-

mitted to an orphanage. She was still in a state of severe nutritional inadequacy and in psychological danger when she was adopted by an
American family at the age of 2½. She was a screaming, terrified child
during the first year in her adopted family. And *nobody could understand
her.* She spoke a foreign language. Perhaps she had the words in her
native tongue to say, "Hold me tight" or "Don't go away; I will be lost
again," but there was no one to understand her in this foreign land.
Which is also to say, in child language, in any tongue, *"Nobody listens to
me!"*

The tirade at the hospital had echoes from the past. There was now
another starving and neglected baby, Beth's own child. This baby, too,
was about to be taken from her mother if Beth could not care for her.
As we reconstruct it, the room at the hospital was crowded with ghosts.
There were, in a sense, two starving babies, Beth and Trudy, and the
past and the present merged, as panic arose in Beth. She was again a
screaming child, "lost and abandoned," and once again "nobody listens to me. Nobody understands me." Mrs. Adelson heard the words
and responded explicitly to these words. In this way the therapeutic
alliance began.

However we do it, it is always the same. The therapeutic relationship
begins with "need" and "a responder to need."

The Assessment Plan

The preceding pages have been a long introduction to the central
theme of this chapter: the clinical assessment of the infant and his parents. However, "the invitation to the parents" and "the initial transference" are crucial aspects of the assessment itself. How the invitation is
given, how the initial transference leads to an alliance with the parents
will, in fact, determine whether an assessment *can* be made.

We have already touched upon the structural aspects of the initial assessment in Chapter I. Typically, the assessment is carried out through
home visits and will include one office visit for developmental testing.
At intake a staff member is assigned as the primary therapist, and this
person will be the central member of the assessment team and the
therapist for the case if treatment at the Child Development Project is
recommended and accepted. In the case of a team assessment, a senior
and a junior member of the staff collaborate in the assessment, and one
of them is designated as the primary therapist. A support team of specialists is also assigned at intake. The assessment period typically lasts

five sessions, but there is no arbitrary time limit. We consider an assessment completed when we have the essential information for evaluating the mental health status of the infant and his parents. In some cases the assessment can be fairly made in three sessions. In others as many as seven may be necessary.

Our plan, then, insures continuity in the relationship between the family and one central person on our staff. The advantages are self-evident. The transference which comes from "need and a responder to need" is a precious gift to the therapist as well as the patient. The practice in many clinics, which is to divide intake and treatment between separate staffs and which results in transfer from the intake worker to the therapist, is a tragic waste of this "gift." For patients like ours, for whom lost and broken relationships, disappointment in love, and rejection are central to their conflicts, the institutionalized clinical practice of separate "intake" and "treatment" becomes one more broken relationship in the chain. Many patients may not pursue the proffered treatment. Since in our work it is the disturbance and disruption of human bonds which has brought babies and families to us, the old clinical model with its own built-in discontinuity becomes a mixed message to the patient. (The clinic says it cares about human attachment; yet the clinic does not practice its beliefs.) It is our hope, then, in the practice which we follow, to give an implicit message to our parents and their children (we have toddlers who can understand) that trust, personal devotion, and steadfastness are qualities which we value and will pursue at all costs in our work, and that these are values which can become their own.

The question may be asked "Why an expanded assessment period?" If the baby is already in great trouble in the opinion of well-qualified colleagues, why do we need five sessions to reach, perhaps, the same judgment? Why not first, an intake meeting and a developmental history; and second, a testing of the infant, a summing up, and recommendations? Indeed, some of our colleagues, when they first meet us and our program, wonder if our expanded assessment is not a profligate waste of our staff resources.

At the close of the assessment period we may, in fact, reach the same judgment as our colleagues, i.e., "The baby is in great trouble." But what we will have learned in those five sessions is *why* the baby is "in trouble," in which areas of functioning adaptation is impeded, in which areas the baby shows affective and cognitive and motor capacities which are age-appropriate and in which areas not. We will have learned where parental capacities and incapacities are affecting the baby, where parental conflicts are impeding the relationship to the baby. We will be able to identify the ego strengths as well as weaknesses in parental personality. And finally, with all this information at our disposal, we will be in a position to consider the best possible treatment plan for the baby and his family.

The five sessions conducted mainly through home visits give us a tremendous range of observations made under optimal circumstances. How can we know in a single visit that change and circumstance have not given us a glimpse of the baby and his parents under the most *unfavorable* circumstances? (The relief check has not come. The telephone is about to be cut off. The baby has a cold. The baby is cranky. The parents haven't slept all night.) In the second or third visit everything may be changed. It has happened in our experience.

As for the developmental history, we consider that there are large advantages in learning the story over several sessions, with no question-and-answer format. If we were to begin with a list of questions, we would place a questionnaire between us and the parents in need. (It is very like being an accident victim in the hospital emergency room while the admitting clerk stands between you and the physician with the crucial questions regarding the maiden name of your mother, your last five addresses, and the name of your insurance carrier.)

If, for example, the birth history of this baby is a traumatic one, too painful to speak about, but the parents are concerned right now about the baby's sleep disturbance, the anguish in recalling that birth will not be experienced right now and we will most likely get a formal response: "Well, it was a long and difficult delivery." A useful fact, by all means, but not as useful as it will be in the third session when the parents trust the psychologist and the event is recalled with tears and perhaps anger against the attendants at that birth. The slow pace of this expanded assessment allows the parents to tell their story in their own way, with guidance from the clinician, of course, but without the intrusion of a formal inquiry. It means that the affectively significant events will be recalled in a sequence that is governed by the affective experience of the parent, and that sequence in itself will tell us a great deal.

"My mother didn't even want to see the baby. She didn't visit me at the hospital. She didn't want Bill and me to marry in the first place.... It was a long labor. It was terrible. And we were afraid ... afraid that ... the baby wouldn't make it.... My doctor didn't make it. I mean, he wasn't there...." Our psychologist is listening with sympathy, and registering the poignant phrases. The mother deserted by her own mother. Her baby rejected by that mother. A young mother, a most difficult labor. (We will get the medical record and details of the birth later, with the parents' permission.) The baby is in danger in the delivery room. (If the mother is right.) The mother "deserted" by her obstetrician. Rejection. Loss. Desertion. That's how the baby came into this world.

By such means we are likely to learn in five sessions much that we need to know of the history of the family and the baby, and we can construct a useful fact sheet and timetable for quick reference in our patient file. But the expanded assessment gives us more than the fact sheet, of course. We will know, finally, how the events recorded there were experienced by the parents and the baby.

Again, to return to the question of whether we can assess a case more economically, we have been asked by some of our colleagues if we could not get all we needed for assessing the baby through the administration of infant tests. And again, it must be said that we feel the most economical approach will only give us part of the story. The Bayley Scales of Infant Development (Bayley 1969), our chief instrument (and by agreement among infant specialists the most reliable of existing infant tests), will give us inestimable help in our assessment of cognitive and motor capacities of the infant but will not be able to identify (except grossly) disturbances in the affective sphere.

There are not yet standard scales for the assessment of the affective ties between the baby and his parents. And since babies are mainly referred to our program for presumed affective disturbances, our judgments of adequacy or impairment must be derived from close clinical observation. We do have available to us from a large scientific literature the indicators of human attachment—a sequence of discriminative and preferential behaviors exhibited by the baby toward his human partners and the expected age ranges during which these behaviors are manifested. Smiling, gaze, vocalization, and motor approaches are the chief indicators in this series. (Later we will discuss our clinical use of these indicators in assessment.) Yet, each of these indicators must also be judged on a qualitative basis. Careful observation may reveal that the baby has these differentiating behaviors in his repertoire but that they are muted or qualitatively thin or rare.

The Bayley testing does not examine the baby's social and affective repertoire as intensively as we require for the clinical assessment of a presumed affective disturbance. Many of the babies examined by us and judged to have a severe affective disturbance fall within normal Bayley ranges in the cognitive-motor assessment. This in itself is an important finding; it speaks for adequacy in these spheres of functioning and is counted as a large plus in our estimate of the baby's potential. On the other hand the finding, in five hours of observation, that these babies rarely smile to the mother, rarely gaze at the mother, rarely vocalize to her, do not discriminate her from strangers—at ages when all these behaviors are in the normal baby's repertoire—becomes the vital clue that "something is gravely wrong in the primary attachments between the baby and his parents."

It is of the greatest importance that these findings—"an absence or paucity of indicators of age-appropriate attachment behaviors"—have been derived from clinical observations over a number of sessions. Thus, if we record in the summary of a particular baby (Chapter VIII), "*rarely* smiles to mother," this statement is more than an impression. We can, in fact, examine the detailed records of five sessions in which circumstances have provided us with the largest range of observations, under the most favorable circumstances, and see that only *one* smile to mother is recorded and that this smile is judged by the observer as "an empty smile." (In a single session, neither we nor any experienced observer of infants would wish to generalize from the finding that there was "only one smile to mother.")

The same principles apply to our observations of parents and generalizations regarding their parental capacities or incapacities. Anxiety in the parents who are being observed may constrict their spontaneity in responding to the baby or in reading the baby's signs. Over five sessions, during which we expect we have reduced the parents' anxieties and elicited trust in us, we should have a good range of observations with which to arrive at fair judgments. In the case of Greg (reported in Chapter VII) we can examine the records of five sessions in the home comprising fifty pages of narrative record and find that in every instance in which the baby signals "need" (hunger, distress), his teenage mother summons his teenage father. In the one instance in which the mother herself responds to the baby's hunger, she cannot find milk in the refrigerator and feeds the baby a bottle of Kool-Aid. Here we can generalize from the evidence of five sessions that the mother is unable to respond, herself, to the baby's signals of need. In social situations in which a mother can seek or elicit responses from a 5-month-old baby (a gaze, smile, vocalizations) we have no observations involving this mother and baby and a number of observations which involve the father and baby. When we are led to say, "Annie *avoids* contact with her baby," we mean that in nearly every circumstance in which a baby or his mother *can* engage in a social exchange the mother absents herself as a partner.

In many other cases we will find ambiguity in the clinical picture of parenting. The record of Nina's assessment between the ages of 7 months and 9 months (Chapter V) shows that Nina's young mother is able to read a large number of "social signs" in her baby—a smile, a gesture, a complaint—but she is unable to read the signs of hunger in her baby! And that baby has been referred to us as "failure to thrive." The ambiguity in this picture will be critical for the clinical diagnosis.

Clinical Illustrations

Our methods of observation and differential diagnosis are best described through illustration. For clarity, we propose to describe two cases, Delia and Sandra, referred to us by social agencies for "assessment of possible neglect." In each case, the referring agency has identified "neglect and emotional deprivation" and has chosen us as an infant psychiatric unit to make the assessment.

Delia and Sandra are close in age. Delia is 3 months old at the beginning of the assessment and Sandra is close to 4 months of age.

How shall we judge "neglect" or "adequacy" in these visits to two babies and their families? Physical care of the child will certainly provide us with some information, but it is possible for a child to be well cared for and well nourished and yet show all the signs of maternal deprivation. Emotional deprivation must be read through other signs.

A 3-month-old baby who is suffering emotional neglect will show the signs of deprivation in the absence or paucity of indicators of human attachment and in a constricted affective range. A mother who is unable to respond to her infant's emotional needs will reveal this through her inability to respond to signs of physical and social need in the baby and through misreading or ignoring these signs.

We expect to see in a healthy baby at 3 to 4 months of age a smile of greeting and response to the human face, a smile already becoming "preferential" for the face of his mother and other human partners, but at this age, ready and available for strangers too. There are vocalizations in response to the smile of other persons or their talk. There is gaze reciprocity between the baby and his human partners. There is motor excitement which we read as pleasure in social interactions (joyful kicking, hands and arms in motion). All of these social behaviors are in the repertoire of the baby *if his partners have elicited them.*

Affective qualities that we expect to see in a healthy, well-mothered baby, judged fairly over four or five sessions, would include a smile that is generous and speaks to us observers as "cheerful," or "joyful," or "exuberant"; vocalizations which are animated; pleasure in tactile contact with his mother (snuggling, molding, touching, and exploring her face or her hands); the ability to be comforted by his mother when he is in need or distress. These qualities are not in the innate repertoire of any baby; when we see them we must conclude that his human partners have given him pleasure and a sense of trust.

The mother's capacities and incapacities in mothering can be read to a large extent through the baby himself, but here we need to exercise caution in judgment. A sick baby, a premature baby, a mentally defective baby, a baby with a sensory or motor deficit, may present problems for his mother which do not fairly test the mother's own capacities. And the baby himself, sick or biologically incapacitated, cannot give fair testimony for qualities in mothering.

Assuming good health and biological intactness in the baby, we can assess the qualities and capacities of the mother through extended observations of mother-infant interaction in the ordinary circumstances of the baby's day. As visitors in the home, we can see a feeding, a diapering, a period of play, or intervals in which no specific childcare is required but a mother and a baby are together in the same room and casual exchanges between them will take place.

Can the mother read the baby's signals of need or social invitation? How does she respond to them? Here we must assume for purposes of clinical study that the infant clinician can read a very large part of the infant vocabulary of signs and signals, and the mother's "reading" of them can be judged on the basis of the clinician's "reading." But there will be many ambiguities, and we ourselves feel that to be on the safe side we should invite the mother to "explain" her baby's signals to us. "What do you think she wants?" A mother may be able to say, "Oh, she's getting fussy and wants to be held for a while." Or, she may say, "He's just spoiled rotten. He thinks he should be held every minute." Or: "He's just mean, like his father."

DELIA

A social worker in a public assistance agency asks us to assess Delia, a 3-month-old baby. Delia's mother is unmarried. The family is black. There is one older sibling, Donna, who is 3 years old. The home is described as unkempt—dirty and disordered. The social worker thinks the baby looks retarded and neglected.

Evelyn Atreya of our staff conducts the assessment. Edna Adelson serves as psychological consultant and tester. The clinical evidence and conclusions drawn from it will be brought together in a full staff review. One session will be videotaped, with the mother's consent, and the tape employed in the full staff review for careful study.

There are then two questions asked of us by the referring agency: "Is the baby neglected? Is the baby retarded?"

How does the mother see the problem? The referring social worker isn't sure. She discussed our project with Miss W and, "Miss W didn't say much. . . . She said it would be 'all right if we visited.' " We are uneasy. Mrs. Atreya, in her intake notes, wonders if the mother was pressured into seeing us. (Delia and her family are among our first cases in the infant mental health program. We have not yet worked out with our referral sources the careful step-by-step process for dealing with parental questions and anxieties about us.)

Evelyn Atreya, in her first meeting with Miss W, becomes the interpreter of our program. "Many times mothers have difficulties, or there are things that concern them when their children are young." She tells her that if there were things that concerned her about Delia, and if she would like our help, we would try to help her. Miss W smiled and said she didn't have any questions.

Not a promising beginning. To herself, Mrs. Atreya registers, sadly, the impression that Miss W is distrustful of our program and that she may already have guessed, correctly, that the public assistance agency questioned her competence as a mother.

The assessment, then, would be conducted within a climate of strain for the mother, and all of our observations must take into consideration the mother's own anxieties.

The home, as described in our record, is indeed dirty and disordered, corroborating the social service report to us. There is thick dust and debris covering the floor and the shabby furniture. Clothes and other objects are strewn everywhere. There is a strong smell of urine in the house. Miss W herself is wearing soiled and tattered clothes.

Mrs. Atreya puts aside the visible signs that the house is neglected and focuses on the children and their mother. Both Delia and Donna are in the room.

From all appearances both children are adequately nourished (no small achievement for a mother on an AFDC budget). Delia is cleanly dressed.

Gradually, in this visit and in the next three sessions, Miss W begins to feel at ease with Mrs. Atreya. The climate Mrs. Atreya establishes is the easy, informal one in which a mother and her visitor are watching a baby and discussing her accomplishments, a climate in which the mother can speak about anything on her mind and trust the clinician. Mrs. Atreya herself engages in simple baby games with Delia. When the baby does something wonderful, Mrs. Atreya and the mother share the delight. And for the mother, who had guessed that her competence was in question with AFDC, Mrs. Atreya does everything possible to show herself as a nonjudgmental, noncritical person who wants to understand a mother's feelings.

In the course of these sessions, Mrs. Atreya is also observing Donna, the 3-year-old. On one occasion she is playing with toys which Mrs. Atreya has brought especially for her. She is manifestly jealous of the attentions to her sister. "Lady," she says reproachfully, "why are you talking to that baby all the time? She can't say anything to you." And, with Mrs. Atreya, she converses in a very respectable 3-year-old English. Watching Donna in pretend games with the new toys, Mrs. Atreya sees good representational play, good language, good problem solving ability for a 3-year-old.

And Delia? I will offer these pictures of Delia, and her mother, Donna, and Mrs. Atreya, which come back to me from the one videotaped session.

Delia is sitting on her mother's lap and Evelyn Atreya is playing games with her with a rattle and a squeaky toy. Delia's smile is radiant; she is obviously enchanted with her visitor and the small talk Mrs. Atreya is addressing to her. She is really more interested in Mrs. Atreya than in the toys that the visitor has brought with her. She makes pleasant vocalizations in "conversational" response to Mrs. Atreya, and we, the viewers, register these as good vocalizations for her age. Good signs. A 3-month-old baby who responds with joy to the sight of a human face and the sounds of the human voice is a baby who has learned to associate these human attributes with pleasure. Someone important to Delia has given her such pleasures. From all evidence it is Delia's mother.

During the four assessment sessions there are hundreds of observations of Delia and her mother covering a wide range of circumstances. These are recorded in the narrative record.

When the observations are organized, this is what we see: In the largest number of observations of mother and baby together, we observe that Delia settles comfortably in her mother's arms. Delia has preferential smiles for her mother. The smiles are radiant, joyful. (We confirm Mrs. Atreya's judgment in the taped session.) Delia has beautiful smiles for Mrs. Atreya when they play together. Delia seeks eye contact with her mother, and gaze reciprocity between them is observed throughout these sessions. Delia vocalizes (with differentiated sounds) when her mother approaches, and vocalizes with animation in social exchanges. Delia seeks tactile contact with her mother in feeding and social situations.

In brief, all the signs of human attachment and reciprocity between a baby and her mother which can be discerned at the age of 3 months are there. Actual neglect would have been read in the absence of these signs. And, of course, no baby can invent this repertoire of attachment signs for the benefit of a psychological examination; they have emerged in the course of many weeks and could only emerge if they had been elicited by the baby's human partners.

The largest number of observations of Delia's mother in caregiving and social exchanges with the baby show that Miss W is able to read and respond to Delia's social signs (smile, gaze, vocalizations) in a natural, unaffected way. There are many instances of shared pleasure between mother and baby. Miss W is able to comfort Delia when she is fussy by holding her, talking to her. There are two instances in which Miss W showed an inability to recognize signs of physical discomfort in Delia (the baby in an awkward posture and needing to shift position) and instances in which Miss W seemed inept in lifting the baby or pulling her to sit. Miss W appears to alternate between holding Delia for her feeding and using a propped bottle. (Mrs. Atreya finds a tactful way to speak to Miss W about Delia's need to feel closeness with her mother in feeding.)

On balance, Miss W appears to be an adequate mother and, while we register as negative aspects of her mothering her inability to read certain motor cues in her baby and her disposition to distance herself through a propped bottle, these deficiencies in mothering do not, as we see it, constitute "neglect" or "incompetence" when placed in the larger context of qualitatively good affective response to her baby.

Miss W's housekeeping constitutes a health hazard for herself and her children. But again, we cannot cite the poor housekeeping as evidence of child neglect.

In the light of these generally favorable findings in the affective sphere, it is now of considerable interest to us that the picture of cognitive-motor development presents some puzzles.

During each of these visits Mrs. Atreya has been giving balanced attention to the cognitive-motor capabilities of Delia. Even before the formal Bayley testing, Mrs. Atreya has been organizing her observations with scale items in her head. The experienced baby clinician can make a fair estimate of the baby's capacities by registering information, obtained in natural circumstance and through improvised games, "ticking off" the scale items in a mental inventory. Such an estimate does not take the place of formal testing; it provides guidelines for the clinician in extending inquiry and integrating these observations with all other observations during the early phase of the assessment.

Balanced attention to both cognitive-motor and affective capacities is necessary in every assessment. This is not only because the question of "retardation" has been raised in connection with Delia's status, but because the assessment of every baby must include all sectors of development.

In this informal assessment of Delia's cognitive-motor capabilities, Mrs. Atreya notes that Delia's gross motor development is very adequate for her age. She has good head control in all postures. She elevates her head and shoulders in prone and enjoys sitting supported and standing supported. She can support her weight in stand. At 3 months, she is already making an effort to sit when in supine position. (These last two items are in advance of her age.) These items speak for neuromuscular adequacy and also, on the experiential side, for adequacy in nurture and opportunities to experiment with postures. (Grossly neglected babies will reflect their poverty in experience through flaccidity in the age-appropriate postures, or severe retardation in the attainment of gross motor milestones—assuming, of course, that there is no biological impairment in these systems.)

Within this picture of adequacy in gross motor functioning, Mrs. Atreya is puzzled as she watches Delia's hands and then is puzzled again as she watches Delia's eyes. As Delia approaches 3½ months in the assessment period, she is not observed to bring her hands before her eyes for visual inspection; she does not use her hands to approach an object within easy reach of her fingers. The hand items should not yet cause us concern. (Median age is 3.8 months for these items; range 2 to 6 months.) But the experienced infant clinician always has his own eyes fixed on the child's hands and the child's eyes, and Mrs. Atreya has been registering another set of observations.

Delia is not tracking well with her eyes. Mrs. Atreya sees an eccentric pattern. She notes: "When an object is held at eye level and is moved horizontally across Delia's visual field, she loses it, usually on the right side but sometimes on the left. The same thing happens when objects are presented circularly. We did observe that Delia can track objects vertically."

Delia shows signs of visual impairment.

Mrs. Atreya, registering this information, has also been observing Donna, the older sister, who brings objects very close to her eyes for inspection. Mrs. Atreya notices that Miss W is wearing glasses with very thick lenses. She suspects a familial ophthalmological disease in the mother and the children.

Delia's rapt attention and joyful response to the human face had nearly obscured the visual defect in the early sessions. But the human face is a large target for this child with visual impairment. It was only when smaller objects, toys, were experimentally introduced into the field of vision that the deficit and the field of deficit could be discerned.

When the Bayley was administered by Edna Adelson at age 0:3:9, Delia failed nearly all the visual and visual-motor items, as we might have predicted. On those vocal and social items where visual discrimination and eye-hand coordination would not impede performance, Delia performed well. Mrs. Adelson chose not to score this test, since the performance of a visually handicapped child cannot be fairly reduced to a score.

On reflection, we can see that there would have been certain risks in assessing Delia on the basis of a single session which included a Bayley testing. Thus, if we had not had an assessment period extended sufficiently to provide abundant clues to a visual impediment, Delia's performance on the Bayley could as easily be read as cognitive-motor impairment due to primary mental deficiency or gross neglect. (The most severely neglected babies we have seen will also fail visual-motor items.)

During our staff meeting we review Mrs. Atreya's findings in the extended assessment, Mrs. Adelson's test findings, and the single video-taped session at home. We have a team consensus in our judgment.

Delia is not neglected. The evidence from our assessment of human attachments (baby to mother, mother to baby) and the qualitatively good social responses in the baby's repertoire speak for adequacy in mothering. The physical care of the child (when we separate this factor from poor housekeeping) is good. Delia's apparent good health and nutrition make their own statement of adequacy in maternal care.

There is no evidence that Delia is "mentally deficient," if we read our observations and test findings fairly. Her failures in those test items which require visual discrimination simply confirm all observations prior to the testing session in which visual impairment was discerned.

In our report to the referring agency these findings are summarized, and we make the strong recommendation that Delia and Donna be seen in our medical center's ophthalmology department for an examination.

There are no indications that the family needs continued service from our program.

In Delia's case, and in many others known to our program, the referral begins with the impression of another clinic or agency that "something is wrong" with the baby. Sometimes a label has already been given the baby, as with Delia—"neglected" or "retarded." The label, right or wrong, can determine the course of the child's life and that of the family. An infant mental health program with a team of specialists can provide an assessment which fairly examines every aspect of the baby's functioning and the family's capacity. There are many cases like Delia's in which our program only needs to provide an assessment, which can in turn lead another clinic in our community into the formulation of a good plan for the baby and his family.

Whether Delia is labeled "neglected and retarded" or "visually impaired; otherwise adequate and healthy" can be a crucial "social intervention," with life consequences for baby and family.

SANDRA: IS THE BABY NEGLECTED?

Sandra is referred to us when she is 4 months of age (exact age 0:4:1). A public health nurse calls us to ask for our help. Sandra "appears neglected." "She is left to herself, with a propped bottle. Always dirty. Mother is unable to show warmth. Has refused help offered by nurse and other agencies." Sandra was premature by one month; her weight was 5 pounds 3⅓ ounces at birth.

There are three older siblings: a girl, Linda, age 5, two boys, Dennis, age 2½ and Eddie, age 18 months.

We learn of a family in chaos. Ken, the father of the first two children, has been long out of the home. He is described as a brutal man. He is now threatening Mrs. A with a custody fight over the children. He accuses her of child neglect. The father of the two younger children is no longer in the picture. There has been a recent eviction by a landlord. The A family is living in extreme poverty. The house is described as filthy.

William Schafer of our staff is assigned to be the primary person in the assessment; Edna Adelson is psychological consultant.

The public health nurse is successful in getting Mrs. A to call us for an appointment. (Our record does not tell us how she introduced us, however.) In her phone conversation with Mr. Schafer, Mrs. A is snappish, her voice has barely restrained hostility, but she herself has initiated the first phone call. Mr. Schafer, in introducing himself, says he understands that Mrs. A is facing some real difficulties; that sometimes we are able to help with such problems and would like an opportunity to meet with her so that she could decide if we could be of use to her.

Mrs. A says in reply that she has certainly been having lots of troubles with the kids and feels that she needs help before she goes out of her mind.

Mr. Schafer sets up an appointment for the first visit.

He finds the house, once a dilapidated old building in a slum, now divided into apartments. No names on the doors. While Mr. Schafer is waiting, unable to guess which door might be the As', three very dirty children come down the stairs. He learns that they are Linda, Dennis, and Eddie. Only Linda speaks. She says her mommy is upstairs getting dressed. From some signs given by Linda, Mr. Schafer gathers that Mrs. A is expecting him and that he can wait in the living room.

The room that serves as a living room is tiny, furnished with two tattered upholstered pieces and a few straightback wooden chairs. The room has a dank smell of urine and dirt.

As his eyes take in this scene, Mr. Schafer sees that on one of the straightback chairs with a cushioned seat, there is a tiny infant, lying on her back. This must be Sandra. Near the baby's cheek, but out of her grasp, is a bottle filled with milk. An old shirt or rag is placed between the baby and the edge of the seat. The seat is tilted slightly toward the back of the chair. The baby is dressed only in a diaper on this cold day.

It is an unforgettable scene and, we fear, an eloquent statement. Sandra is "introduced" to us as a solitary, unprotected infant, positioned on a precarious seat with a bottle out of reach. The mother is heard in the next room, apparently the kitchen. Since she is expecting Mr. Schafer, and the question of child neglect has already been introduced in the custody fight between her former husband and herself, we reflect to ourselves that Mrs. A may already be making a confession to us.

Mrs. A makes an appearance at last. She is haggard, looks much older than her age, greets Mr. Schafer with a "Hi," and asks him if he would like a cup of coffee. He accepts.

During the rest of that first visit Mr. Schafer listens as Mrs. A speaks of herself and her problems, and the three older children move in and out of the room, approaching their mother warily, moving away after sharp reprimands and orders, and, from time to time, a hard slap from their mother. Dennis and Eddie are never heard to utter an intelligible word in this session or any that follow in the assessment period. Linda, the eldest child, is not manifestly retarded in speech, but she is an alternately frightened and defiant child whose lack of school readiness has already alarmed her kindergarten teacher.

Mrs. A sees her problems, she says, as the two oldest children, Linda and Dennis. But, having said this, she never indicates in the rest of the hour *how* they are problems. The story of her desertion by her first husband and his threats to gain custody of the children are woven into a story of brutality toward herself and the children and the mother's own anxieties about the outcome. Linda, we learn in passing, misses her father very much, and as Mr. Schafer attempts to pursue this important thread, the story gets lost and cannot get disentangled from a maze of contradictory statements in which Ken, the father, has "not seen Linda since she was 3" and "when he last saw her a few weeks ago he beat up Linda."

During this outpouring, in which the past and the present are hopelessly entangled, Mr. Schafer listens attentively to Mrs. A and also observes the children. Sandra, the baby, who is our primary patient, the child who is suspected of being grossly neglected, is rarely mentioned spontaneously by the mother. During the entire hour of this first home visit, she lies mainly unattended, unwatched, in her precarious chair bed.

When Mr. Schafer attempts to elicit information about Sandra, Mrs. A gives some background regarding Sandra's birth—a difficult labor—and about an illness at 2 months in which an iron deficiency was diagnosed. But Sandra is no problem, her mother says. "She is a very good baby who never cries at all."

During the entire session, as Mr. Schafer watches Sandra, he never sees a smile, and outside of a few "fussy" sounds, there are no vocalizations. Sandra does not seek eye contact with her mother or anyone else in the room. There are no observations in which the baby brings her hands together at midline. Nor is there anything to occupy those hands. There are no toys in the room, no place in the room that has been set aside for the baby as a safe place or a play space.

At one point Sandra needs a diaper change. Her mother changes her, picks her up, and holds her on her lap. During the lap interval Mr. Schafer notes that at no time is the baby held in a ventral position; she is held away from her mother and always in a position where there is little or no opportunity for the baby to fixate her mother's face or for the mother to make eye contact with her baby. There is only one observation in which the mother "notices" the baby and briefly engages in a vocal invitation (a clucking to the baby) to get the baby's attention.

The baby looks uncomfortable on her mother's lap. In supported sit she appears for a few moments to hold her head up well. However, after a brief interval, she becomes noticeably fatigued in this posture, and her head begins to droop.

It is a sobering first session. The question "Is the baby neglected?" which brought us to this family should not yet be answered on the basis of a single home visit, but there are ominous signs that this baby is neglected and severely retarded. And just as ominous in this session are a large number of observations of the other children, which we have excluded in order to focus attention on the baby. These suggest that all four children are emotionally endangered.

In the three sessions that follow, the observations of Sandra and her mother follow a consistent pattern. Baby alone and unattended. Or, as in one session, baby crying desolately with no one responding to her cries. Baby placed in a playpen among a heap of rags with a propped bottle. The playpen itself positioned behind a sofa so that baby has no contact with anyone in the room. Baby clad in a diaper in a cold apartment.

When Sandra is 0:4:26 (that is, 25 days older than our first observation at 0:4:1), our observations in the areas of human attachment, cognitive and motor development can be summarized on the basis of four sessions.

In the area of human attachments, there are no observations which show that Sandra recognizes her mother or discriminates her from other persons. There are no smiles for mother, there is no visual regard of mother's face, there are no vocalizations in response to mother, and no reaching for mother or any anticipatory motor responses upon approach of mother. Her cries are weak and disconsolate, without expectation that they will summon another person. There are, in fact, no smiles, no vocalizations, no gaze exchanges or motor approaches to *anyone* in the family. (There is recorded one faint smile to Mr. Schafer when on one occasion he is able to elicit a response from the baby.)

The dominant mood of the baby is solemn, joyless, detached.

At an age (4 to 5 months) when a normal baby seen over a four-week interval will demonstrate a full range of preferential behaviors for his mother—smiling, gaze, vocalization, motor approaches—there is nothing in Sandra's repertoire that speaks of human attachment or pleasure.

Sandra's cognitive-motor attainments at 4 to 5 months are equally sobering. Formal testing is not employed. Sandra's repertoire is so meager that we will not gain more information from the Bayley than we have in the home observations. Gross motor development is severely retarded. She cannot yet control her head in a supported sit. (It is no longer easy to judge whether there is a primary neurophysiological defect or whether experiential poverty has deprived this child of opportunities to "practice" head and trunk control. A child who has spent her entire short life mainly supine can present the picture that Sandra gives us.)

Sandra, informally tested by Mr. Schafer for visual following, attempted reach, or reach for objects, is grossly retarded. Her visual tracking is jerky. Her hands have not attained midline organization. There is no attempt to reach for an object. Is there a visual deficit? Probably not. There is focus and brief attention to the object presented but a jerky tracking of the object as it is brought across her field of vision, a pattern more likely associated with extreme experiential poverty. And since Sandra fails the early items on visual regard and midline organization of the hands (no mutual fingering, no hand regard) the items of reaching and attaining which should emerge at 4 months are beyond her capacity. Thus the Bayley item "closes on dangling ring" (median age 3:8) is failed by Sandra at age 0:4:20.

Sandra's one observed smile to the examiner at age 0:4:20 would be credited on the Bayley at 1:5. She fails the earliest vocalization items in social response (2:1) and in vocalization of two different sounds (2:3).

Sandra at 5 months of age is functioning at the level of approximately 2 months of age in her cognitive-motor development.

From all the evidence derived from four home visits, Sandra is suffering most extreme neglect, in both the physical and emotional sense of the term. Can Sandra be helped through our program? Here we need to examine the mother's capacity to nurture her child and to use our help.

The clinical assessment of Mrs. A and her parenting capacities can also be derived from observations over four home visits as well as one visit which took place in the hospital when Sandra was admitted with pneumonia.

Mrs. A is overwhelmed in the face of extreme external pressures and the sense that she herself is an abandoned woman. Although she knows that Mr. Schafer is coming to talk with her about the children, she mainly speaks about herself. Her grief at abandonment by the two men in her life comes through in each of these visits. She is, herself, without emotional sustenance. She is depleted, exhausted, harried by poverty and by threats of a court fight over the children. She is fiercely protective of her rights to her children; she wants them and will not give them up, she says. But there are only rare glimpses of a capacity in her to respond to her children's needs. Her own needs for sustenance are paramount, and she is manifestly grateful for the emotional sustenance she receives from Mr. Schafer. But her own exhausted resources can barely be mobilized for her children.

In four home visits there is only one social exchange between mother and baby (the tongue-clucking game reported earlier), and Sandra's sober response to her mother's overture suggests to the observer that this is an unfamiliar experience for the baby. In all other instances we see the mother unable to register signs of the baby's needs, or, if the signs become intrusive, the mother's most typical response is to ask Linda or a visitor to go to the baby. In the rare instances of caregiving (a diapering, a repositioning of the baby), the attention to the task is wholly mechanical. Sandra is placed "out of view" in a playpen behind the couch. Sandra is fed by means of a propped bottle. It is, in fact, the paucity of examples of caregiving or social exchange with the baby that sobers the observer and the reader of the detailed observations during four sessions.

The circumstances of these home visits, with children and neighbors constantly in and out, do not give us the opportunities to fully explore the dimensions of Mrs. A's conflicts. We see depression—we think a very severe depression—in Mrs. A, but the external chaos of her life, the hopelessness which to some measure derives from the circumstances of extreme poverty and actual desertion by the men in her life, make it difficult in these early sessions to reach a discriminating diagnosis of depression. (Mrs. A herself attributes her physical exhaustion, her lethargy, her lack of appetite, her difficulties in sleeping, to external circumstance.) In the fairest balancing of external causes for depression and "internal" causes for depression, it seems to us that they coalesce, that one feeds into the other. The sense of being unworthy, unwanted, without hope for herself, which appears to go deep into her personality, is confirmed by circumstance, perhaps even reenacted with the materials of circumstance which are always available to the poor. We cannot yet know in these initial diagnostic sessions whether the label "severe depression" can be applied with clinical exactness.

We catch one glimpse of Mrs. A's ability to mobilize herself on behalf of Sandra when Sandra is hospitalized with pneumonia. Her anxiety for her baby is real. She gladly accepts Mr. Schafer's offer of transportation to the hospital to see the baby. Mr. Schafer sees moments of awkward tenderness in holding and feeding the baby. And there is one extraordinary moment after leaving the hospital when Mrs. A speaks of the visit and says with surprise, "She knows me!" Why was she surprised? Mr. Schafer asks her. (Sandra was 0:5:11 on the day of this visit.) Well, Mrs. A explains, she "couldn't expect that such a small baby would know her mother."

Mrs. A's innocence and ignorance regarding babies and their needs is sobering to all of us. Mrs. A is puzzled and quite unbelieving when Mr. Schafer becomes the tactful interpreter for Sandra, for what she might want, what she is needing. She sees Sandra as "a very good baby," "no problems." She is "too young to have problems." It's when kids get older and can talk that they begin to get problems, she explains.

At the close of the assessment period our staff agrees that Sandra, and indeed all of the A children, are in the most extreme danger because of maternal neglect. We are reading the signs of this danger through the emotional poverty, the absence of age-appropriate signs of human attachment, and our estimate of mental retardation in Sandra and all of the children.

We also know that none of these signs of gross emotional neglect would constitute evidence for neglect in our courts! In the absence of manifest brutality or abandonment, no court in our state would regard Sandra and the other A children as neglected.

We agree that we must take on the A family for treatment at the Child Development Project. We will do everything possible to provide help for Mrs. A in meeting the needs of her children, in learning about children and their needs, and in the process providing necessary psychological support for the mother herself. We are not sure whether we can help Mrs. A on behalf of her children. And, as a last agonizing thought before we accept the As for treatment, we wonder if we can help Mrs. A in time to help the baby who must be brought to adequacy as soon as possible in this critical period of her development. Some of the extraordinary problems in Sandra's case, and our decision making, are discussed in Chapter III.

III

Treatment Modalities

SELMA FRAIBERG

VIVIAN SHAPIRO

DEBORAH SPITZ CHERNISS

WHEN our infant mental health program was first instituted in 1972, we described our new project to our colleagues and invited their collaboration. "A mental health program for babies?" one of our friends said. "That's great . . . but what do you *do* with them?" Other responses were more forthright. When a two-line announcement appeared in our local newspaper that a professor in the department of psychiatry had received a grant from the National Institute of Mental Health for an infant program, an irate taxpayer promptly wrote a letter to the editor demanding to know why the taxpayers should be asked to support a crazy woman professor who wanted to put babies on a couch and psychoanalyze them.

The Baby as Patient

All of this has given us to understand that the notion of a baby as a psychiatric patient is hard to assimilate. A baby has none of the conventional attributes of a psychiatric patient. He can't talk about his problems. He can't form a therapeutic alliance. He has no capacity for insight. Such patients are usually labeled "not suitable for treatment" in the language of psychotherapy.

The forms of treatment we describe in these pages are also unconventional. The treatment takes place mainly in the baby's home, with one or both parents present. The baby is at the center, and everything that transpires in the treatment is either centrally or peripherally addressed to the problems of this patient, who can't talk. If treatment takes place in our offices (which can also happen), the baby is brought in for the office interview.

The parents, who are our collaborators in treatment, are also our patients, of course. They are the patients who *can* talk, and the family sessions will in some ways resemble conventional psychotherapy of the kind that takes place in a conventional office, except that the setting will be a family kitchen or living room or a playroom of the Child Development Project. Since the parents are talking about their baby *and* themselves, what is it that the baby brings to the therapeutic session? Wouldn't it be easier (and more tranquil) if the parents left the baby at home and came to our office for their treatment sessions? Does it make a difference that the baby is present?

We are convinced that it does make a difference, but we didn't know why until we were well into our work. The baby, physically present in the session, was not part of a "therapeutic design." While we were working out adaptations of conventional psychotherapy and developmental guidance for an infant-parent treatment program, we were open to many variants in method and explored them. But "the baby in the room" idea evolved from our earlier work, our study of the early ego development of infants blind from birth. Since infant observation and infant-parent interaction were central to that study, the baby *was* always in the room unless he was napping. We soon discovered that the presence of the baby was not only necessary for our study of development, but the baby in the room became a partner in the ongoing dialogue. He was intensely, emotionally *there* and gave import to all exchanges between the parents and us. Parents discussing a baby who happened to be napping in another room could, we found, distance themselves in their report to us, and their communications might screen out emotion. Then, perhaps a few moments later, when a wakeful baby was brought into the room, there was a heightened emotional climate. If there were tenderness and deep love for the baby, the presence of the baby evoked the most poignant expressions of love. If there were conflicting emotions toward the baby, the conflict seemed to surface with his physical presence. The physically present baby touched off a chain of emotions in the parent which often led to revelations of feelings in words, or to the formulation of painful questions to us, as if the sleeping baby had aided repression or denial in the parent and the wakeful and present baby broke the barrier against feelings.

We also saw that the baby, as the patient who couldn't talk, could nevertheless engage in an eloquent dialogue with his family and with us. Without words he could tell us how he was feeling about the world and himself, whether he was valued, understood, satisfied, whether he was going through a rough time, whether he was facing problems of an ordinary or an extraordinary kind. And since his parents were engaged with him—talking, smiling, holding, feeding, bathing—or perhaps not engaged with him, the "dialogue" between baby and parents could be read by us as experienced observers and clinicians.

It was natural for us, then, when we began the new program for babies who were mainly biologically intact but suffering from emotional disorders, to follow a pattern in "interviewing" that had become congenial to us. The baby "belonged" in the interview, and has remained there in our work, except for those times when parents have needed privacy and their own space for periods of difficult therapeutic work. (When the baby is beyond the age of 18 months, we begin to modify the pattern of visits, reserving intimate discussions with the parents for private sessions. The child who has begun to understand language may find his parents' outpourings of grief and anger confusing and disturbing.)

In our new work, the baby and his parents were not research subjects but patients, and the privilege of inquiry was given us by the nature of our work. As our earlier work had been concerned with a developmental study of blind infants, we felt we did not have the privilege of making intimate inquiries into the parent-child relationship except under unusual circumstances. We provided developmental education to facilitate the blind baby's development, and this represented the decent limits of a contract with our parents, in which they permitted our visits so that we could learn and help them and other parents through what we had learned.

In the new infant mental health program, we had another kind of understanding from the outset. There was a baby in trouble, and the family had come to us to find out what was causing the problem and asking us to bring help to that baby and to them. In order to help, we needed the privilege of entering their intimate lives.

With this privilege, we were no longer only observers in a family living room. We were therapists, saying in effect, "Tell us how it is for you and the baby." And what emerged, typically, was a dramatic "telling"—and in fact "showing"—us, with the baby and the family enacting their sad story in the family theater. And it mattered that the baby was there, in the center of the story. He was "telling" his own story, of course, but he was also at the crossroads of dialogue and entering into the dialogue.

For example, in the story of Jane and her mother (Chapter VII) we witness a 5½-month-old baby screaming disconsolately in her mother's arms. Her mother makes no move to comfort her and stares off into space, as if she has not heard her baby's cries. The mother's face reveals her own depression and hopelessness. In this interval of noncommunication, mother and baby are both making an eloquent statement. Jane is telling us that there is "no one there" to bring comfort in great need. Her mother is telling us, without words, that her own inner anguish is unbearable. She closes off the registration of her baby's anguished cries, even as she closes off the cries which rise within herself.

In moments such as these (and they proliferate in our records) we learn more by observing a baby and his parents together than we might learn through many sessions in which a parent, in conventional therapy, speaks *about* his child. How would Jane's mother report this to a therapist if the baby were not present in treatment? She might say, "She's a fussy baby. She cries a lot." And the magnitude of the interlocking solitude and grief of mother and baby could not be discerned in any way.

Six-month-old Billy (Chapter VIII) and his schoolgirl mother must tell their story together. Kathie, his mother, is concerned about only one problem in her baby. "He spits up all the time." Billy's doctors and our staff are gravely concerned about Billy's growth failure during the past three months. Billy, who is one of the most silent babies we have ever met, makes his own eloquent statement of the problem. He is tense, solemn, with large vacant eyes. Not once in the first five sessions does he look at his mother, smile to his mother, or vocalize to his mother. He occupies himself in solitary play. Once, when the therapist asks if Kathie would like to hold Billy and sit in our rocking chair, Kathie complies. She holds Billy limply in her arms and rocks. And as the rocking continues, Kathie seems oblivious of the circumstances in which she is holding a baby, and rocks slowly, rhythmically, with a distant look upon her face—the mother is a child, rocking herself.

We have seen that Billy avoids his mother. Kathie, in every observation we make, avoids physical contact with him. And if we encourage her to hold Billy, we see that she creates psychological distance in the very circumstance of holding him. We watch Kathie's depressed face. We watch the tense, solitary Billy and see him, at moments, on all fours mechanically rocking himself. Our fears for Billy grow with each observation.

If Kathie were in treatment for herself in a conventional psychotherapy, if we did not see Kathie and Billy together, we would see a depressed 17-year-old girl. She would speak about herself, perhaps, and speak about her unhappy marriage. She might speak about her baby who "spits up all the time," but she could not tell us that her baby was in extreme psychological peril, because she would not know that. In this hypothetical treatment, the therapist would deal with Kathie's feelings of emptiness, isolation, inner rage, and—if we were lucky—within two years the depression might lift and Kathie might have resolved some of the adolescent conflicts that were impeding her growth. Her capacities to mother her baby would certainly be larger with these benefits of treatment.

But, in two years, the 6-month-old baby would be 2½ years old. Growth failure would probably have followed its typical course, with repeated hospitalizations for Billy. The cumulative severe nutritional deprivation and emotional deprivation would most likely result in a crippling of the child's potential in health and personality. The most devoted mother might not be able to undo the effects of early impoverishment in nutrition and experience for Billy.

No baby can wait for the resolution of a parental neurosis which is impeding his own development. He must have our help too. And we have learned in our work that it is possible to give help to the baby and help to the parents concurrently, with great benefit to both, and that the baby can be brought to adequacy even when his parents have not yet resolved their own personal conflicts. This sounds like a contradiction, but in our presentation of case reports in this volume, we will document this point and offer our own explanations.

When a baby is at the center of treatment something happens that has no parallel in any other form of psychotherapy. We have a consensus among our staff on this point. We often see changes in the baby and his parents as early as the first weeks and months of treatment. But if a baby's mental health status shows positive change a short time after intervention begins, we must fairly say that our therapeutic work and guidance on his behalf have been aided by the strong developmental currents which are present throughout the early months of life. Undo the impediments to forward movement, and the baby takes off! It's a little bit like having God on your side. But it's not so easy to explain the changes in his parents which have occurred during the same time. The changes are not yet fundamental changes in personality, but they represent changes in the capacity to nurture and relate to their child. (For example, four months after our work begins with Jane and her mother, Jane has reached adequacy in nearly all aspects of development and her mother has become nurturant and caring, despite the fact that her mother is still, clinically speaking, "depressed.")

Such changes in parenting capability within a short course of therapeutic work cannot be attributed solely to the gifts of the therapist, since in other psychotherapeutic circumstances the same therapist, with the same gifts, does not see, or expect to see, such radical positive shifts in any aspect of personality in a few weeks of treatment. We think another factor is facilitating this rapid development: the baby.

The baby can be a catalyst. He provides a powerful motive for posi-

tive change in his parents. He represents their hopes and deepest longings; he stands for renewal of the self; his birth can be experienced as a
psychological rebirth for his parents.

The baby, in fact, evokes profound memories and feelings in his parents which normally lie deep in personality. This need not lead to
pathological disturbance. To be in touch with the deepest reservoirs of
feeling in oneself can lead to a binding together of the elements of personality, a form of self-healing. When the stirring of old conflicts does
lead to grave disturbance in the parents (as we see in many of our patients), we find that we are still advantaged in our work. The powerful
conflicts which have led to this crisis have broken through into consciousness, or near consciousness, ready, as it were, for our help in resolution and healing—perhaps more ready than at any other time in
adult life.

If there are strong currents at work to bring developmental progression for the infant, there are also strong currents at work to bring developmental progression for the parents. Nearly every parent who has
suffered in his own childhood wants something better for his child.
Nearly every parent knows heartbreak when the baby is not doing
well. So it happens that many parents who would never be "motivated" to go to a psychiatric clinic for themselves, and who may, in fact,
be initially fearful of us at the Child Development Project, or hostile
toward us and all helping persons, can be brought to trust us and con-
fide in us. Because we are the people who care about their baby and
them. The baby becomes the bond which unites us; we are their partners and their allies in bringing their hopes for the baby to fulfillment.

The Therapist in an Unconventional Therapy

There cannot be a more alien setting for psychotherapy than the one
encountered in Edna Adelson's story of Beth and Trudy (Chapter IX).
Beth's living room in a slum apartment is furnished with two crumbling and soiled mattresses on the floor. The therapist sits crosslegged
on one. And maintains her professional composure. Beth sits on the
other mattress. Trudy, the baby, is lying in a heap of rags beside her.
The therapist is listening to the 17-year-old mother tell of being found
as an abandoned child fifteen years ago on the streets of a war-torn
city. The mother is not listening to the whimpers which come from the
baby beside her. The baby is in a critical nutritional state and a critical
psychological state. Another "abandoned" child. Beth does not remem-

ber her early years, of course. She has only dreamlike memories of a trip by plane to the United States and the meeting with her adoptive family. She remembers almost nothing, but she is repeating the past in the present, and the repetition—dreadful to watch—has caught a baby in its morbid path.

In this alien setting, then, therapist and patient sitting crosslegged on the dirty mattresses, the work of therapy is begun and will continue for many months to come. It is a therapy that moves from the mother's communications to the baby's, then back again from the baby to the mother. The method employed in this therapy is an adaptation of the method of psychoanalytic therapy, united with developmental guidance on behalf of the baby. The therapeutic work for the mother is one of listening, observing, giving permission to feel and to remember that which can be remembered, examining the past in the present, undoing the painful effects of that past, giving hope and the prospects of new solutions to old problems. The therapeutic work for the baby is one in which the mother is helped to recognize the baby as a symbol of her abandoned self, to find pathways to understanding the sorrows of early childhood (her own and her baby's), to find pathways of feeling which can unite the mother with her baby in hope instead of futility.

And concurrent with the therapy which leads to remembering and insight and positive identification between mother and baby is the form of treatment we have called "developmental guidance," in which the therapist becomes a nondidactic educator of the mother as to the physical and emotional needs of her baby and the ways in which a mother can provide these needs. It is guidance in nutrition and in child development, and it is unobtrusively introduced into every session.

The therapist may also take an active role in providing concrete help. Sometimes, as in the case of Beth and Trudy, there is no food in the house for the baby. (Management of an AFDC budget is beyond Beth in the early period of treatment.) The therapist arranges for emergency food supplies. If the baby is sick and must see the doctor, the therapist may offer to drive mother and baby to his office. Altogether an unconventional form of psychotherapy.

In a single session the therapist is helping Beth to unravel her past and to see the past in the present, the therapist is providing nutritional guidance for a "failure to thrive" baby, the therapist is guiding the mother into new ways of nurturing the child's emotional development, and the therapist may need to provide emergency aid or transportation to a doctor. (The therapist in this case is a clinical psychologist who once sat in her own quiet office and listened to a single patient in a single hour.)

How shall we classify the treatment of Beth and Trudy? "Intensive psychotherapy," most certainly. But "developmental guidance" and "supportive treatment" are equally central to the work. "Crisis intervention" just as surely, if we were to read the record and witness the therapist helping the 17-year-old schoolgirl mother to cope with lost welfare checks, evictions, unpaid bills, and the hazards of slum living. The admixture of methods and services in every case which we describe are almost too numerous to catalogue. A few vignettes may enlarge the picture.

Vivian Shapiro, the project's chief social worker, arrives at the home of an 18-year-old mother who has just come home from the hospital with a new baby. It is a visit to welcome the new baby and to do all those things the therapist can do to promote the bonds between the frightened adolescent and her baby. The treatment at this point can be called "developmental guidance." When the therapist arrives, she finds there is no food in the house. The relief check has not arrived. After welcoming the baby and conveying to the mother what one can do under the circumstances, the therapist goes back to her office to arrange for money from our project's emergency fund and spends the rest of the day on the telephone tracking down the lost relief check. Today's treatment now includes "crisis intervention." It also requires "the provision of concrete services."

Dr. Carolyn Aradine, our nurse consultant, is visiting a young woman who is about to deliver her second child. The patient is in a panic. She suddenly decides that she will not deliver the baby in the hospital, or if she does, she must go home the same day. The nurse consultant, who has been providing guidance and preparation of the mother for delivery, is confronted with a hysterical young woman who cannot be reached by reassurance or through the strength of the nurse-patient relationship. Since Dr. Aradine is trained in psychotherapy, she registers the depth of the anxiety in her patient and places it within a context she already knows: This young woman had undergone the most terrifying experiences in a hospital as a child. The nurse raises a question, which is also an interpretation. "This is terribly frightening to you," she says to her patient. "Tell me, is it *this* hospital that frightens you, or is all this mixed up in your mind with the hospitals you knew when you were little?" Suddenly there is a rush of tears and the patient makes a crucial link with her past. There is relief, finally, through crying and through talking. At the close of the session, the patient, with insight, says she is now ready to go to *this* hospital. In a single session, the nurse has provided "guidance," "crisis intervention," and a form of psychotherapy that gives insight.

When Edna Adelson, a clinical psychologist, arrives to visit Jane and her mother for one of their therapeutic sessions, she finds Jane feverish and crying with pain. Her mother is in a panic. Jane must get to the doctor quickly. The therapist drives Jane and her mother to the hospital and spends the morning with both of them as they go through the various examinations and procedures.

In the terms of classical psychotherapy, the therapist has "stepped out of her role." How can the same therapist who listens to Jane's mother and helps her disentangle the past from the present become the active helping person in a situation like this? What happens to the transference when the therapist is both the "mother figure" in the transference of the past and a kind of "mother substitute" in a time of crisis? These are proper therapeutic concerns and must be dealt with in the treatment process. But clearly *not* to drive a sick baby and her mother to the hospital would be the height of folly and a misguided psychotherapy all by itself.

We appear to be "bending the rules," and since each of us at the Child Development Project conducts conventional psychotherapy as a conventional psychotherapist, this bending of the rules must be explained. A good number of the advantages in psychotherapy, we concur, come from adhering to the rules. We much prefer conducting psychotherapy in our offices. We are vastly advantaged in dealing with transference issues when we can maintain our professional distance. We treasure the privacy of the office for our patients who need it for examination of their problems. And, to be candid, we would rather hear about a domestic crisis in our office than literally walk into one in a family living room or witness a shrill marital fight while a hungry baby is crying for breakfast.

The unconventional therapy we describe in these pages, however, is addressed to the needs of a baby and family who must be seen together, and this in itself is an unconventional circumstance. Once a therapist *must* visit his patients in their home, he has modified his professional role. This does not mean that he modifies his professional *behavior*, but in the eyes of the adult patient the therapist has become a guest in his home, whereas in conventional therapy the patient is a visitor to the therapist's office and everything in that setting (the desk, the chairs, the couch, the books on the shelves) speaks for "the profession" and defines it.

When the therapist leaves the office setting to become a therapist in the family living room or kitchen, he must define himself for the patients. He is a guest, but he must be a professional guest. The reasons for his being in this living room are clear to the patients from the start. He does not speak about himself and his life, as an ordinary guest or neighbor would do. He addresses the parent as Mr., Mrs., or Miss unless the parent is a teenager, in which case he follows the wishes of the parent. He maintains formal address for himself.

But none of us are distant or remote, and we are not blank screens. One of the patients is a baby, and when you are talking to a baby and telling him how lovely he is and how clever his tricks are, it's preposterous to put on your professional shrink manners. The other patients are the parents, who probably have had no experience with the arts of psychotherapy (and may have successfully dodged the practitioners of the art for years). The neutral mask of the psychotherapist would be read by them as "indifference," "coldness," and "hostility." What they need and want is a face and a voice that speak for caring, compassion, devotion, and professional wisdom.

Yet with all of these modifications in therapeutic role, we shall see in the clinical reports which follow that transference to the therapist and transference as a vehicle for therapy are significant aspects of each treatment mode and are central to the work in intensive treatment cases. The therapist, it is true, is not and cannot be the distant and neutral conductor of conventional psychotherapy but becomes a transference figure for the adult patients, the parents, even while he retains his real and substantial aspect for the patient. Thus while a mother named Annie eventually comes to form a strong therapeutic alliance with Mrs. Shapiro, and Mrs. Shapiro is demonstrably Mrs. Shapiro when she makes her visits to Annie and her husband and baby in the family living room, we see many sessions in which Mrs. Shapiro is transformed into the "witch-mother" of Annie's childhood, and Annie must be helped to see the repetition of the past in this transformation (i.e., the transference).

At the same time, the positive transference, the relationship of trust which is painstakingly built with Annie, who has rarely known a trusting relationship, becomes the vehicle for the work on behalf of Greg, the baby. Annie, who has never known mother nurture herself, is initially without resources to mother her baby. Even after the first period of treatment in which her conflicted feelings toward her baby are brought to the surface and illuminated, we see that Annie is limited in her capacity to mother her baby. Annie is without stable traditions in mothering and can offer little more than mechanical care. The therapist's "psychological nurture" of Annie enables her in turn to begin to respond to her baby. But Annie cannot read her baby's signals (and often misreads them as though he were an adult) and must learn through the therapist the most elementary facts about a baby's needs, how he communicates his needs, how his mother is special to him. All this is interwoven into the fabric of the sessions, as Annie and Greg are together with the therapist.

But none of this can be assimilated unless there is trust in the therapist. For many of our parents there will be mistrust, doubt, and even outspoken hostility in their first visits with the therapist. The label "uncooperative parent" would be unprofitable. If we see mistrust and hostility in the context of transference, there are pathways open to the therapist for modifying these attitudes and bringing about a therapeutic alliance. If we speak directly to the feelings of "not being able to trust" or "anger toward people who do not help," there may be relief and readiness to begin to trust.

In this way, too, the transference becomes the context for offering developmental guidance. There will be many times in the course of treatment when a parent finds himself unable to use our suggestions or openly negates them. If we ask ourselves, "What is happening within the relationship between therapist and parent?" and examine the transference, we will find almost without exception that negative feelings toward the therapist are intruding. If we deal with the negative transference and bring about or restore a positive alliance, the guidance which had been spurned or hotly negated can be accepted and tried out—often before our eyes.

In this way the transference opens up pathways for the parent for examination of his conflicted feelings, frees the baby from the conflicted past of the parent, and becomes the vehicle for the concurrent guidance we are providing on behalf of the baby. This "transference cycle," to coin a phrase, will appear again and again in the course of the work—with a single family.

A Brief Overview of Treatment Modes

In the chapters that follow, we have grouped the cases in three sections, according to the treatment mode predominantly employed: brief crisis intervention, developmental guidance-supportive treatment, and infant-parent psychotherapy. While each of the principal types of treatment in our work can be distinguished in terms of problems and objectives, the methods (which we will describe later) have much in common and frequently overlap.

Whether a case at intake will eventually come under one or the other of these classes of treatment will depend upon our clinical assessment of what is needed to bring about the most favorable outcome for the baby and his parents. In other words, the treatment provided is, to the best of our judgment, the best alternative or "the treatment of choice," to borrow a phrase common in clinical usage. This judgment is based on an assessment of the problem in terms of its dimensions (chronic or acute, reactive to external events or intrapsychic conflicts), and of the parents' psychological capacities and needs in treatment.

In *brief crisis intervention*, the problem is brought to us as a family crisis involving the baby. This mode of treatment is chosen when in our assessment the problem is largely reactive to a circumscribed set of external events and when the parents' psychological capacities suggest that they can make use of a brief focused intervention. In such situations it is possible, and sometimes necessary, to accomplish a great deal in a limited time (as few as three sessions) and this, then, becomes our objective.

These situations often involve an emergency. For example, a young woman has been abandoned by her husband just prior to their baby's birth and comes to us distraught with grief and in a precarious financial condition. Her problems must be dealt with as quickly as possible in order to assure the baby adequate health care, food, and shelter, and also to make possible the bonding between mother and newborn. Brief crisis work is also an important mode in somewhat different situations, where the problem is not some emergency demanding immediate action but is nevertheless both acute and specific. In the case of Gretchen (Chapter IV) we meet two young parents who live in terror that something bad will happen to their 4-month-old baby. In three sessions we learn that their fears are related to unresolved grief over the loss of their first baby. In a brief period of work the parents find the crucial connections between their fears for Gretchen and the loss of their firstborn. For another mother whose baby's birth has intensified her mourning over a recent death, a few sessions connecting these events alleviate the symptoms of postpartum depression for which she had been referred.

Thus in brief crisis intervention the problem may involve or directly affect the baby, but it is caused by specific situational factors. In this mode, our treatment objective is to bring about a favorable resolution of the situation within a limited time. Therefore, its choice as a treatment mode is based on an assessment of the specificity of the problem, the problem's acuteness, and the parents' abilities to respond to brief work. When the problem is a more chronic one, and/or the causes are more diffuse and related to intrapsychic issues rather than to external events, a choice between the treatment modes of developmental guidance-supportive treatment and infant-parent psychotherapy is made.

The choice of *developmental guidance-supportive treatment* is made in two kinds of situations. In one, the parents may be judged by us as having good parenting capabilities but neonatal complications or the baby's chronic illness may be straining these capacities to an intolerable degree (Robbie, Chapter VI). In other cases there may be signs of grave emotional impairment in the baby and serious problems in the parents, but our diagnostic appraisal of the parents' limited capacity to deal with internal conflicts leads us to choose a treatment that does not focus on these conflicts (Nina, Chapter V). In both these kinds of situation our objective is to provide emotional support and to strengthen parenting capacities, while simultaneously providing developmental guidance in the form of information and discussion about the baby's needs.

Thus, both the depressed teenage mother of a failure to thrive child and a well-functioning couple with a handicapped child can benefit from this mode of treatment. While the young teenage mother cannot tolerate exploration of her intrapsychic conflicts, whereas the couple has no need for it, in their different ways they can both make use of information about their babies that is provided with acknowledgment of their own feelings and needs. In sum, the choice of developmental guidance-supportive treatment is made when a problem is seen as chronic and interpretive work is either not possible or not indicated. In both such situations, we choose a treatment that is mainly ego supportive and ego strengthening, combining with it the provision of developmental information, discussion, and advice to facilitate healthy development in the child, and the strengthening of the parent-child bond.

In *infant-parent psychotherapy* the problem is seen by us as a grave conflict within the parents and between the parents and their baby. It is one in which the baby has become the representative of figures within the parental past, or a representative of an aspect of the parental self that is repudiated or negated. In some cases the baby himself seems engulfed in the parental neurosis and is showing the early signs of emotional disturbance. In treatment, we examine with the parents the past and the present in order to free them and their baby from old "ghosts" which have invaded the nursery, and then we must make meaningful links between the past and present through interpretations which will lead to insight. At the same time, in the course of parental treatment, we maintain the focus on the baby through the provision of developmental information and discussion. We move back and forth, between present and past, parent and baby, but we always return to the baby.

This mode is the treatment of choice for situations where the past has invaded the present and is endangering the baby's development. The choice is dependent, however, on the parents' ability to make use of such a focus, and it may be contraindicated in certain situations. For example, there may be ego impairment in the parents which cannot sustain inquiry into causes and motives, or the teenage mother still living in the midst of real family conflict may find it too threatening and overwhelming to engage in such inquiry. *However, our experience with a large number of gravely disturbed parents has shown us that this is a form of psychotherapy which can be used in the treatment of a broader range of cases than those described in the adult psychotherapy literature.* The caveats of the textbooks regarding interpretation and the dangers of stirring old memories have not always been justified in our experience. In illustrative cases in this volume, we see that adolescent patients, "acting-out patients," depressed patients, and "borderline" patients are among the patients who have profited from these methods. The level of education of the patient, the ability to verbalize, and the capacity for introspection were factors which did not impede the use of this method of psychotherapy, although they are factors often cited by psychotherapists as contraindications for the method.

The above classification of our cases is useful only if we also appreciate how much they overlap. The classification is descriptive for the mode if we mean that it identifies the central focus and objectives implicit in a given mode and in the main distinguishes this mode from another. But in the vignettes we offered earlier in this chapter, and in the case illustrations in the chapters that follow, we will see that supportive treatment and developmental guidance are incorporated into each of the treatment modes, including infant-parent psychotherapy, and that crisis intervention does not restrict itself to the cases labeled "crisis intervention" since crises, daily or weekly, generate themselves in all of our work.

THE TREATMENT OF CHOICE

Our choice of treatment mode is based in each case upon our clinical assessment of the problem as summarized in our discussion of the three primary treatment modes. It is a choice governed by no other criterion than "the best possible alternative" our program can offer. The only external restrictions in taking on new cases are the size of caseload and practical limits for each staff member and trainee. We do not charge fees and we do not recover costs of service from Medicaid, Blue Cross, or any insurance program. This is our own wish. The costs of service have been covered by the terms of our NIMH grant for a demonstration-research program and our Grant Foundation funds for training. If we had been dependent on private fees or insurance for support, we could not have provided long-term help for those children and families in need of intensive treatment. Nina, Jane, Greg, and Billy, whose stories appear in later chapters, were all children of poverty. So were the largest number of children who came to us. Medicaid in Michigan would have covered a limit of ten sessions for these children. We know that in many clinics today "the treatment of choice" cannot be made on the basis of clinical judgments, but must be made on the basis of the patient's ability to pay a fee or on third-party payments. "Brief treatment" (which *can* produce good results when it is the treatment of clinical choice) may be prescribed in many clinics because it is the only alternative that can be offered to patients of limited means, and the criterion of patient need does not enter into the decision.

We have been greatly advantaged, then, in our program by the freedom given us to conduct treatment on the basis of need only. It was our wish, but not our wish alone: NIMH wanted from our work, among other things, an assessment of patient needs in this new field of infant mental health. If we had burdened our study with fee and insurance requirements, we could not have begun to answer the questions "Who is out there in need of these specialized services?" and "What kinds of service and treatment are required?"

Moreover, if we had charged fees or collected insurance, we could never have reached many of our parents and their endangered babies! Initially many of our parents did not see that their babies were in trouble. Someone else did. And we did. Often it was necessary for us to make dozens of house calls in order to present ourselves as decent and caring people and to invite the parents to share their concerns with us. One cannot send a bill for services that have not been solicited. Often, too, in the course of treatment there were innumerable appointments that were never kept, were rescheduled, not kept again, in a pattern that we have learned to live with patiently. If we were dependent upon fees or insurance reimbursement, approximately half of our work time would not be reimbursable. All this is the way of life in "outreach" therapy. There is no way in which a program such as ours can send a bill for services: "Outreach ten visits; Nobody home: $400.00."

We record this experience because it may be useful to our colleagues in planning other programs for infants and parents. But in the context of this discussion, it is important to note that we were uniquely advantaged in offering "the treatment of choice."

We should not close this topic without discussing a last, very important point. Sometimes the treatment of choice is *not* our infant mental health treatment. In certain cases foster home placement may be the recommended treatment. Thus, in the case of Sandra (Chapter II) the severe mental disorder of the mother was beyond the help of our program. Following a six-month period during which no progress was made, we considered that the baby and, indeed, all four children were in great danger, and we recommended placement. We have rarely needed to recommend foster home placement in our program, which is an interesting fact in itself when we consider the large number of neglect and abuse cases in our treatment caseload. But in the case of Sandra, for example, there was no way we could help the mother in time to protect the baby's development and that of the other children in the family.

Today, with several years of experience behind us, we might not wish to wait six months to make the painful decision that we made for Sandra and her family. In the first years of our work we had learned that many cases described as "hopeless" could be helped through our treatment. How could we know that a Sandra and her mother could not be helped until we tried? We did, in fact, serve a protective function for the family, that is, we were standing by to see that the children would not be physically harmed, and we were providing all the help we could give to keep the family together. But the baby made no developmental progress during those six months. And a baby cannot sustain such severe emotional deprivation without great danger for further development. Today, with the wisdom of years of work, we would probably have recommended placement after the first exploratory work with the family (including assessment) led us to identify the dangers for the baby and the severity of the mother's mental disorder.

Are there other instances in which treatment in our program should not be considered "the treatment of choice"? We can think of some. In the case of a child who is suffering from mental retardation which is not related to the quality of parenting, there are other programs in our community that can better serve the child and his family. The special education services which these programs offer and which will have continuity into the school years will better serve the child and his family than our services. In such cases we will offer an extended assessment to the family and work with another program in the community toward long-range educational goals. Similarly, with respect to handicapped children, we have expertness among us in work with blind infants but none in the field of deafness, for instance. In such a case we might consider that other programs in our community have more to offer than we do.

In short, the "treatment of choice" in our program or any other is made on the basis both of need and the resources of the program.

Treatment Methods

The description of our treatment methods presents us with extraordinary problems in exposition. The methods are better revealed through the clinical case reports that follow. In reading them, we see that the methods of psychotherapy and the methods of developmental guidance are interwoven through every case and in fact are united in any single session.

But in this chapter we want to provide an introduction to the methods, and in order to do this we have to take apart an integrated structure and examine the components. The moment we do this we are dissatisfied. How shall we show the overlap or the coalescing of the methods in a single hour? If we take apart the structure for study and exploration, will we add anything of value?

We will try.

For purposes of exposition, we will treat the methods of developmental guidance and the methods of infant-parent psychotherapy *as if* they can be regarded separately. And for fairness, we will sketch in the overlapping features in each section. In order to keep the methods from coalescing (which is their natural tendency in practice) we will identify their characteristics through *emphasis* or *modal characteristics*, and as the exposition leads us to the margins of fusion, we will note it and quickly erect a dam before our readers (and we) slide over into the common territory. It will be a neat trick if we can do it. If we fail, the clinical reports in the following sections (which make no pretense of separating methods) may give the better picture.

THE METHODS OF DEVELOPMENTAL GUIDANCE AND SUPPORTIVE TREATMENT

The term "developmental guidance" in our work refers to a mode of education of the parent that is integrated with psychotherapeutic work. Since the term is widely used in various infant intervention programs to mean various things, there may be some confusion about just what we mean and do not mean when we describe it as a treatment method. In many infant intervention programs it means "cognitive stimulation" or "modeling the correct behavior for the parents" or "teaching the parent about child development." And it may even mean all of these things in one program. The "intervenor" in these programs is in effect an instructor. In many such early education programs there may be an "infant curriculum," that is, a sequence of tasks which the baby and mother perform together under the guidance of the intervenor.

Our own form of developmental guidance grows out of the circumstances in which a baby and his parents are suffering with either emotional disturbances or chronic external stress, and the relationship of baby and parents is in grave danger. It is a form of education which is guided by the therapist's clinical understanding every step of the way. On the one hand, we provide an ongoing, nondidactic education to facilitate the development of the parent-child relationship and to lead parents into an understanding of their baby's needs, and the ways they, as parents, can promote development. On the other hand, we also address the feelings and psychological stress the parents may be experiencing as they attempt to respond to the infant's developmental needs.

The differences between our methods of developmental guidance and the methods of other intervention programs are mainly those that reflect the extraordinary problems in infant-parent relationships which are brought to us, and the psychotherapeutic principles which guide us in our work. If, for example, the problems which came to us simply reflected the parents' innocence or ignorance of the needs of babies, an educational model might serve as well as any other. But our babies and their families come to us with disorders in the development of human attachments (or neonatal impediments to functioning), and the parents come to us with psychological conflicts which are distorting their relationship to the baby (or are immobilized with grief and anguish in reaction to a tragedy at the time of the child's birth). It is true that many of our parents do not know the "language" of babies, have limited knowledge of normal child development, and that they too could be called "innocent" when they come to us, but innocence and ignorance are often compounded by the psychological impediments to parenting that we see in many of our parents, and developmental guidance for these parents must move on two tracks simultaneously: helping the parents learn the language of babies, and finding the psychological impediments to that learning.

With our patients, then, developmental guidance must promote and enhance the parent-infant bonds and educate the parents in understanding their child and in finding new pathways in child rearing which will bring optimal development in every area of personality. The three vignettes that follow illustrate the range of use of developmental guidance. Detailed case reports of three of these children are in this volume—Nina (Chapter V), Robbie (Chapter VI) and Greg (Chapter VII).

Nina: Guidance to Promote Mother-Infant Bonds:

Many of our parents do not come to us with the idea that babies can love and that parents are central to the development of love. Many of our parents have not known in their own childhood the kind of love and protection which we want to help them achieve for their own children.

Karen (Chapter V), the 16-year-old mother of Nina, is genuinely surprised when her therapist remarks on the ways in which 7-month-old Nina shows preference for her mother over the therapist, how "special" her mother is to her. She's telling us, says the therapist, that her mother is the most important person in the world to her. Many months later, Karen tells the therapist what those words meant to her. It is the first time in her life that anyone has told her she is important to someone.

At every opportunity when Nina, Karen, and the therapist are together, the therapist comments on this special relationship. "That smile was special for Mom, wasn't it, Nina?" "Are you tired now, Nina? Are you telling me you'd rather get into Mommy's lap?" Nina cries when her mother is about to leave the room for a moment. Karen thinks she is "spoiled." The therapist says, "Mommy will be right back, Nina," and to Karen, later, "When you love someone very much, it's so hard to see them go away. It will be easier when Nina is older." Karen is surprised again. (The long daily separations from mother while Nina is in the nursery are very painful to Nina.) The therapist guides the discussion into the subject of separations, how a baby of Nina's age does not yet understand that a mommy is "someplace" even when she is not present, and what ways Karen might think of to make things go better for Nina during these long separations.

In a subtle way, Nina's behavior, which Karen sees as "spoiled," is interpreted as it should be: a normal reaction in a baby to loss of a loved person. Karen's theory, "spoiling," will lead to no good solutions. The understanding of the behavior which the therapist offers can lead to new and good solutions.

Nina, otherwise bright, is severely retarded in language development. Karen, when we first meet her, rarely talks to Nina. The whole topic can be opened up indirectly. The therapist always talks to Nina. Karen thinks it's a little odd to talk to a baby who, after all, can't understand English. But watching the therapist, she begins to get the point. Nina obviously responds to this talking. And the pathway is opened to a discussion of "how babies learn to talk." (In a few months Nina is positively garrulous!)

Within the context of love between a baby and mother, nearly every area of infant development becomes accessible to developmental guidance. For Karen, who has not known love and understanding in her own childhood, learning to understand her baby's need for love and her baby's "language" leads her into discoveries of her own unsatisfied longings for love. When these longings can be acknowledged by Karen they are translated into new ways of mothering for Karen. Karen can read longing and grief and the wish to be understood, and she can respond with feeling.

Robbie: Guidance to Sustain "an Unrequited Love"

Robbie's parents (Chapter VI) *do* know how babies learn to love. Their anguish is that the love being held in readiness for a baby has become a kind of unrequited love. The long-awaited baby is born very prematurely (at twenty-seven weeks gestation) and goes through recurrent life-threatening illnesses. He remains in intensive care for the first 4 months of his life. During the first 2 months, his parents, devoted, very capable young people, can only visit him through the small glass portholes of his isolette. The heartbreak for the parents, who live with constant anxiety for the life of their newborn, is compounded by the fact that the life-giving intensive care of the hospital has deprived them of their baby and their own parenthood. The baby "belongs" to the hospital, not to them. Circumstances beyond the control of the parents—and beyond human control—create impediments to attachment for Robbie and for his parents. If there were no help for the parents at this point, the estrangement of the parents and baby could have effects later. The baby might go home still seeming to be a stranger when finally reunited with his parents.

The treatment methods employed by the therapist grow out of her assessment of the impediments to attachment, which are real and circumstantial. They are in no sense impediments of personality; the anguish and the anxiety of the parents are the reactions of two basically healthy people living in a nightmare. (We would have more cause for concern if there were not pain and anxiety under these circumstances.)

The therapist at first becomes the "bridge" between the parents and their baby. She is the stable, dependable person who listens, who helps them speak of their pain and their anxiety, who visits with them in the hospital intensive-care unit and becomes the "interpreter" for the silent, mainly unresponsive baby who lies in a glass cubicle. She helps the parents understand the hospital system. She provides the encouragement they need to seek more information and express themselves more directly to hospital staff. The staff are thus enabled to become collaborators in fostering the attachment between the two parents and their baby.

When Robbie is able to leave his isolette, the therapist often accompanies his mother on visits to the nursery. At each visit there are signs of response for the parents, which the therapist comments upon and weaves into her own commentary on the development of Robbie. Robbie's parents begin to feel the rewards that all parents need. These are parents with large resources of love for their baby, which has been closed off literally and metaphorically by a glass porthole. The skill of the therapist lies in freeing that love and sustaining it during a period when the premature and sick baby can not return the gift in the lavish and whole-hearted way that healthy and physiologically mature babies reward their parents. When Robbie, at last, is united with his family in his home, he is very much a person, treasured by his parents. He is not a stranger. In the many months of work that follow, the therapist brings her knowledge of nursing and infant development to the unique task of fostering the bonds between an infant and parent when the baby cannot utter sounds because the last of the life-saving measures in the hospital has been a tracheostomy.

Greg: Guidance When A Baby is Endangered by His Mother's Past

But now, if we move to another group of examples, the work of developmental guidance becomes more complex. How shall we promote and facilitate the bonds between parents and a baby when the parent has turned away from his child, avoids the baby or is repulsed by him, and cannot even minister to his physical needs? And what can we offer the baby, as patient, who avoids his mother, is fearful of her, and has taken refuge in solitude?

Annie (Chapter VII) avoids Greg, her baby, and 4-month-old Greg avoids his mother. He rarely looks at his mother, rarely smiles to her. He does not turn to her when he is in distress. Annie avoids touching the baby or holding him and turns over his care to her husband. It will not help to encourage Annie to hold her baby or to provide her with techniques for engaging her baby. By the time we meet Annie and Earl and Greg, public health nurses have already acknowledged discouragement and defeat in their attempts to bring Annie closer to her baby.

In our own observations during the initial assessment period, Annie's avoidance of her baby can be pieced together through our observations and her communications to us. Annie is afraid to get close to her baby. She is afraid of her own destructive feelings toward him; afraid she might kill him. When Annie is helped to talk about herself, we learn of a childhood in which brutality, sadism, and repeated abandonment constituted the largest part of what she knew of parenting. When the therapist reaches Annie through her memories of pain and intolerable fear, Annie, for the first time, reaches out to her baby and holds him.

It is at this point that developmental guidance united with psychotherapy can begin for Annie to foster the bonds between her and Greg. Annie, who had never known protective love, finds ways to give such love to her baby.

But bereft of the experiences which would lead to understanding a baby, interpreting the "language" of a baby, and unable through any tradition to confer "personhood" on a baby, Annie must learn all of this with the help of the therapist. Psychotherapy alone will not give her this knowledge. In Annie's tradition, a baby doesn't know anything and doesn't yet have feelings of his own. In Annie's tradition, a 6-month-old baby who annoys his parents with his fussing is "just plain spoiled" and before the spoiling takes over and has permanent effects in personality, "you let him know who is boss" and reinforce it with a smack that he'll remember. The therapist, watching Greg with Annie, helps Annie to look for causes in the "fussing." (In the same way, the therapist is helping Annie to look for causes in her own feelings and her behavior.) The cause might be discomfort in one position, or the loss of a toy over the rim of the high chair, or just wanting some sociability. It all makes sense some place. It is a new way of looking at a baby, and it is hard work for Annie. But she trusts her therapist. And she learns a lot.

The quick smack which Annie had in her traditional repertoire has to come under scrutiny in the sessions with the therapist. The therapist, witnessing one such episode, draws Annie's attention to the fear on Greg's face. Annie sees it, as if for the first time. "Is this what we want, Annie?" the therapist asks. The words are intended to have a double meaning for Annie. Annie had been remembering her own childhood and the frightening aspects of her mother and her stepfather. And she says, in a low voice, "I don't want my child to be afraid of me."

INFANT-PARENT PSYCHOTHERAPY

In infant-parent psychotherapy, the familiar methods of psychotherapy are modified to serve the unique requirements of our work. Our objectives are to identify those aspects of parental psychological conflict impeding the development of stable bonds between parents and baby or impeding development in the child in other specific areas, and to resolve those conflicts through a process in which the sources of parental conflict are illuminated and interpreted. The baby is liberated, as it were, from the distortions and displaced affects which have engulfed him in the parental neurosis. This is therapeutic work which moves from the present to the past and from the past to the present.

It differs from conventional psychotherapy in its focus on the infant and the parental conflicts which have been visited upon the baby. This means not only that concurrent developmental guidance is part of the infant treatment but that the therapeutic work itself is to a large extent "selective" in its areas of work.

When we say "selective," we do not mean that we are not attentive to any and all material that the parent, as patient, brings to us. But, in analogy with "the patient's definition of the problem" in all psychotherapy, there tends to be a clustering and proliferation of patient communications in the area defined as the problem, and in our cases the problem, of course, is the baby. As therapists, we too are "selective" in highlighting and exploring those aspects of the parents' communications that illuminate the conflict with the baby.

Our methods in this infant-parent psychotherapy are clearly indebted to psychoanalysis. The therapeutic alliance, which is indispensable to all therapeutic work, is given strong impetus in our work with parents by the parents' hopes for their baby. If impediments to this alliance appear either at the beginning of the work or at any point in the work, we look for causes in the relationship between parents and therapist, that is, we see the obstacle in therapeutic work as a manifestation of negative transference. The negative transference is examined as a defense against painful memories or feelings, transferred, i.e., reexperienced with the therapist. In the course of examining these transference repetitions, the disturbing memories and affects are given voice and given meaning (through the therapist's interpretation). The patient's insight gives him the possibility of finding new solutions to old conflicts.

The repetition of the past in the present becomes a key to the understanding of seemingly inexplicable attitudes and actions in the patient. (Many of our patients have lost control over their lives because the past and the present have merged, as in a nightmare.) The therapeutic work of unraveling the past becomes a form of "undoing" the past, of diminishing or abolishing its power to invade the present.

When there is a baby at the center of such a psychotherapy, we are given extraordinary insight into the repetition of the past in the present, one in which the baby himself is endowed with attributes and qualities, and sometimes malignant influence and malevolent intention, which *cannot* belong to a baby and *must* belong to other figures in the parental past.

It is as if the baby has become a transference object.

The phrase "the baby as transference object" is unsettling. How can a baby be a "transference object"? In the language of psychotherapy, we speak of the therapist as transference object, meaning that he is a screen upon which is projected the figures of the patient's past with the reevoked attitudes and affective connotations of those past experiences. However, in life, it is not only a therapist who is capable of evoking the figures of the past. A positive aspect of a beloved parent can be transferred to a lover or a friend or a teacher. A negative aspect of a parent can be transferred to a lover or a mother-in-law or an employer, even with minimal cooperation on the part of the partner who is elected for this role.

But how can a baby become a transference object? We will have more to say about this in Chapter VII but this may be the place to introduce this alien notion.

"The Monster"

"He is a monster!" a young mother is telling us, and she has called him "a monster" in each of the sessions in which she has been invited to tell us how she sees the problem. "The monster" is 11 months old. He has the face of a cherub (in repose). "The monster" has severe temper tantrums in which he flails about, screams, and often cannot be reached either through his mother's voice or the therapist's. "The monster" also wakens several times a night, screaming in terror. "He won't leave me alone for a *minute*," the young mother says. "I can't even go to the bathroom without his *pestering* me . . . he wants everything I have. If I'm eating, he wants *my* toast, *my* coffee, or *my* orange. . . . He gets his *own* way all the time. . . . He *deliberately* tries to get my goat."

The mother and "the monster" engage in frequent contests in our playroom. In a "no-no" contest, "the monster" usually wins.

On one occasion the mother and "the monster" are quarreling in our playroom (if a nonverbal partner can be said to quarrel). Turning to the therapist, the mother says, "Did you see? *He started it, he did it first!*"

The therapist has the eerie feeling that she has been transformed into a mother, invited to referee a quarrel between her two children.

None of this can make sense if we look at the facts. An 11-month-old baby cannot be a monster who tyrannizes a grown woman. His cognitive capabilities (even if they are good for his age) are not up to the complex mental gymnastics that are required to execute a plot against his mother or to imagine a victory in which he triumphs over her through a war of attrition.

It is no help, as the therapist finds, to offer developmental guidance only, to divest the baby of his monster attributes through tactful explanations to the mother of his actions, or to suggest alternative modes of handling everyday problems. In the last instance, this mother always reports, "I tried it and it doesn't work."

Finally, it is more profitable to ask the question "Who is the monster?" If it cannot be a baby, then the baby must represent another figure in the mother's past.

We are struck by the phrasing of the mother's complaints. There are the phrases that a child uses in bringing a sibling dispute to a mother. "He gets into all *my* things. He won't leave me alone. He pesters me. Did you see? He started it! He did it first!"

As the therapist encourages the mother to talk about herself, the original "monster" emerges from the mother's childhood. That "monster" was the mother's brother, two years older than she. And as the mother remembers him, he was a bully and a tyrant who reduced her to utter helplessness and inconsolable crying in her room. And that "monster" was *her* mother's favorite. He could do no wrong.

In the course of a few sessions, the mother's rage and heartbreak emerge as she recalls the first "monster" and the mother who gave a small girl no protection against tyranny and openly sided with her favorite child. The therapist, listening with sympathy, finds the moment after each revelation and outbreak of feeling to help the mother see the connections between the "monster" of her childhood and her own baby, and between the mother's mother who she felt could not be trusted and her fear that the therapist could not be trusted. The mother saw all this with wonderment, and the monster attributes which she had given her own baby (13 months old by this time) begin to recede.

Now the mother can see her baby as a deeply troubled child. She can look at her child with the therapist and consider, for the first time, that a small boy who flies into rages during the day is the same small boy who has night terrors, and that the two aspects of the child must be looked at together. When the monster returns to his original abode in the remote past we very clearly have a little boy who suffers from overwhelming fears. Now we can help!

At this point the therapist offers suggestions to the mother, always united to an understanding of the meaning of the child's behavior. (Here we shift back to developmental guidance.) The child who is "understood" by his mother begins to reward her. The no-win contests come to an end. The night terrors diminish, then disappear.

Since we are examining our psychotherapeutic methods in this section, the "monster" story serves nicely to illustrate "selection" of the areas for therapeutic work. The "monster" in this mother's past was by no means the only figure who had played a decisive role in shaping her troubled personality. There were many tragedies in that childhood and, for that matter, many monsters. If the mother were in individual psychotherapy, the whole tangled web of childhood griefs and fears would be opened up over time. In our infant-centered psychotherapy we start where baby and parents are most in need of clinical understanding. In the case cited, the problem first brought to us is a particular "monster" in the past who is exercising a morbid influence upon a baby and his mother. If there are other monsters or other ghosts who have invaded the baby's nursery, we will meet them in our work with the same thorough scrutiny. But in this story, we were favored by the circumstances in which only one of the many monsters in the mother's past chose to take up residence in the baby's nursery.

"The Intruder"

The baby as "transference object" can be explored in the clinical studies presented in this volume. Billy (Chapter VIII) is another baby who, at 5 months, is the unhappy victim of an unsettled quarrel in his mother's childhood. The baby is starving, and the 17-year-old mother cannot feed him. Nor can she love him! Billy has turned away from his mother and his father. The baby's life is in danger, and the therapist, in almost daily visits, is doing two things at once in every session. She is present at feedings to give practical help in establishing adequate food intake, and she is trying to understand the mother who can only give mechanical compliance with the good advice and often forgets it.

There is a litany of complaints against the baby. "Whenever we are eating, he *pesters* us for food," says the mother. The therapist says, "Could he be hungry?" and the schoolgirl mother says, "How could he be? He just ate!" The therapist asks, "How much could he eat if we gave him all he wants?" The mother says, fighting angry tears, "If we gave him everything he wants, he'd eat us out of house and home!"

The mother is hungry. The father is hungry. They are living in poverty. Billy, we learn, has "spoiled everything." If all the lamentations could be compressed into a single sentence it would come out like this: "He has taken everything away from me, all the good things I wanted for myself."

How can a 6-month-old baby "eat us out of house and home"? Even in desperate hunger themselves, few parents could say this—and mean it.

The irrational fear must be understood. And while the therapist is keeping a watchful eye on food (for the baby *and* the parents) and giving emotional support to this child-mother, her eyes and her ears are searching for a clue to the mystery.

In the full clinical report, we see a rapid unraveling of the love-hate conflicts in the mother which have been visited on her baby.

There was another baby in this mother's life who took all the good things away from her, another intruder who "spoiled everything." It was a baby sister, and in the language of childhood, that baby had stolen food (love) from her "hungry" sister.

When the young mother makes the astonishing connection between past and present, Billy becomes *her* baby and the first intruder and despoiler moves back to the mother's childhood, where she can safely "pester" and carry on old quarrels (and she does for a while), but she can no longer invade this baby's life with his mother.

And Billy begins to thrive!

Not the end of the story, of course. From time to time old ghosts appear in new disguise, but now the therapeutic work can move freely between developmental guidance and parent psychotherapy.

Reenactment of Tyranny

In the case of Annie and Greg we see another form of transference in which the baby is caught up in the morbid past of his mother. We have touched on this story at several points in this chapter.

Annie, the mother, as we have seen, avoids her baby because she is afraid she will harm him. And this is not an unrealistic fear. Her rage, indiscriminately directed toward everyone (including the therapist), could result in physical harm to Greg, as we see when it breaks through from time to time.

Annie herself, we learn, had experienced terrible brutality in her childhood and repeated abandonment by her mother. She is now a mother who is driven by forces beyond her control to reenact her own tragic childhood.

What is repeated is the tragedy of a helpless child (her baby now) and a dangerous parent (herself). What is *transferred* to the baby is one part of herself, the helpless and crying child, and this aspect of her childhood self she does not remember at all at the beginning of treatment. She only remembers herself as tough. How Annie took over and identified with the dangerous and brutal aspects of her parents is a part of the story that is better told in the clinical narrative in this volume.

We hypothesized that if Annie could remember her childhood terror and helplessness, she could move protectively toward her baby. But it is just *this*, the overwhelming anxiety of her own childhood, that has undergone repression.

The therapeutic work in Annie's case must help Annie recover the emotional experience of childhood helplessness and terror in the safety of the therapeutic relationship. When Annie remembers and reexperiences the anxiety, she does begin to move protectively toward her baby.

Abandonment Reenacted

In two other cases, Jane and Trudy (Chapters VII and IX), two mothers who had experienced abandonment in early childhood have psychologically abandoned their babies. In each case, the baby has become the representative of a childhood self which is not remembered. "The abandoned child," long buried in memory, is revived, reborn, given another name. And as if a diabolical stage manager had contrived this hideous drama, there is now another abandoned child and the old one is now the abandoner, watching like the observer in a nightmare as a distantly familiar horror story is reenacted and the observer is helpless to stop it from happening.

In each of these cases the therapist becomes, so to speak, the awakener from the nightmare. When we join with the mother to protect the baby from abandonment, we reach out in the same moment to the other abandoned child: the mother as child. We speak directly to the heartbreak for each. Long before the mother is helped to remember her own childhood terror at abandonment, we help her to name it, and the awakening from the nightmare occurs at just the moment when the therapist names it, and does what no one had done in the first abandonment: offers human sympathy, lets the tears come, helps to find the words, and stands by as symbolic protector for that lost child as well as the new baby.

When the nightmare ends, the therapeutic work has only begun. But the mother has already joined us in an alliance to protect the baby from the old nightmare. And then we see, in each of these cases, that the mother (still not understanding all that she will need to free herself and her baby from the past) turns to her baby and returns the gift which she has received from the therapist. She can find sympathy and understanding for her baby, can find words for the child who has no words, and can become the protector of her child.

"The Lost Baby"

Finally we should mention that not only the childhood conflicts of the parents may be reenacted with the birth of a child. In our brief crisis intervention papers we see how uncompleted mourning for a beloved dead person, in the period before the birth of the baby, can profoundly affect the parents' capacities to bind themselves to their child.

Gretchen (Chapter IV) is brought to us at 4 months of age because something is terribly wrong with her. "She is turning away from us. She doesn't seem to like us," the parents tell us. And Gretchen gives eloquent confirmation of her parents' fears. She literally turns away from them. Also, we learn that Gretchen is an inconsolable baby who cries for hours at a time. We hear her disconsolate wail in our office. Gretchen's cries are intolerable to her parents. The mother pleads with the baby to stop her crying.

The therapist "hears" something in the parents' story that is not communicated in their words or in their feelings. There was a firstborn son who died some years before Gretchen was born. (Cause of death was Sudden Infant Death Syndrome.) The parents, in telling this tragic story, are unable to summon grief in the telling. They are sad, but detached.

In the course of three sessions, the therapist helps the parents to speak of their tragedy, to recover the memories of the first baby, to relive the moment of his death, and to feel the relief of tears at last. They had never been able to speak to each other about the dead baby; they had never, until these sessions with the therapist, allowed themselves to cry. There had been no mourning allowed until this time.

Gretchen's disconsolate wail, unendurable to the parents, represented their own inconsolable grief, which could not be endured and could not be expressed. Their fears for Gretchen, their almost obsessive concern that something would happen to her if they were not watchful, their fear that if they should become strongly attached to Gretchen, some cruel fate would intervene, could all come together now in the course of this belated but necessary mourning.

The story, as we will later see, has a very good conclusion for Gretchen and for her parents.

The therapeutic methods in this brief form of treatment are very similar to those which we employ in the intensive treatment cases reported later in this volume. The therapist identifies an unresolved conflict in the parents which belongs to another time and another baby, a conflict which has reformed itself around this baby and is endangering the infant-parent attachment. By following the affective routes which lead back to the first baby, the therapist helps the parents and the baby find new solutions.

IV

Brief Crisis Intervention:
Two Cases

SELMA FRAIBERG

VIVIAN SHAPIRO

VICKI BENNETT

JEREE PAWL

IN THIS CHAPTER we present two clinical examples of a form of crisis intervention on behalf of a baby and his family in which circumstances limit the number of visits and the time span of the work. By chance, two of the most instructive of our cases in this group, Neil Yates and Gretchen Raab, have certain factors in common. Both babies are just under 4 months of age. The mothers of both babies are depressed, and the depression of each is related to the loss of a loved person in a period antecedent to the birth of the baby. In the case of Neil's mother, earlier griefs are compounded by a hysterectomy shortly after Neil's birth. In both cases the families are getting ready to move to another community, and the time limit imposed by the moving date gives us only three visits.

While the therapist responds to the crisis, we see, as early as the first session for each family, that old ghosts in the parental past have invaded the nursery and are interfering with, or are in danger of interfering with, parental bonds to the baby.

The repetition of the parental past in the present, mentioned in the previous chapter, is a subject we shall treat at length in Chapter VII. In the two clinical stories to be reported in that chapter, the "ghosts" have taken up residence in the nursery, and the parents are locked in a morbid conflict with their babies, a conflict of such magnitude that many months of intensive treatment are required to abolish the ghosts and free the baby from the parental neurosis.

But whether or not the ghosts take over and imperil the baby depends to some extent upon the parents' own resistance, their ability to see the "ghost" as alien, an intruder upon their joy in their baby, and, we hope, to seek help in banishing the intruder from their lives. They may not be able to name the ghost when they arrive in our consulting room—there they will need our professional help. But to say "Something is wrong, something is happening that we don't want to happen," as the Raabs and the Yateses say when they come to us, is far removed from the kind of "statements" that we get from Mrs. March and Annie Beyer in "Ghosts in the Nursery," which are, "I am defeated by forces which I cannot control" and "I don't know why I am here or why I was sent here because there is no help for people like me."

Thus we are advantaged in our work with Neil's parents and Gretchen's parents from the outset. And this, in addition to the skill of the therapists, accounts for the benefits of treatment in these two cases in which good and important work was accomplished in only three sessions. When brief treatment can be effective, it is usually because some special advantage in circumstance or in the psychological constitution of the patients combines with a high degree of skill in the clinician. It would be a mistake, we feel, to generalize from these experiences and argue that brief treatment is "better than" or "just as good as" intensive, long-term treatment. Three interviews with Mrs. March or Annie Beyer, the two mothers of the "Ghosts" chapter, would have left two endangered babies with two seriously depressed mothers, one of whom was already afraid that she would kill her baby. The "undoing" of the past which was essential for the work with Mrs. March and Annie proceeded slowly, because these two women were drowning in the past. Depression in each was severe, had endured for many years, and had been further compounded by the birth of a baby.

In contrast, the depression in Mrs. Raab and Mrs. Yates was reactive to circumstances of tragic loss. The necessary psychological work of mourning had been closed off. But both women gave evidence of intactness of ego functioning and devotion to child and husband which spoke well for the capacity to love if a burden were lifted from them.

The therapeutic techniques employed in these two illustrations of brief treatment are, in several ways, adapted from our work in the intensive treatment cases which are described later in this volume. In our intensive treatment work we had seen how defenses against affect (isolation, partial repression) had operated to dissociate memories from their attendant affects. So it was that the patient could recall the loss of a loved person in fine detail, but could not experience the loss, grief, anger, or guilt. The buried affect emerged in depressive symptoms or a pervasive sense of guilt "without knowing why," or it might erupt in anger toward a baby "without any reason."

All this has long been illuminated in psychoanalytic literature and in the practice of psychoanalysis. The work of therapy is to bring together memory and affects and to help the patient reexperience with the therapist the emotional import of an experience in order to master it and find new and more favorable adaptive routes. In our adaptation of the psychoanalytic method for the intensive treatment cases, we provided "a safe place" in which to remember, to feel, and to understand. We spoke to "feelings" as therapists and in our detailed narrative notes we see the phrases: "How sad that must have been for you . . .," "How that must have hurt. . . ." We were giving "permission to feel," and we gave such permission at every moment we saw the struggle to defend against painful feelings. As affect emerged, we helped the patient find the lost links to both the past and the present experiences of painful events.

In the two examples of brief treatment which follow, we see the therapist in each case finding the affective routes into the experience of tragic loss so that grief could find words and tears, and the work of mourning and healing could be accomplished.

We also see a small-scale model of our work as represented throughout this volume. The baby is present in the family interview; the therapists' eyes move back and forth between the baby and his parents. The baby as the patient who can't talk is carrying on his part of the conversation in eloquent language of his own. Gretchen consistently turns away from her parents' faces and their voices, and we witness the heartbreak for the parents. Gretchen breaks into disconsolate wailing which pierces the climate of the room at the moment that her mother is struggling with words to speak of her own inconsolable grief. Neil, the child of a depressed young mother, should, by all of our expectations, be a sober, distant baby. But he is full of joy, and his long, ecstatic vocal accompaniments to his parents' sad story must be listened to, also. He is saying, "Look at me! *I'm* fine. *I* have no complaints." And the therapist, eyes on Neil, then on the mother's face distorted with grief, has received an important communication from the baby: This mother, in spite of her own anguish, has been able to give her child love and devoted care.

Neil

Neil Yates is 4 months old. A pediatric nurse calls to ask if we can offer help to Neil and his parents at a critical moment for the family. Mrs. Yates appears to the nurse depressed, and the baby, who is "overfed" in the nurse's opinion, vomits frequently and suffers from constipation. The family is about to move from our state to another, three thousand miles away. The mother's anxiety and depression have deepened as she anticipates the move. She is in near panic as she tries to make the necessary plans.

The date of the move will give us, at best, three sessions.

The nurse, who has known the family since Neil's birth, feels that Mrs. Yates's depression is a reaction to a series of tragedies in the past year. We learn that Mrs. Yates had had a hysterectomy when cervical cancer was diagnosed shortly after Neil's birth. The operation was performed soon after the diagnosis, and with little time for Mrs. Yates to prepare herself psychologically. Following the operation, Mrs. Yates reported panic states, fear of dying, and fears that she was going crazy. She "can't get things done." (That is, she is disorganized in managing her daily life.) She is afraid at night and has to have a light on in her bedroom.

But there is more. Both of Mrs. Yates's parents died last year. The father died of cancer; the mother, following post-surgical complications.

Mr. Yates is an itinerant workman. Both Mr. and Mrs. Yates were reared in Appalachian mountain villages, where education was limited and ancient superstitions guided the ways of life.

We learn that this is a second marriage for Mrs. Yates. An earlier marriage ended in divorce. There is one daughter, Doris, age 10, from the first marriage, who lives with her mother and stepfather.

FIRST SESSION

Vivian Shapiro became the therapist for the Yates family, and the first meeting took place in our office within three days after we agreed to see them on an emergency basis.

Both Mr. and Mrs. Yates were present at this session. (A session with Neil present was to be scheduled.) Mrs. Yates looked sad and depressed, and it took some time for Mrs. Shapiro to register that this was indeed a pretty woman, because grief and anxiety distorted her face. Mr. Yates, tall, blond, with a look of strength in his face and his carriage, was manifestly concerned about his wife and tried throughout the session to help her talk to the strange woman. In spite of excellent preparation given by the nurse, both parents seemed confused about the reason for referral to *this* clinic. Perhaps it was the label on our door—The Child Development Project. It took a bit of time for Mrs. Shapiro to help Mr. and Mrs. Yates to understand that we work with babies and their parents, that we understood that they were going through a troubled time, and that we would like to help them in any way that we could. We knew, of course, that the family would be moving within a very short time, and we would use this time together to see in what way we could best help.

Mrs. Yates found it hard to speak. She said there was really no problem with her husband, it was just herself. She thought that she was going to die. She was frightened of being alone. "I'm just depressed," she said, "and I don't know why." Mr. Yates said that he, too, did not know why. Mrs. Shapiro said, with sympathy, that she knew that many sad things had happened to the Yateses during the past year and that there might be a good reason for feeling depressed. To help out this nearly inarticulate young woman, Mrs. Shapiro said that she knew that Mrs. Yates had lost her mother and father in the past year, and that she had had a baby, found out she had cancer, and had a hysterectomy a few weeks ago. She said it was quite understandable that Mrs. Yates would feel depressed and have worries about dying.

This seemed to come as a complete surprise to Mr. and Mrs. Yates. Incredibly, it seems it had not occurred to either of them that the events they had experienced during the past year might have some relationship to Mrs. Yates's anxiety and depression. Mrs. Yates, registering surprise, asked Mrs. Shapiro in all innocence if that could be part of the explanation for her feelings. The therapist said that it might certainly be so.

(To herself, Mrs. Shapiro registered this as an extraordinary communication. If, in fact, Mr. and Mrs. Yates had made no connection between loss through death, cervical cancer, and a hysterectomy, what mental mechanisms had made it possible for Mrs. Yates to say, "I feel depressed and I don't know why"?)

But Mrs. Yates now seemed ready to talk, and Mrs. Shapiro guided her into speaking of loss. Mrs. Yates spoke of her father who had "died of cancer in the neck." There had been surgery and a period of recovery. Then, in a way that Mrs. Yates could not describe or understand, he was rushed to the hospital and died.

Shortly after Mrs. Yates's father's death, her mother, who was grossly obese (weighing about 340 pounds), elected to have a shunt operation in order to lose weight. But her mother had also had long-standing liver and kidney problems. She was not able to tolerate the operation and died of complications.

Mrs. Shapiro registered for herself that here were two experiences of family members who had undergone surgery with expectations of success and had died.

But Mrs. Yates's story had been told factually and without manifest affect. Here we begin to get the answer to the question that was raised earlier. She was depressed, but she didn't know why. She could remember the events but she couldn't experience grief, or loss, or anxiety. This was not to say that Mrs. Yates was "without affect" or incapable of profound feeling. As Mrs. Shapiro saw it, the painful affects had undergone dissociation from experience and transformation into depression and phobic symptoms.

Here is a dilemma for the therapist. In a therapy that gives us the necessary time for the work that must be done, we may need many weeks or months before the patient is capable of uniting the buried affect with his experience. The question for this treatment, which must be brief, was whether the affective experience of loss, of many losses, would be available for this limited work. There was no question, of course, that we were going to need help for Mrs. Yates in her new community, but to create a meaningful bridge between this crisis intervention and a referral she would need to have some glimmer of understanding that there was a "why" in her depression and that it was linked to real events. It was not "something in her head" alone. The Yateses, we remember, were a couple with limited education. They were not people who would normally seek psychiatric help.

Mrs. Shapiro asked Mrs. Yates if she could remember her feelings around the time of the death of her mother and her father. Mrs. Yates said that when her father had died unexpectedly, her mother had called, weeping on the telephone. Mrs. Yates remembered that she said to her mother, "Mama, why are you crying so much? All you ever did was fight." And her mother said to her, "But you don't know how much we really loved each other."

Mrs. Yates then went on to say that when her mother died, she felt as though the event was not real. She was called back home—it was totally unexpected. Soon after her mother's death, she married her husband and they moved to the Midwest. Mrs. Yates became pregnant. It was a terrible year. She was completely depressed. She missed her home town. She had fears of being alone. She would not go down to the basement of her house by herself.

Mrs. Shapiro, voicing great sympathy for Mrs. Yates, reflected upon these terrible losses and then said that of course she would be missing her mother, especially at this time with a new baby and her own surgery. Mr. Yates, who was able to follow Mrs. Shapiro very well, then joined in to say that his wife had always wanted to have a friend who would be like her mother, overweight and older. In fact, the woman who had helped take care of his wife's mother had come to help take care of Neil when Mrs. Yates went into the hospital for the hysterectomy.

This led to the story of the hysterectomy. In the small rural hospital in which Neil had been delivered there had been a routine Pap test following delivery. Six weeks following the birth of Neil, Mrs. Yates received a letter saying that the Pap smear had been positive. The family had never had a personal doctor. There was no one to turn to. Mrs. Yates called the hospital to speak to "someone," and there was no one to tell her what a positive Pap smear meant. Finally, in an incredible tale of lost connections, and no one there, Mr. Yates drove his wife to the hospital and demanded to see the doctor who had delivered the baby. He was the only doctor they knew, and it was that obstetrician who told Mrs. Yates that she did indeed have cancer, that she had a kind of cancer that was 99 percent curable if the uterus and cervix were removed. The Yateses went home and talked about it for a night. Mr. Yates said he did not want his wife to sacrifice her life and felt that they had already been lucky to have a baby. Mrs. Yates entered the hospital immediately for a hysterectomy.

Once again, Mrs. Shapiro asked Mrs. Yates about her feelings. Mrs. Yates said that she didn't think about it until the day it happened. She added that since then, however, she had been worried about dying, and she was afraid of being alone in the house.

(Again Mrs. Yates had made no connection. She had "no feelings" about the hysterectomy but she could remember that her fears of dying and of being alone were somehow uncertainly connected.) Were these fears recent or had she in fact had them before? Mrs. Shapiro asked. Mrs. Yates could remember times in the past when her "nervousness" made it hard for her to manage.

Then Mr. Yates, again following Mrs. Shapiro's questions with an intuitive understanding, said, "I think there's one other thing you should know that might be related. My wife had a twin sister who died suddenly at the age of 4 years." And as he said this Mrs. Yates began to tremble uncontrollably. Mrs. Shapiro encouraged her to tell her more about this. Mrs. Yates said that she and her sister had been very close. One evening the two girls were dancing when her sister became suddenly sick. In the village in which Mrs. Yates lived there may not have been doctors, or if there were, one did not go to them. Mrs. Yates's aunt came over to put a poultice on her sister's chest. Her sister grew worse. By the time they got her to the hospital, she could barely breathe. "They couldn't get the oxygen machine connected fast enough and she died."

Could she remember her feelings then? Mrs. Shapiro asked. Mrs. Yates could remember the family huddling together and that she herself was somewhere in her room. She really did not have any memory of her feelings at the time. (In the next interview we are to see much more of her feelings.)

Mrs. Shapiro noted to herself the extreme anxiety in Mrs. Yates when she talked about her sister. Again, Mrs. Shapiro said that she could understand that the death of her sister may have been still another place where feelings of loss and fears of loss might come from. There had been so much for her to cope with. Anyone in her situation would have felt overwhelmed.

With this, both Mr. and Mrs. Yates responded with relief. Mrs. Yates had thought that her feelings were crazy. And now she thought they were "not so crazy." (That is, there were reasons.) She asked Mrs. Shapiro what could help her feel better. She was afraid to leave with her husband for his new job. Mrs. Yates would need to go down a week earlier to find a trailer. She did not want to go. If only she could see a doctor and he could tell her what to do to feel better, then maybe she could go a week or two later. Mrs. Shapiro explained as sympathetically as possible that although she indeed thought that Mrs. Yates needed help, there was no help that would go as quickly as that. But there would be help that we would arrange for her if she would like us to in her new community. And again Mr. and Mrs. Yates relaxed visibly upon hearing this.

Toward the end of the session, Mrs. Shapiro asked if the Yateses could tell her a little about Doris, the 10-year-old daughter. Mr. Yates had said earlier that Doris had never quite accepted him as a stepfather. Often she would kiss everybody else in the room good night but not Mr. Yates. He was quite pained as he said this. When Mrs. Shapiro asked how he understood this, he said that he thought Doris really wanted her own father back. (This was a father who had literally disappeared for years.) Mrs. Yates said that Doris never talked about Steven, her father, and that he had not called for three years. Doris had never once mentioned him. (Mrs. Shapiro reflected to herself that Doris's way of handling pain seemed to be very close to Mrs. Yates's way of not thinking about things, of putting them out of mind.)

When Mrs. Shapiro asked if they would tell her a bit about the baby, Mr. Yates said that Neil was a beautiful baby, and Mrs. Yates said that he looked very much like his father. Generally they thought that Neil was a happy baby. The six weeks after the baby's birth were the best Mr. and Mrs. Yates had known. And then had come the news about cancer. Mrs. Shapiro said she thought it was very important that the baby had been a comfort to Mrs. Yates and that she had been able to mother him.

At the close of the session, Mrs. Shapiro spoke of the immediate crisis. It was now Friday and Mr. Yates was leaving the following morning. Mrs. Yates said that she was afraid to stay alone. Mrs. Shapiro asked her what plans she could make to ease the fears. It took some help on Mrs. Shapiro's part to get Mrs. Yates to anticipate and plan for a separation that was already giving her great anxiety. But with close attention to the topic and guiding the couple step by step, she finally helped Mrs. Yates to arrive at a sensible plan. She would invite somebody to stay with her, a close friend. Mr. Yates said that he would call his wife every night and would come back as soon as possible. Mrs. Shapiro offered her own home telephone number, in case of need. Also, the nurse who had befriended the Yateses and had referred them to our program would be available. Mrs. Yates was temporarily shored up against her terrible fear of being alone.

Mrs. Shapiro said that she would like to see Mrs. Yates and the baby on Monday and offered an appointment. Mrs. Yates welcomed the appointment.

SECOND SESSION

Mrs. Yates arrived with Neil. She seemed pleased to see Mrs. Shapiro, but again the therapist registered a look of pain and sadness in her eyes. Neil, at 0:3:22, was a beautiful, blond baby who did look exactly like his father, Mrs. Shapiro noted. And while the therapist and Mrs. Yates talked, Mrs. Shapiro's eyes moved from mother to baby and baby to mother. An extraordinary story was disclosed in this observation.

In spite of the fact that Mrs. Yates was still uncomfortable following her hysterectomy, she was able to hold the baby close, to rock him, to talk to him. This meant to us that a seriously depressed young mother had resources within herself to mother her baby. And the baby himself, as we shall soon see, gave testimony to the quality of their affectional ties. But Mrs. Shapiro also observed that when Neil was fussy Mrs. Yates's most common mode of comforting him was to feed him his bottle. Neil, as we already know, was in fact overweight, and Mrs. Shapiro reflected to herself that if Mrs. Yates was overfeeding him it might be related to her own emotional exhaustion, that the easiest way for her to comfort her baby was to feed him.

But Neil himself was full of smiles. There were special smiles for his mother, and he turned to her frequently and to the therapist frequently. He was quite active. He was able to reach his toes with his hands. He was able to turn over and was also vocalizing frequently. Mrs. Yates held him for most of the visit and was in touch with him constantly.

This meant to us that in every area but feeding this was a mother who was responsive to her baby's needs and his signals. And the baby himself, adequate in all areas of development, and with preferential behaviors toward his mother, gave independent testimony of the love that he was receiving from her.

Observing all this, Mrs. Shapiro praised Mrs. Yates for her capacity to be in touch with her baby despite the fact that she was not feeling well. Mrs. Yates said that after her operation she felt it was harder to respond to her baby's cries. Mrs. Shapiro said this was understandable. It was as if Mrs. Yates needed someone to respond to her *own* cries.

At this point, Mrs. Yates became extremely sad. Mrs. Shapiro asked her if she could tell her what she was thinking. She missed her mother, she said. How much she wanted her mother. How lonesome she was. How frightened she was. When the therapist asked her what she would want to tell her mother, Mrs. Yates's fears flowed freely. Weeping, she said that she wanted to tell her about the hysterectomy. She wanted to tell her mother that she could have no more children. It was indeed a sad moment for the therapist to witness too. Mrs. Shapiro told her that it was a very sad time and of course she would want her mother and of course she needed her mother. Mrs. Yates said that she didn't know if she could take "one more thing going wrong." She didn't know if she could survive.

Mrs. Yates then went on to say that she had been thinking about her twin sister. In Mrs. Yates's village there was a saying that if you lost a twin sister you were locked in death with that sister forever. She said that she had heard that saying but had never known what it meant. It had haunted her all these years.

Mrs. Shapiro suggested another way of looking at this. Mrs. Yates had said that she had often been very fearful of dying. The therapist wondered if maybe once before she had lost "part of herself" when her sister had died. Mrs. Yates began to tremble once again and a look of great sadness came over her face. Now she spoke more about the circumstances of her sister's death, how they had been playing and singing together when suddenly her sister became sick. After the death of the sister, Mrs. Yates's father began to drink and became an alcoholic. Her mother began to gain weight, and other illnesses followed. Mrs. Yates said that she had slept with her mother since her sister's death.

But there were other losses too. And this led Mrs. Yates to talk for a while about her first husband. She had become pregnant at 16 and decided to marry Steven. Shortly after Doris's birth, Steven had a series of affairs with other women which finally led to divorce. Many hard years followed while Doris stayed with her parents and she tried to support herself through work. And then she and Chris Yates found each other and got married.

Suddenly Mrs. Yates thought of something else. For the first time this weekend (following the first session with Mrs. Shapiro) Doris had talked about her father. She said she had wished that her mother had remarried Steven instead of Chris. This hurt Chris, of course, but it brought up the whole subject of fathers, and Mrs. Yates said they had a talk for the first time.

Throughout this visit, Mrs. Shapiro observed the intensity of Mrs. Yates's emotions as she recalled painful memories. It was a good sign, of course. We are not always so rewarded in brief treatment by the patient's ability to link affect and memories, but when patients come to us at a point of crisis, buried affect may become available to us in ways that we cannot anticipate. In the first session we had seen that memories and their attendant affect were isolated. But in this second session, in response to Mrs. Shapiro's "permission to feel," memories and affect were reunited in a significant way.

Mrs. Yates herself seemed to feel this. She asked the therapist if it were really possible to feel better through talking. Other people had told her that time would take care of things. Mrs. Shapiro asked her what she thought. Mrs. Yates said, with marvelous wisdom, "You have to be able to ask the right questions. Chris tries to help me but I don't think he has the right questions." It was a beautiful insight, Mrs. Shapiro thought. She pointed out that it would be very difficult for a husband, no matter how hard he tried, to be really able to act as a therapist for her. What Mrs. Yates needed was someone who had knowledge and understanding and who could help her put into perspective all that she had suffered.

Mrs. Shapiro guided the discussion now at the close of the session to the subject of the impending move. Mrs. Yates said that she now *wanted* to rejoin her husband as quickly as possible. (Her terror of moving had abated.) This led to further discussion of the kind of help that Mrs. Yates would need when she rejoined her husband. And Mrs. Shapiro said that she herself was trying to get in touch with a therapist in Mrs. Yates's new community and would be able to tell her more about it next time.

THIRD SESSION

This would be the last session with Mrs. Yates before she left to rejoin her husband.

Unbelievably, there was another medical crisis. Mrs. Yates had just returned from her visit to the doctor and began the session in an anguished voice. "Now the doctor tells me there is a chance I will get vaginal cancer. It's a rare chance but there is a chance." And she started to cry. "If one more thing happens, I don't think I can survive. But I need to survive, because who will take care of my children?"

Beneath this outpouring, Mrs. Shapiro discerned muted rage toward this doctor, toward all doctors, perhaps. And when Mrs. Shapiro suggested that Mrs. Yates might have many feelings of anger toward the doctors because of what had happened to herself and to her family, the rage burst forth. There was rage toward the doctors who had recommended surgery for her mother and the doctors who had sent her father home "all right" only to discover there were medical complications that brought about his death.

Mrs. Yates went on to speak of her fears of death. And this brought further memories of her dying mother. The doctors had called Mrs. Yates "to ask if they should bring down the machines" to keep her mother alive. She remembered that she was angry at the call. It was not a question she thought she should answer. She had not wanted her mother to have the operation at all. Her mother hadn't needed it. She had loved her mother fat. Why had she needed it? And now they wanted to know whether to keep her mother alive. And when she asked what that would be like, "they" told her it would just be keeping her alive; she could never really recover brain functioning. Mrs. Yates then made the decision "not to keep the machines going." Mrs. Shapiro said that some of these decisions were too hard for humans to bear. Mrs. Yates then went on to describe her dying mother, swollen and beyond recognition. She went to her mother and repeated, "Mama, Mama, I'm here. You didn't die yet. You can't die. You have to stay. Don't leave me." She said that her mother looked at her and smiled. But it was no use. Her mother was dying. Her mother had looked awful. Her mother was not her mother. And when her mother died, the terrible thought began to come to her that maybe she should not have made the decision to let her mother die. Here Mrs. Shapiro supported Mrs. Yates. There really had been no hope for her mother to survive as a person.

Mrs. Shapiro, throughout this outpouring, had discerned an inarticulate anger toward the mother who had died, and tried to find a way to put this into words. Finally, she said gently that sometimes people feel angry at those who die when they still need them, and that this sometimes made a person feel very guilty. The therapist wondered if Mrs. Yates was puzzled by her angry feelings toward her mother.

Suddenly Mrs. Yates became quiet and composed. She said that she had never thought about it that way. She supposed that maybe she had been angry. And she reiterated that she had loved her mother fat. Her mother had not needed to have the operation. Mrs. Shapiro sympathized with the anguish for Mrs. Yates.

As Mrs. Yates talked about anger toward her mother and the doctors, Mrs. Shapiro noticed that the trembling had ceased and Mrs. Yate's depression seemed to lift. The therapist commented upon this to her. She said one could see that as Mrs. Yates could talk about these things she seemed to be in better control of herself. And with some surprise, Mrs. Yates agreed with this.

It was now close to the end of the hour, and Mrs. Shapiro used the time to bridge the move from our community to rejoin her husband and to find help for herself in her new community. Mrs. Shapiro already had made the necessary contacts and was able to give Mrs. Yates the names of doctors who would be able to help her.

In closing, Mrs. Shapiro told Mrs. Yates that she had really done quite well in all that she had had to cope with. It was too much for anyone to bear without feeling sad and without grief. She hoped that Mrs. Yates would get further help if she needed it and she would very much like to hear from Mrs. Yates.

For all this Mrs. Yates thanked Mrs. Shapiro warmly and expressed gratitude to the nurse who had been so helpful and had referred her to our program.

CONCLUSION

There was no further correspondence from Mrs. Yates, and we do not know whether she got in touch with the doctors whose names were given to her when she rejoined her husband.

All of us would want to know how things turned out for the family.

Can we know whether our brief crisis intervention had any effect beyond these three sessions?

We can only offer this much of an estimate of the work that was done during this critical period. A young mother, with a reactive depression and many phobic symptoms, suffering with insomnia and fears of death, had come to us thinking that she was "going crazy" because she had not been able to understand the meaning of her depression. She had closed off painful affect and was left with memories but no access to them as meaningful events. The therapist, through giving Mrs. Yates "permission to feel," helped the patient recover the feelings of grief, loss, and anger toward those whom she had loved and lost through death or betrayal (if we think in this last instance of her first husband and "all the doctors"). Through the help given her, she found relief in discovering her own feelings and in understanding something of herself. We would hope that some measure of this self-understanding might stay with the patient and that, whatever new trials may lie before her, she might not be immobilized and might find better adaptive solutions.

For the baby, Neil, who had been marvelously protected from the mother's own real and internalized conflicts, we feel that if we have helped his mother find a path which may lead to recovery from depression, we are protecting his own future.

Gretchen

In the case of 4-month-old Gretchen, extraordinary circumstances also gave us only three sessions in which to offer a form of help to the family. Happily, we later learned, this work brought positive and enduring changes for the baby and her family.

THE PRESENTING PROBLEM

A public health nurse called to ask if we could provide help for Gretchen Raab and her two distraught parents. The nurse had known Gretchen and her family for three months. In the last few weeks there had been increasing difficulties in feeding and sleeping. Mrs. Raab had had considerable difficulty in breast feeding and had recently begun to wean Gretchen to formula. The baby was irritable, crying frequently and inconsolably, and both the parents and the nurse had felt that Gretchen was not a "social" or "responsive" baby. She smiled rarely.

In the course of the intake discussion, the public health nurse offered her own valuable reflections about the possible causes of tension and anxiety in the parents which might have disturbed their relationship to Gretchen.

Five years ago, the Raabs' first baby had died suddenly. From all available information, the cause of death was Sudden Infant Death Syndrome. (It should be noted that at that time SIDS was a medical mystery. As we reflect upon the circumstances now, it is likely that no physician or nurse could have offered an explanation which would have alleviated some measure of the guilt of the parents.) Indeed, the nurse told us, both mother and father felt that their grief and anxiety over the death of the first child had interfered with their relationship to Gretchen. The mother seemed to be feeling guilty about her inability to feel comfortable with Gretchen.

The parents wanted help urgently. But the father was about to change jobs, and the family would be moving in two weeks to another region of our state five hundred miles away.

Vicki Bennett, then a graduate student of social work in our training program at the Child Development Project, had received this call while she was on intake rotation and, following our practice whenever possible, was assigned as therapist for the family. In consultation with her supervisor, Dr. Jeree Pawl, two, or possibly three, visits would be planned immediately before the family move, and we already knew that if the family needed continued support or help they were moving to an area where graduates of our state infant mental health training program would be available to them.

In a return call to the public health nurse, Mrs. Bennett offered our plan to see Gretchen and her family the following day if the family wished. The nurse said that she would call the Raabs immediately.

Within five minutes, Mrs. Bennett received a phone call from Mrs. Raab herself, having just heard from the nurse. She was eager to see Mrs. Bennett. Both she and her husband wanted to talk with Mrs. Bennett as soon as possible. And did Mrs. Bennett want to see the baby too? Yes, Mrs. Bennett said, this was the way we liked to work. What might be the best time during Gretchen's day to arrange the appointment so that she would be awake and alert? Mrs. Raab laughed ruefully as she considered the problem of finding a "good time" for her irritable baby with irregular patterns, and then thought that perhaps early afternoon might be the best time of day.

THE FIRST SESSION

When Mr. and Mrs. Raab and Gretchen arrived for their appointment, Mrs. Bennett could read anxiety on their faces in the moment of their greeting. Mrs. Raab seemed close to tears. Mrs. Raab was holding Gretchen on her lap, and as Mrs. Bennett stooped to say hello to the baby and held out her finger in greeting, Gretchen returned a wide-eyed, expressionless stare. Mrs. Bennett's first impressions of Gretchen were: "A tiny baby. Appears to be well-nourished, with a very pale complexion and wisps of brownish-red hair. She was bundled in a warm and woolly snowsuit." Mr. Raab reached over to Gretchen with an offer to carry the baby upstairs to Mrs. Bennett's office. Once in the office, Gretchen remained on her father's lap for approximately the first twenty to twenty-five minutes of the visit.

During introductory conversation, in which Mr. Raab spoke of his new job, he held Gretchen sitting up on his knee, with one of his hands in front of her chest and the other patting her back. Gretchen seemed to be contented, but Mrs. Bennett registered an infant face that seemed dazed, almost stuporous.

Mrs. Bennett said she had understood that both Mr. and Mrs. Raab seemed concerned because Gretchen was more upset these days than she should be. Mrs. Raab said yes and began to speak of Gretchen and her irritability from the earliest days on. Now, the mother said, since she was being weaned from the breast, her fretful crying and her inconsolability were even worse.

Mrs. Raab spoke of the problems that she had had with breast feeding, her concern that Gretchen was not getting enough milk and that she was crying much of the time, apparently out of hunger. They had tried many things: different schedules, different postures, and, although Mrs. Raab rarely offered supplementary bottles, Gretchen had vigorously refused to take formula from a bottle. And now that Mrs. Raab had begun weaning Gretchen from the breast, the introduction of the bottle had become very difficult. Mr. Raab said that Gretchen cried furiously when Mrs. Raab tried to give her a bottle, and she was really only willing to take the bottle without too much fuss from her father.

Even more painful to both parents were signs that Gretchen was turning away from her mother and her father. Mr. Raab said, "She doesn't look at us very much either. She seems to avoid looking at us!"

Mrs. Bennett, who was noting to herself this "turning away" and avoidance of visual contact between Gretchen and her parents, could feel the hurt and the sense of rejection that both parents were experiencing. She said, sympathetically, "I imagine that makes you feel pretty bad and anxious too."

It was at about this point that Mrs. Bennett coughed briefly and Gretchen, who had been staring off in the direction of the window, now turned suddenly and looked at her with wide eyes. Mrs. Bennett said, to Gretchen, "You're nice and alert, aren't you? You heard that cough." Mr. Raab said that sometimes Gretchen was very alert and would turn her head toward noises, but sometimes she wouldn't. Sometimes she would "just ignore you when you were trying to get her attention." Mrs. Raab said that this bothered her too and that whereas at first she had been concerned about Gretchen getting enough food, now she was worried about whether Gretchen was withdrawing or not. Mrs. Raab smiled sadly and added, "If it's not one thing, it's another."

Mrs. Bennett responded sympathetically and said, "I do hear that you have a lot of concerns about Gretchen." And at this point Mr. Raab began to speak about their first son who had died.

He said that he didn't know if Mrs. Bennett knew or not, but maybe one reason they were so anxious had to do with their baby who had died five years ago. Mrs. Bennett said sympathetically that she did know that they had had a baby who had died suddenly and that that must have been very, very painful. It was understandable how those memories could influence the degree to which they would be anxious now about Gretchen.

Mrs. Raab seemed sad and near tears, and both parents were silent for a few moments. Mrs. Bennett repeated sympathetically, "It must have been so terrible," but neither parent could yet find words. Mrs. Bennett asked how old was the baby who had died. Mrs. Raab said that Len, the baby, had been 4 months old. Mrs. Bennett said, "You could hardly help but worry about Gretchen and whether she will be all right." Both the Raabs nodded without words.

Perhaps at this moment, in a private session with the parents, tears would have come, memories might have come, and fears and painful feelings would have been put into words. But just at this moment

Gretchen, who was becoming fussy, now broke into a full-fledged cry. Mr. Raab patted her and bounced her on his knee gently for a few moments, then picked her up and held her over his shoulder where she cried for a few more moments before quieting down. Mrs. Raab said that this was typical. Gretchen would fret, begin to cry, and couldn't be comforted. It was really very hard for her to take, said Mrs. Raab. Mrs. Bennett said, "At those times it must seem as though nothing you can do pleases her." Mrs. Raab agreed.

We register, as readers, the poignant juxtaposition of events in the room. The parents themselves are speaking of their inconsolable grief at the sudden death of their first baby, they are struggling with their own tears, and the baby begins her inconsolable crying. The two parents find the baby's cries nearly intolerable. For all parents a baby's inconsolable crying is hard to bear. But for these parents the disconsolate baby echoes their own inconsolable grief, *their* cries and *their* suppressed tears. It can be an agony to tend to a crying child when the longing to weep yourself is so powerful within you. And then there must be something else. The inconsolable crying of the baby is a terrible reproach to a parent. It is as if the baby is saying, "You are not good parents. You can't make me feel good."

All this can be seen before one's eyes in parent-infant psychotherapy when the baby is present for this kind of family interview. And while the therapist who has the luxury of interviewing parents in the privacy of his office would have been able to follow the inquiry into parental feelings about a dead baby without the interruption of a new baby's cries, Gretchen's cries, which interrupted the sequence of her parents' story of another baby now dead, were not really "an interruption" when we consider how much is revealed or can be revealed at such a moment.

Gretchen's cries now lead us into another part of the story, but we will see that in the end the pathways lead back to the first baby.

Gretchen's crying subsided a bit while her father patted her, then was renewed. This time, Mrs. Bennett got up from her chair and got a mirror with a rattle on it. She handed it to Mr. Raab so that he could show it to Gretchen. (Mrs. Bennett was simply providing a distraction.) At first Gretchen paid no attention. Mrs. Raab held the mirror out to Gretchen and said, "There's an ugly baby in there, a crying baby." Mrs. Bennett reflected in her notes, "It was painfully obvious at this point how difficult it was for her to hear Gretchen cry." After a few moments, Gretchen did settle down once more after father bounced her up and down gently on his knee.

(We are registering how much of the comforting of Gretchen comes from her father, but we do not see this as an indictment of the mother.

Something in Gretchen's cries is wounding Mrs. Raab and we can only guess where all this hurts.)

The interview moves in another direction for a while, with some questions from Mr. and Mrs. Raab about our program, and Mrs. Bennett sketches the nature of our work, giving special emphasis to our concern with big problems and little problems and our wish to help parents and their babies to feel close to each other. At one point, when Mrs. Bennett is speaking about individual differences in babies and how this too has a lot to do with how parents and babies get along, Mr. Raab smiles and says, "Right. That's what we would like to know. We would like to know about how much of this has to do with our anxiety and how much of it has to do with Gretchen. I mean, maybe she's just a quiet baby or something and then we won't worry about it so much. But we just want to make sure that if she *is* withdrawing, it doesn't get any worse." Here Mrs. Bennett gives strong agreement and support of the parents in their wish to understand so that things could go well for them and their baby.

Then Gretchen begins to cry again. Mrs. Raab reaches out and takes the baby from her husband and sits her on her knee. She bends over and says, "No, no. Don't do that. No!" It is a plea to the baby, as if Gretchen were an older child, as if Gretchen were doing something wrong. Again, Mrs. Bennett registers to herself the suffering of this mother when she hears Gretchen's cries. Gretchen does not settle down so Mrs. Raab picks her up, holds her over her shoulder, patting her on the back. Now Gretchen does calm down considerably and stops fretting altogether. Mrs. Bennett notices this and speaks of it. She says that when Mrs. Raab holds Gretchen *very close* that seems to help a lot. This is the first time in the session that Mrs. Raab holds Gretchen in a close ventral position and it *does* bring the baby comfort. (We are left with the interesting question "Since the mother does have ways of comforting her baby, what is it that normally distances her?")

Gretchen is quiet now, and then, in a circuitous way, the path of the interview returns to the first baby, Len.

There had been some talk about labor and delivery (which was normal in all respects for Gretchen), and Mrs. Raab adds spontaneously that all this had been very different with their first baby, Len. Len had been born prematurely and weighed only 3 pounds 8 ounces. Mrs. Bennett, mindful of the anguish that all parents of premature babies experience, listens sympathetically. Mrs. Raab adds that he had to spend the first six weeks of life in the hospital. Mr. Raab says it is funny, but in many ways they had been less anxious about Len than they were about Gretchen. Once Len came home they thought that he was all right. Mrs. Raab says, "But it was hard to feed him. He didn't like formula either and he had projectile vomiting." Mrs. Bennett again expresses her sympathy for the parents and their dilemma and then says she thinks this could be very worrisome, that Len and Gretchen had similiar eating problems. Mrs. Raab looks very sad and says yes. And because Mrs. Bennett senses that Mrs. Raab wants to say more, she now asks, very gently, under what circumstances Len, the first baby, had died.

Mrs. Raab says that they had been driving to visit her family and the baby died on the way. She says that she had fed him, then put him down in his car bed, and when they stopped at the next stop they found the baby dead. As Mrs. Raab tells the story, she seems far away and expressionless. Mrs. Bennett, listening to the story, records that she herself wants to cry for the parents. To the parents she says, "It must have been so very hard." And then she asks Mrs. Raab if there had been anyone she could talk to after the baby had died. Had she had a chance to talk about what that was all like? No, says Mrs. Raab, in fact she tried to shut it out of her mind; she tried not to think about it very much. Mr. Raab explains that they had been in the process of moving to their first home at the time the baby died. Mrs. Raab says that she had not been able to go back to the apartment but that her husband had gone back and packed up all of the baby's things and put them away.

Mrs. Raab then goes on to say that for five years she had tried to get pregnant again and had been unable to. She describes visiting doctors and taking fertility drugs.

Nothing worked and finally they were sure they would not be able to have any children again. The following year Mrs. Raab discovered that she was pregnant. Mrs. Raab says that "physically" the pregnancy had gone well. But psychologically it had been a difficult time. She was very moody and irritable and quite depressed at times. Mr. Raab smiles sympathetically and says, "It was a difficult pregnancy for you." Mrs. Bennett says that it would be very hard to go through the experience of the first baby's death and not feel anxious and frightened during the second pregnancy. She wonders, she says, if it might not have made Mrs. Raab very anxious to even think about having another baby. Both Mr. and Mrs. Raab agree.

At this point, Mrs. Bennett, glancing at Gretchen, reaches out her finger and says, "Hello," and suddenly there is a little smile on Gretchen's face. It is the first smile that has appeared in forty-five minutes. Mrs. Raab says, "She's smiling at you. Maybe it's just *us* that she doesn't like to look at." Mrs. Bennett says, "I'm sure not. I think that right now you're just more aware of Gretchen's irritability and fussiness and that makes it hard."

Mr. Raab, picking up on the theme of special concerns for Gretchen in contrast to the first baby, says that he finds himself so much more "possessive" of Gretchen, so much more worried about what would happen to her if she got a cold or if she gets around somebody with a cold. He even remembers feeling angry toward his mother-in-law when she came down to visit the baby. He wanted her to get away from *his* baby. And that, he says, was odd because his mother-in-law is really a very nice person. Mrs. Bennett says that one thing she thinks she is hearing today as she listens to both parents is that they are always watching, always alert to find that something could be wrong with Gretchen. Mr. Raab nods and his wife looks sad again. Again, Mrs. Bennett connects this with Len, the first child, and how they had felt pretty much that he was all right and Mr. Raab interrupts to say, "Yes, that was right." They hadn't worried about something being wrong with him. And it had been so sudden. As they talked on, it is clear that both parents have little knowledge about Sudden Infant Death Syndrome, except that there really were no signs beforehand, no indication that something was wrong.

Mrs. Bennett, in preparation for closing this session and planning for the next, brings some of her reflections together for the two parents. It is so hard to know, she says, how much of their concern for Gretchen is real and belongs to Gretchen and how much belongs to the past and to their great sadness. She suggests that Gretchen and her parents meet with us again, perhaps twice before the date of their leaving. They will talk together and observe Gretchen together and perhaps do a developmental assessment of Gretchen with videotape so that she and they could look at Gretchen together. They might see in what ways Gretchen's development was proceeding well, in what ways the parents could help her, what made her like other babies of her age or in what ways she was different. Both parents seem very much interested. And Mr. Raab, nodding vigorously, says they want to know what they can do to make sure that Gretchen "develops right" and doesn't become a "withdrawn baby." It is at this point that Mrs. Bennett hears him murmur something about "autistic" and, in following this up, finds it clear that both parents are afraid Gretchen might be autistic. Mrs. Bennett records in her notes that she herself does not have a sense, in watching Gretchen, that she is a "withdrawn" baby, but she does seem to be "a quiet baby." Somehow she manages to communicate to the Raabs that she herself does not have the impression that Gretchen is autistic.

In sketching plans for the next two visits, Mrs. Bennett also manages to create a bridge for the Raabs to their new home and to the infant mental health specialist we had in mind who would be able to offer further help to the Raabs if they wished.

In leaving, the parents seem to be relieved of some of their anxieties and, as Mrs. Bennett pats Gretchen's hand in farewell (and gets the tiniest tentative smile), Mr. Raab says, "We'll be able to come back and see that nice lady again, Gretchen," and both parents thank Mrs. Bennett with warmth.

CASE CONFERENCE

In the case conference between Mrs. Bennett and Dr. Pawl, the diagnostic and therapeutic implications of this session were discussed. It was clear that mourning for the lost baby, Len, had never been "worked through." Following this terrible experience there had been no one to help the Raabs, and the two grief-stricken parents, each dealing with private pain, might not have been able to help each other. But their grief was still capable of expression as we saw when Mrs. Bennett touched upon their feelings, and it was offered to Mrs. Bennett as a plea for help. Neither she nor Dr. Pawl could be sure how much of this grief could be worked through in the two sessions that remained, but if it were possible to help the two parents experience their pain with a sympathetic and understanding listener and to get some glimmer of the relationship between mourning for their first dead child and the anxieties for Gretchen which were disturbing their relationship, even this much could be a positive help to the parents and would leave them, we hoped, able to seek help from an infant mental health specialist in their new community.

Both Mrs. Bennett and Dr. Pawl were impressed by a striking repetition of circumstance for the Raabs at this point in their lives and at another point in their lives just before the death of Len. First of all, Gretchen's age (4 months) was very close to the age of Len when he died. And this time, too, the family was about to make a trip, in fact to the same city, in repetition of the circumstances under which the first baby had died. Both Len and Gretchen were babies who were "hard" to feed. The mother had been unable to breast feed Len, of course, since he was hospitalized for six weeks after birth. The mother was unable to breast feed Gretchen successfully. Clearly, many earlier circumstances were evoked for the Raabs during the first weeks of Gretchen's life and gave poignancy to old memories.

SECOND SESSION

This session was planned both for developmental assessment of Gretchen and for further discussion of the parents' concerns. As is customary (when our families give consent), we videotaped the developmental testing.

In general, Mrs. Bennett was satisfied that Gretchen demonstrated adequacy on the Bayley Scales of Infant Development. But it was indeed painful to witness with the parents the videotaped record of Gretchen's avoidance of eye contact with her mother and her father. In one sequence, the tape reveals the pathos for Mrs. Raab. She is speaking to Gretchen in an animated voice, her own smiles and her face almost beseeching Gretchen for a response. Gretchen not only avoids looking at her mother's face but actually has to shift her trunk in order to turn away from her mother's wooing. In thirty minutes of continuous taping, there is not a single instance in which Gretchen seeks contact with either of her parents or, when she is seated on a parent's lap, touches or explores him or her with her hands. Once, when Gretchen is crying, her mother pats her absently on the back. Gretchen has her hands stretched out in space, not seeking her mother for comfort.

The parents were reassured that Gretchen was not retarded. And the question with which they had entered the first session, "Is it Gretchen or is it us?" received a partial answer.

Mr. and Mrs. Raab said that after the first session they had done a lot of thinking and a lot of talking to one another. They discovered that they had never really talked about the death of the first baby together. They alluded to it. It was always on their minds. But they never really talked about what it felt like. Mrs. Raab made the point that at the time Len had died she had lost contact with everyone who could have helped her. She was no longer seeing her obstetrician. The pediatrician was no longer interested once the baby was dead. And there really wasn't any person at all to help with any part of their feelings.

Together the parents spoke to Mrs. Bennett of their memories of Len's death. They talked about how desolate, how bleak and how lonely the landscape was at the truck stop where Len had died. They talked about feeding the baby and then putting him in the back of the car. Then pulling into the truck stop and finding that he was dead. Mrs. Raab seemed to emphasize the grayness, the bleakness, the fact that the leaves were gone from the trees. It was a truck driver who called the state police, and the baby was then taken by them to a rural hospital where he was declared dead.

Anxiety for Gretchen, and the name of the fear, could now be put into words. Mrs. Raab described her own sleeplessness. She was both disturbed when Gretchen cried and worried when Gretchen was asleep that she wouldn't wake up again.

Both parents now needed almost no help in seeing the connection between their anxieties for Gretchen and the death of Len.

THIRD SESSION

The third session had been scheduled two days before the Raabs were due to make their move. But an impending blizzard made it necessary for them to leave one day early, and Mrs. Raab called to see if Mrs. Bennett could schedule her final appointment with them that very afternoon.

In this session, as Mrs. Raab brought in more memories of the death of Len, she was able to cry heartbrokenly for Len and for herself and her husband. For the first time, we believe, she truly experienced the grief that she had been unable to feel or to express five years before.

And as the mother spoke on, she was able to make the connections with Mrs. Bennett of her fear of getting close to Gretchen. She was afraid that Gretchen might die too. Mrs. Raab had also discovered that even though she experienced relief when Gretchen would fall asleep, she felt she needed to wake up the baby. She didn't know which was worse, having to tolerate Gretchen's crying or being frightened all the time when she was asleep.

And she spoke of her sense of failure because she had not been able to breast feed Gretchen. She had not been so aware of this sense of failure with her first baby, now that she thought about it, because he was premature and in an isolette. Then, too, since the Raabs had done some reading about Sudden Infant Death Syndrome, they knew that breastfed babies were less at risk for SIDS than bottlefed babies. Weaning Gretchen from the breast reactivated these anxieties too.

During this session, Mrs. Raab also told Mrs. Bennett about a recurring dream she had had when she was pregnant with Gretchen. Time after time she would dream that she would have a baby, but when the baby was born he would already be walking and talking. Mrs. Bennett suggested that Mrs. Raab was dreaming of a time when the baby would be older, and the critical time period when the new baby was small, and when their first baby had died, would be over with and past.

The relief of crying and talking about the first baby, of discovering many similarities between the past and the present, seemed to mobilize new energies in Mrs. Raab. At the close of this session, she seemed more composed, and even her planning for the move showed orderly and thoughtful precautions and plans. Whereas in the first session the Raabs had planned to drive separately with Mrs. Raab and Gretchen in one car and Mr. Raab in the U-Haul, the Raabs now thought that it would be much more sensible for the three of them to drive together in one car and to arrange for someone else to drive the U-Haul. (It was a better plan and, perhaps, a symbolic statement of the fact that things go better when a family is united and close to one another.)

There was another shift in feeling. Whereas in the second session, Mrs. Raab thought she could hardly bear the interval between the last visit with Mrs. Bennett and the first projected visit with the infant mental health specialist in her new community, by the third visit Mrs.

Raab said that she was still eager to "see the specialist" but didn't think it had to happen immediately. She could wait.

Mrs. Raab, thanking Mrs. Bennett for her help, said thoughtfully that she herself would like to work with and help parents who had experienced what she had experienced. Without such help she knew that the death of a baby could be an interference with the relationship to a new baby.

FOLLOW-UP

There were letters from the Raabs and a communication from the infant mental health specialist in their new community. Mrs. Raab did call the mental health specialist a few weeks after they arrived in their new community, but it was not so much a call for help as a following up on an agreed-upon plan. The specialist made a home visit and found the Raabs and Gretchen manifestly doing well. They did not feel they needed further help.

In January, approximately two months after Mrs. Bennett had last seen the Raabs, Mrs. Raab wrote a touching letter to her. In the letter she sounded like a competent and relaxed mother. Everything was going well for all of them. Gretchen was smiling and eating well and developing at a good pace. They were happy in their new home and their new community and had made new friends.

In her letter Mrs. Raab said, "Our whole life has shifted into lower gear. It's as if a burden had been lifted from our shoulders."

And in July of the same year, when Gretchen was 11 months old, the Raabs wrote and asked if they might visit Mrs. Bennett with Gretchen. They brought a radiant, vocal, social, and altogether delightful Gretchen as a "gift" to Mrs. Bennett. The parents had asked for another developmental testing (though they weren't worried about what would be found) and Gretchen performed very well indeed.

The parents showed no special concern for Gretchen's development and described no special problems. Mrs. Bennett saw Gretchen's appropriate preferential behavior toward mother and father and appropriate reserve with her as stranger. She saw that Gretchen, who had once been the "inconsolable" baby, now turned to her parents when she needed them and could be comforted by them.

SUMMARY

Much work took place in the three sessions with the Raabs and Gretchen. The parents were able to speak to a sympathetic and understanding therapist of their anguish for the baby who had died. Before they left the first session, they had already discovered with Mrs. Bennett's help that anxiety which belonged to the first baby had impeded their spontaneity and joy with the second. They also discovered in this session and the two that followed that their "inconsolable baby," Gretchen, had stirred up for them their own inconsolable grief. They saw the repetitions between the past and the present that had led them to tremendous anxieties for Gretchen. The "burden that was lifted," which Mrs. Raab spoke of in her letter, was the pain and the mourning for the first child as well as the intolerable anxiety for Gretchen. The mourning was, in a certain sense, completed through talking with Mrs. Bennett, allowing the grief to be renewed in order to be mastered, and the parents became free to love and to enjoy Gretchen.

V

Nina: Developmental Guidance and Supportive Treatment for a Failure to Thrive Infant and Her Adolescent Mother

DEBORAH SPITZ CHERNISS

JEREE PAWL

SELMA FRAIBERG

NINA was 7 months old when she was referred to us by her pediatrician. At that time she was hospitalized for failure to thrive. Nina had not gained weight in four months but during her stay at the hospital she ate well and made normal weight gains in response to excellent nursing. Studies conducted at the hospital revealed no organic basis for growth failure. The pediatrician and hospital staff concurred in their opinion that the primary cause of growth failure was "maternal and emotional deprivation." Karen, Nina's mother, was 16 years old and unwed. Mother and baby were supported by AFDC and were allowed, grudgingly, to live in the home of the maternal parents. While Karen attended high school, Nina spent her days in a private nursery for young children.

We were asked to make an assessment of Nina and Karen in order to explore the possibility of providing continued treatment through our program.

Nonorganic Failure to Thrive

The term "failure to thrive" describes infants who show growth failure in the absence of any organic cause. In strict usage, it is employed for infants whose weight has fallen below the third percentile. It is almost universally associated with the impairment of the mother's capacity to nourish, both in the material and in the psychological sense of the word.

The typical course of medical treatment for a failure to thrive infant is hospitalization with intensive one-to-one nursing care. With nurse-mothering and the introduction of a good nutritional regime, the baby begins to thrive. When his nutritional state is stabilized, he returns to his home. Typically, these gains are lost within a few weeks and the baby may return to the hospital again—and the cycle renews itself.

It is the mother who is the key. Whether or not the baby will thrive outside of the hospital depends upon the mother's capacity to follow the medically prescribed regime to insure adequacy in caloric intake for her baby and to provide the psychological nutriments for growth and development. But the dietary advice given by the hospital and later guidance that focuses only on caloric intake and bypasses the emotional center of the maternal-infant conflicts are not successful. (Whitten et al. 1969.) There is usually a discontinuity between the health services provided when the baby is an in-patient and the services offered after the baby is discharged to his family. There may, in fact, be little follow-up or support for the baby and his family after discharge.

Follow-up studies of babies hospitalized as "nonorganic failure to thrive" are sobering. Using the criterion "weight adequacy" only, over 34 percent do not attain weight adequacy in the extended period post-discharge (Leonard et al. 1966; Shaheen et al. 1968; Glaser et al. 1968; Whitten et al. 1969; Evans et al. 1972; Fraiberg and Bennett 1979 and Fraiberg and Bennett 1978).

Equally ominous are the follow-up reports indicating that whether or not the failure to thrive baby attains weight adequacy, 80 percent of the children who have been diagnosed as "nonorganic failure to thrive" show residual effects of their nutritional poverty and emotional deprivation in serious to severe personality problems, learning disorders, and mental retardation (Glaser et al. 1968; Evans et al. 1972).

All reports agree that the families of failure to thrive infants are difficult to reach and to maintain continuing contacts with. However, Shaheen and associates report than when the hospital can engage the family in a close collaborative relationship and provide continuity of care in the period following discharge, the outcome, using weight adequacy as a criterion, is more favorable. (78 percent of their population had sustained weight adequacy at follow-up.)

In our own work with failure to thrive infants at the Child Development Project we have seen our task as twofold. We must try to bring every baby both to sustained *weight adequacy* and to *psychological adequacy*. We see failure to thrive as a problem for the infant mental health clinic in which pediatric and psychiatric services must be united to insure the future development of the baby and the harmony of infant-parent relationships. Our experience and our results are reported in Fraiberg and Bennett (1978) and Fraiberg and Bennett (1979).

Three clinical reports of failure to thrive are included in this volume: Nina, who will be described in this chapter, Billy (Chapter VIII), and Trudy (Chapter IX).

In the story of Nina and Karen which follows we will describe the interlocking aspects of a severe eating disturbance in a baby and her mother.

Nina and Karen: The Initial Assessment

The period of our initial assessment covered a span of five weeks, including hospital observations of baby and mother, office visits in which mother and baby were both present (Karen's mother would not permit home visits), observations at Nina's nursery, and a session for developmental testing. (During the same period there were eleven consultations with Nina's pediatrician, nursery personnel, our staff pediatrician and nurse, and the case supervisor.)

The first meeting of the therapist with Nina and Karen took place in the hospital. Karen had given passive consent to the recommendation of the hospital that she might wish to talk with someone at the Child Development Project about Nina's feeding problems.

The schoolgirl mother and her baby presented a striking picture. Karen gaunt, terribly thin, hair disheveled, her face pinched and sad;

Nina long and thin, eyes dark and wary, face somber, a pacifier in her mouth during most of the session.

A hospital creates the most unfavorable circumstances for making observations regarding the quality of parent-child relationships. In the case of a failure to thrive baby, we can fairly assume that the mother already knows her competence as a parent is under scrutiny, that a starving baby who gains normally in the hospital is seen as an indictment of the mother, and that maternal neglect is the unspoken question (or sometimes the explicit question) which will guide future decisions.

Karen had no reason to trust the therapist. Her passive consent to that first visit appeared to us later, as we came to know her, as a characteristic surrender to circumstance. And she was afraid, as most parents are when parental competence is questioned, that if she did not comply, the baby would be taken from her.

In the course of that first visit in the hospital, the therapist saw fear and mute distrust in Karen (masked typically by a frozen smile). There was no formal history-taking at this meeting. (Everything we need to know will emerge gradually in the course of many sessions.) The important issues for this meeting were to establish a relationship that might lead to trust, to observe mother and baby together in order to make judgments regarding the qualities of the mother-child relationship, and to assess the potential for using our help.

Nina was very much in the center of this session. The therapist made friendly vocal overtures to the baby and Nina scrutinized her warily, as we should expect at this age. But she sought her mother's eyes from time to time and reached for her mother on several occasions. The therapist registered this information and throughout the session mentally recorded all the information she needed to be able to assess the nature of the attachment between baby and mother, mother and baby. In all her observations of Nina during this session the therapist saw clear differential and preferential behaviors toward her mother, in gaze, smiling, and motor approaches. In only one area was there a marked deficit: Nina rarely vocalized to her mother. In fact, Nina's vocalizations were limited to the range of a 3-month-old—small grunts and squeals. In moments of discomfort or distress, Nina sought comfort from her mother in an accustomed, expectant way that told us her mother was a source of comfort. There were marked differences in Nina's attitudes toward her mother and the stranger. Once, for example, when the stranger offered her a toy, Nina refused it. When her mother offered her the same toy, she accepted it readily.

The therapist offered a running commentary on these observations. To Nina: "You really know your mommy, don't you?" And to Karen she underscored the meaning of these behaviors. "She's telling us that her mom is the most important person to her." Karen, prepared perhaps for a lecture from the stranger, began to relax, even to smile shyly in response to the therapist's comments. (Later, we were to learn from Karen herself that the therapist was the first person who had come into Karen's and Nina's life who gave Karen the feeling that she could be a good mother.)

Karen, the therapist observed, seemed mainly responsive to signals from her baby and seemed to read the social signs of Nina fairly: responding to gaze, to a smile, to hands uplifted in a "pick me up" gesture, to sounds of distress.

There were many signs of a positive and reciprocal attachment between Nina and her mother. But there were also many puzzles, both in this first session and the sessions that followed. The social signs of attachment were there, for example, but the affective quality of these exchanges was muted, depressed. There was a joylessness and distance between these two even in moments of seeking each other. The sadness on Karen's face was mirrored in the sadness on Nina's face.

Feeding was another puzzle, and a vital clue to it emerged during this hour. At one point in this first session at the hospital Nina uttered a complaint and turned to her mother. Karen decided that Nina was hungry and she arranged for a bottle to be brought to her. Karen then held Nina in her arms and Nina settled comfortably. After a few sucks she refused the bottle. Karen seemed at a loss and could not interpret the refusal. When the therapist asked when Nina had last had a feeding, Karen said, without making any connection for herself, that Nina had had breakfast one hour ago!

This was the first of a number of clues that began to emerge in the early work with Karen and Nina. Karen, who seemed able to read the social signs of her baby could not, at least in this instance, read the signs of hunger or satiation in Nina. Later, the examples proliferated.

The therapist made mental notes to herself without commenting to Karen or giving her advice. Instead, she turned the discussion to feeding in general. She asked Karen in a neutral way how she understood when Nina was hungry. Karen said that Nina's cry was "different" when she was hungry; it was stronger, she thought. (Which was all right, of course, except that in the episode observed by the therapist, Nina's cry was a small complaint, possibly seeking comfort, and Karen had read the cry as hunger.) On the other hand, since Nina's nutritional state must leave her in a state of chronic hunger, could Karen read the signs of hunger in her baby when they were present? These were questions which could be mentally registered by the therapist and explored through further observations.

The therapist then guided the discussion into other areas of feeding. What did Nina like to eat? Karen provided a varied list of foods: meat, vegetables, fruit. From the description it appeared that Nina should have an adequate diet, but from the evidence of Nina's nutritional state, she was actually severely malnourished. Was Karen being untruthful? The therapist thought that the story was much more complicated, that something in feeding Nina was caught up in a personal conflict for the mother. Karen might be distorting the picture of Nina's diet, but she was not intentionally concealing something. The therapist continued to listen without offering judgments or criticism.

She guided the discussion of feeding to "Nina's day" at the nursery. Nina, she learned, had breakfast and lunch at the nursery each day. And who was it who usually fed Nina at the nursery? Karen spoke vaguely of "people" at the nursery who took over feedings, and a picture emerged of Nina's being fed by "anyone handy" in a rotation of staff and volunteers. The therapist asked if Karen thought it made a difference whether she herself fed Nina or whether others did, and Karen said ingenuously that it didn't seem to make any difference who fed Nina. Exploring this a bit, the therapist realized that Karen had no notion of the centrality of a mother for her child or the meaning to a baby of feeding and intimacy with the mother, and that she had given a candid statement of her beliefs—"It doesn't make any difference who feeds Nina."

Here, for the first time, the therapist offered some of her own thoughts. She said that everything she had seen today in the hospital visit had shown her that Nina felt that her mother was the most important person in the world. For all babies, the pleasure of eating was tied to closeness with the mother, being held and fed by the most special person.

Clearly, this was a novel idea to Karen. She struggled to understand it. The therapist asked Karen if she could think of ways in which she could be present for mealtimes in the nursery. This might be one of the ways in which we could begin to help Nina with her feeding problem. Karen, still puzzled, said that she thought this could be arranged at the nursery.

The therapist sketched for Karen the ways in which she would hope to help Karen and Nina. She would like to visit Karen and Nina at home. But here Karen said sadly that she knew her mother would not allow home visits. Her mother did not like social workers and psychiatrists and did not approve of Karen's coming here. She would not stop Karen from coming here if Karen wanted to, but she herself did not want to be involved. The therapist accepted this limitation with some foreboding. Would Karen and Nina like to meet at our office then? That would be all right. The therapist asked Karen's permission to work closely with Nina's pediatrician, and Karen agreed. And would Karen permit the therapist to visit Nina's nursery, to observe her and to talk with the nursery staff in order to understand the situation bet-

ter? Karen agreed without hesitation. Our assessment program, including psychological testing and videotaping the test, was described, and
Karen was asked if she would give her consent. Karen agreed. The con-
fidentiality of all information was stressed and Karen understood clearly that as Nina's mother she was invited to be our collaborator in helping her baby.

In this way the assessment began. Karen understood that at the close
of the assessment period (approximately five to seven visits) the therapist and she would hope to have a good understanding of Nina's problems, and if we felt that continued help through our program was the
best plan, we would discuss planning at that time.

THE PATIENT-THERAPIST RELATIONSHIP

Karen's passive compliance during this session and the sessions that
followed should not be read as "a positive attitude toward help" or
"highly motivated to seek help."

While there were nine visits in five weeks, there were seventeen appointments that were changed, canceled, or forgotten by Karen. Since
we have had long experience with parents who begin their work with
us through a series of broken appointments, we were neither dismayed
nor discouraged by the unpromising beginning. Following each
broken appointment, the therapist phoned Karen to express regret that
they had not been able to meet and to suggest another appointment
time. There were no reproaches or criticisms.

Karen began to understand that the therapist was a person who did
not become angry, did not lecture, never wavered in her concern for
Karen and Nina and her wish to help. For a teenage girl, seventeen
broken appointments constitute a good test of the ego strength of the
therapist under stress. It is useful information for a girl who is reluctant to give her trust. And if you are a girl who is afraid of anger, who
expects anger from adults (and we will learn about this shortly), the
unconscious provocation of persons in authority under ordinary circumstances will bring about objective confirmation of inner belief. If
she had succeeded in provoking the therapist, Karen would have had a
real, and not imaginary, fear of the therapist and she would, of course,
have taken flight from the assessment and from treatment.

Between the forgotten and the broken appointments much work was
accomplished. The relationship between Karen and the therapist
moved toward a positive alliance; the diagnostic questions were clarified and led to treatment formulations. Work in the area of Nina's nutrition was begun as early as the second visit.

Here it is important to note that, because of Nina's alarming nutritional state, it was imperative to begin nutritional guidance during the

diagnostic period even though we did not yet understand the complexities of the mother-infant relationship which were generating the nutritional problems. We will describe these guidance measures at several points in the summary of the assessment period that follows.

THE DIAGNOSTIC QUESTIONS

As early as the first visit, which we have summarized, a number of diagnostic questions and puzzles had appeared. The hospital judgment that Nina was "suffering from maternal and emotional deprivation" was in large part an inference from the medical findings. A starving baby who gives no evidence of organic disease and who with expert nursing (i.e., substitute mothering) gains weight rapidly during hospitalization gives presumptive evidence to the medical team that the child is suffering from maternal deprivation and gross neglect.

For the infant mental health team, the diagnostic issues are highly complex. Gross maternal neglect and abuse can be read through the behavior of both the baby and the mother. Some of the signs are subtle; some are blatant. The grossly neglected infant of Nina's age (7 months) will show in eloquent terms the absence of human connections with her mother. Wherever there should be age-appropriate signs of discrimination and preference for her mother, we will see nondiscrimination, nonpreference, and—even more ominous—avoidance by gaze, smile, voice, motor behavior. The grossly neglectful mother will reveal the absence of maternal feeling for her child through avoidance, through nonregistration of signs of need in the baby, through misreading the baby's sign language, and even through the attribution of malevolent motives to her baby's behavior.

At the close of the first session with Nina and Karen, the therapist had registered a number of ambiguities in the mother-infant relationship which gave rise to the first diagnostic questions. Nina had demonstrated preferential smiling and gaze for her mother and initiated contact with her through reaching. Nina was appropriately wary of the stranger, but warmed up to her as the hour progressed. She sought her mother for comfort and was easily quieted by Karen. But vocalizations were sparse and undifferentiated. In a rough assessment of Nina's developmental accomplishments during this first observation, it seemed to the therapist that Nina was at age level in all areas except language. The signs of human attachment and developmental adequacy were present in Nina, but Nina's *mood* was somber, subdued. There was more to worry about in the qualitative aspects of emotion than in the indicators of attachment, but we would need to be careful. This was a hospital visit and Nina had experienced separation from her mother.

Karen as a mother posed more ambiguities. She was manifestly unable to provide the nutritional needs of her baby, but we had no evidence in that first session that she rejected or harbored malevolent and destructive wishes toward Nina. We were struck by the fact that she could read Nina's social signs and respond to a smile, a glance, outstretched arms, complaints. But on the one occasion that we witnessed a feeding, Karen had misread a small complaint as hunger, and when the baby refused the bottle (she had been fed only an hour before), Karen seemed at a loss. We would need more observations to examine this issue fairly.

KAREN'S STORY

Karen's story emerged gradually in the sessions that followed. Karen and Nina were living in the home of Karen's parents. Both Karen and Nina were supported by AFDC. There were a younger brother and sister in the home.

The household was chaotic. There were violent quarrels between Karen's parents, frightening to witness. As fighting erupted, Karen would hide in her bedroom with Nina—just as she did throughout her childhood when she and her siblings huddled together while the parental fights rose to a climax (often ending with the mother leaving home).

Karen was still a child in her own family. She was dependent, compliant, timid in reproaching her parents for the violence and chaos in their household. Karen said wistfully that she wished she and Nina could leave her parents' home and live in an apartment. But she was afraid of being alone. What would Karen be afraid of? "Of spiders, of noises, of burglars."

Nina's father was mentioned once by Karen. He had been a schoolmate. Nina was conceived in a casual encounter. There was no bond between them; in Karen's narration he was nameless and faceless.

Karen had not known that she was pregnant until the fifth month. She had lost weight steadily during a two-year period and weighed a little over 80 pounds when she conceived. Since she had not menstruated for many months prior to conception, neither she nor her doctor had suspected that she was pregnant. When her parents learned of her pregnancy they insisted that she give up the baby for adoption. Karen, in a rare instance of self-assertion, insisted that she would keep her baby, and the decision brought further bitterness and fighting in the household where the parents each blamed the other for the pregnancy.

Since the birth of Nina, Karen and her baby were unwelcome members of the household, given grudging shelter. Nina's crying was an annoyance to the grandmother. There was no help in the way of childcare from the grandparents. In the rancorous climate of the home Karen's decision to keep the baby was seen as an act of stupidity.

Everyone in the household joined in a chorus of complaints about Karen as a mother. She was told that she spoiled Nina. She was criticized for her ineptness as a mother. There was sarcasm from her own mother. "*You*, a mother! What do you know about taking care of a baby?"

When Nina was 1 month old, she had begun daily attendance at a private nursery serving young children. There was a small regular staff, but for day-to-day program aid the nursery depended on volunteers interested in early childhood development.

The nursery did not seem to have a sense of the needs of young children or their young parents. Nina either had an unpredictable series of caregivers or was assigned to a withdrawn, depressed young woman. While initially arrangements had been made for Karen to return to the nursery to feed Nina lunch, the nursery began providing feedings without consulting Karen. They were also critical of Karen's care of Nina, saying on a number of occasions that she did not react promptly to Nina's illness. On several of these occasions the nursery staff called the pediatrician without consulting Karen and asked for medication changes. Karen's response was to "forget" the medication, thus confirming the staff's sense of her irresponsibility.

Whether she was talking about home or nursery, past or present, there were no tears and no reproaches as Karen told her miserable story. In the moment that the therapist thought a painful emotion was about to emerge, Karen would stare into the distance with a vague, fixed smile.

We were attentive to Karen's story of weight loss during a protracted period prior to conception. We registered in each session the masking of emotion and the characteristic defenses against affect. The picture of the sad, gaunt, 16-year-old girl spoke eloquently to the therapist. "Depression" is the word that describes what we saw. How severe? How pervasive?

The weight loss in the period that preceded conception needed to be understood. The therapist explored this further, and a sobering story emerged: Karen was, and had been for years, severely anorexic. Food was repulsive to her. She ate barely enough for sustenance. Anorexia and a sharp decline in weight had preceded conception by many months. Karen had been under a physician's care and there were no identifiable causes for weight decline and anorexia. But Karen had always been thin, for as long as she could remember. She had never enjoyed food. In fact, she said, her mother said that she herself had been a poor eater as a baby and that Nina was just like her.

As the picture of Karen enlarged during the initial assessment period we saw signs of serious depression. In the absence of medical findings, the anorexia appeared to be associated with a depressive syndrome. Karen's defenses against affect were powerful. Encouragement to speak of her feelings brought only blankness or a characteristic frozen smile. Karen's overall functioning was impaired. She was an indifferent student in school; she had no goals for herself. She had no close friends.

Karen had affection for her baby, but her own resources were depleted by inner conflict and the actual conflicts in her home.

In every session when the subject of food came up—food for Karen, food for Nina—there was vagueness, inattention. When snack foods were provided for Karen and Nina, Karen might nibble at a thin carrot stick for an unbearably long time. Watching the undernourished girl and her starving baby, the thought occurred to the therapist "If Karen can't read her own signs of hunger, how can she read hunger in her baby?"

KAREN AS MOTHER

Karen, as we have said, had affection for her baby. And remarkably, when we consider the inner rage Karen had to control through her symptoms, there was no evidence that anger or rage was visited upon her baby. A baby who has known brutality will show fear and avoidance of her mother. A baby who has known gross neglect will not turn to her mother in need. A mother who is inflicting her own rage upon her child cannot conceal this from experienced clinicians during seven observational sessions.

Yet Karen was uncertainly a mother. There was no claiming of her child in a firm, maternal, protective sense. One of our staff members viewing Karen and Nina on tape remarked: "Karen is like a friendly teenage baby sitter. It's as if she were taking care of someone else's baby for an hour."

She was a schoolgirl, surprised by pregnancy once, surprised by motherhood still. And, schoolgirl that she was, she was lamentably ignorant of most of the elementary aspects of baby care. She literally did not know how much a baby should eat at Nina's age, or what an ideal weight might be for Nina. To Karen, Nina looked "chubby." (Innocence, and also the morbid intrusion of her own anorexia. The anorexic patient characteristically distorts size, weight, body image for himself. Karen was distorting her image of her baby.)

Karen had no idea what one should expect of a 7-month-old child. She was puzzled that Nina wasn't yet walking; worried that Nina still couldn't understand the meaning of "no" at 7 months; ready to begin toilet training of Nina at 8 months because it was already getting a little late. A dozen people taking charge of Nina in the nursery? But why would that matter?

Thus in the course of our assessment the scope of the problems to be addressed had come to extend far beyond the initial concern of nutritional adequacy, including the diverse psychological and physical needs of both mother and child.

BAYLEY TESTING OF NINA

The Bayley Scales of Infant Development were given to Nina in our office when Nina was 0:7:26. Her performance was slightly above age level with a Mental Scale age equivalency of 8:1 months (Mental Development Index: 110) and a Motor Scale equivalency of 8:8 months.

Nina's general performance on the Bayley would not have distinguished her as a psychologically impaired infant. While the Bayley is an invaluable tool to the infant clinician, it cannot serve as a screening instrument by itself. The personal-social items in the Bayley inventory are few in number and do not give us the discriminating attachment behaviors we need to assess affective development. However, an analysis of the language clusters in the Bayley would, in Nina's case and in others we have known, give us important clues regarding adequacy or deficits in this crucial area of social development, since language, in itself, is linked to human attachment.

Thus Nina failed *all* expressive and receptive language items at her age level, e.g., she *failed* "says 'dada' or equivalent" (7:9 months), "listens selectively to familiar words" (7:9 months), "vocalizes four different syllables" (7:0 months). During testing and in all naturalistic observations made during the assessment period we heard no vocalizations higher than a 3-month-old level. She was mainly silent, uttering an occasional grunt.

Our clinical observations of Nina during testing were also sobering. Under moderate stress (e.g., frustrated in a task or in problem solving) Nina typically fell back into a posture of resignation, passivity, and withdrawal, staring off into space with an empty look on her face. We noticed that she startled easily at sounds which could have been predicted, such as the sound of a block upon impact with the table surface.

There was poor integration of sensorimotor schemas. Nina employed "one mode at a time" in approaching tasks, e.g., she would look at the object but not touch it; she would touch the toy but not look at it; she would hold the toy but not explore it.

Fine motor development was poor (although her actual performance on motor items was adequate). She employed a clumsy, flat-handed approach to toys, with fingers rigidly extended, and the index finger was employed in distorted and inutile postures.

TREATMENT CONSIDERATIONS

The therapist had reflected to herself, early in the assessment, "If Karen can't read the signs of hunger in herself, how can she read the signs of hunger in her child?" Karen's anorexia was the key to Nina's own deteriorating nutritional and psychological status, but the internal conflicts of this adolescent mother which were represented in anorexia and depression were not at this time accessible to treatment. Each of the therapist's attempts to elicit affect led to denial, blankness, and withdrawal in Karen. The defenses against affect were formidable, and we read them as "fear of loss of control," the ego's anticipation that if inner rage and grief should be liberated they would engulf the personality or lead to acting out against parents and perhaps against her child.

The precarious equilibrium of adolescence added its own weight to the conflict. In all therapeutic work with adolescents, the therapist moves carefully in the realm of defense analysis, liberating affect in tolerable measures, mindful of the relative weakness of the ego in modulating drives and the demands of external reality (Freud 1946).

Under favorable circumstances, the therapeutic work with a depressed and anorexic adolescent girl might take many months or even years of work to alleviate symptons and to bring about favorable resolution of the underlying conflicts. But this adolescent girl was a mother, and the baby's growth failure was enmeshed in her mother's profound revulsion against eating and in her depression. And Nina could not wait until her mother's symptoms and adolescent conflicts were resolved.

On the positive side of the picture we saw that Karen cared for her baby and was trying desperately to protect Nina from her own conflicts. And in spite of the draining depression which Karen lived with every day, and the external strains of her tumultuous home, she tried to summon resources to care for her baby. But depression of such magnitude cannot be heroically overcome. There were poignant pictures of Karen and Nina in our record, clinging together when Nina cried; they both seemed to be sad and hungry little girls. We could not, for the present and immediate future, reach Karen's inner conflicts through therapy, but we thought we could strengthen her capacities to function and her abilities to mother her baby through supportive treatment. We could not modify the family situation in which mother and child found themselves, but we thought Karen could profit from a stable relationship with a therapist and a refuge in the therapeutic situation in which she could speak of her sorrows and gain relief through being heard, being understood. And since Karen was bereft of a model for mothering, the relationship with the therapist might provide an alternative model which would offer rewards to both mother and child.

We also saw how the psychological conflicts of Karen as mother were compounded by innocence and ignorance of the needs of babies. We have already seen in the assessment period that Karen was surprised each time the therapist commented on Nina's signs of preference for her mother, and of the centrality of the mother for the baby who is learning to love. Even if we acknowledge fully the place of Karen's own conflicts about eating in her inability to provide nutritional adequacy for her baby, there still remained a large measure of ignorance. As we have seen, Karen literally did not know what constituted an average daily food intake for a 7-month-old baby. Nor did she know what Nina had eaten in the two meals each day which were provided in the nursery so that she might plan the evening meal at home. Karen had passively surrendered responsibility for the nursery diet to the several aides and volunteers who rotated in the nursery. As a child herself, she had conferred authority upon them, "the grownups." But the nursery organization, with serial caregivers, did not have a system for recording each child's food intake, and a mother who did not request an oral report could not know what her child had eaten, or whether, in fact, she had refused meals.

We saw Karen's innocence in her unrealistic expectations for a baby of Nina's age. She was surprised that Nina was not yet walking. She was eager to begin toilet training with her 7-month-old. She rarely initiated "conversations" or games with Nina. Nina's silence and her primitive vocalizations (which we registered to ourselves as ominous) did not appear remarkable to Karen, who had no expectations for a baby of Nina's age and no notions about how a baby learns to talk. In fact, like many innocent mothers, she did not confer personality on Nina; a baby was not yet a person in Karen's view.

We would need to build into our treatment a vast amount of developmental information for Karen. From our experience we knew that this education of a mother must not be intrusive or didactic. Karen, in fact, had had courses in child development in high school. Remarkably, none of this information had been assimilated by her. She could not apply information from the class or textbooks to her baby because of her own profound conflicts about mothering, and very possibly, too, because she had never learned to be an observer of her own baby.

Within the framework of the therapeutic relationship, with Nina as well as Karen central to the work, each session could provide the circumstances for observing Nina, for playing with Nina, for raising questions, finding the meaning in a puzzling piece of behavior, placing the behavior in a developmental framework, finding solutions.

The Initial Phase of Treatment

The first phase of treatment, roughly a seven-month period, was seen by us as the critical period of the work. Nina's deteriorating physical and psychological state required that we move as fast as possible to bring her to adequacy. In fact, by the time Nina was 14 months old, she had reached weight adequacy, and her psychological status placed her well within optimal expectations for a baby of her age.

The work was focused on mother-infant attachment and nutrition, with full understanding on our part and Karen's that the two areas of concern were intimately related.

ATTACHMENT

In every session with Nina and Karen, the therapist found ways to enhance the relationship of Karen and Nina and demonstrate the centrality of a baby's attachment to her mother. Every sign of preference Nina showed to her mother was commented on. "It's mommy you really want, isn't it, Nina?" "That smile is special for mommy." "Mommy knows how to make you feel better." And to Karen (who once had not believed that babies knew how to love) the therapist commented on each of the signs of preference, the special smile, the fretfulness that could only be soothed by Karen, Nina's signs of comfort and relaxation in her mother's arms, her distress when her mother left the room momentarily, her pleasure at reunion. Karen, almost unbelieving as she saw her baby through the therapist's eyes, began slowly to register the meaning of these signs of love in her baby. In videotapes of this period we see a new animation on Karen's face when she is together with Nina; tenderness and solicitude appear in her gestures, and a sense of claiming her baby, of feeling that she *is* Nina's mother, comes through in a number of taped vignettes.

The therapist initiated games with Nina and introduced Karen into the games. The games themselves were commonplace: the introduction of a toy, a "conversation" with the baby about the toy, praise for the baby who made such fine music on the toy xylophone. All this seemed new to Karen. There were no traditions in Karen's family for playing with a baby. Karen herself, in her reticent way, began to enjoy the baby games. For all adults there is a healthy regression that is allowed in playing with babies and small children. Karen, who seemed not to have known a playful side of her nature before she came to us, took the permission of the therapist to enjoy baby games, to allow herself the occasional silliness that is the privilege of parents.

"To talk to a baby" seemed odd to Karen (and to many parents we have known). We have no way of knowing what Karen thought when she witnessed "serious" conversations (and sometimes "silly" conversations) with Nina, but she did discover that Nina responded by "talking." The therapist needed to do little more than initiate the "conversations" to bring Karen into the spirit of this discourse. Karen herself began to initiate "conversations" with Nina. The therapist made some tactful comments to the effect that "this is the way Nina is learning to talk," and Karen grasped the essential principle. Predictably, Nina's language began to develop rapidly.

Karen, who had once believed that a 7-month-old baby should know the meaning of "no" and respond instantly (otherwise she might become "spoiled"), had frequently engaged in contests with Nina. Now, watching the therapist, she saw that conflict could be avoided through the offering of substitutes for forbidden objects. In discussion with the therapist, she began to understand that a child of Nina's age could not yet assimilate the meaning of "no," that this would take time and many developmental advances; gradually we saw how Karen herself began to take over the relaxed and deft handling of conflict in her baby which she observed in her therapist.

NUTRITION

Every session sustained a dual focus on human attachments and nutrition. While we could assume that the strengthening of the attachment between baby and mother would affect Nina's capacity to enjoy food, Karen, the provider of food, had great difficulty in assimilating essential information on the nutritional needs of her baby. Her own revulsion toward food distorted her perception of hunger in Nina and her ability to translate concrete nutritional information into meal planning for her baby (as well as herself). Since every decision about "what to feed the baby" was caught up in emotional conflicts we could not yet deal with in Karen, we tried to circumvent conflict by means of a daily menu which Nina's pediatrician worked out for Karen. The daily menu, with recommended quantities, might, we hoped, take decision making about food out of the realm of conflict. Karen was invited to discuss the diet with the pediatrician and with us, and the pediatrician recommended that Karen keep a daily record of Nina's food intake and her preferences.

Karen was never able to keep this record. However, Nina began to gain weight steadily, and our best guess is that the menu with recommended quantities did give Karen the kind of factual information she could translate into meal planning and, further, that the issues of quantity and quality were easier to deal with when "someone else" made the decision, so to speak. This plan, combined with the work in the area of human attachments, brought about favorable changes in Nina's nutritional status within a matter of weeks.

RELATIONSHIP WITH THE THERAPIST

Throughout the initial treatment period we saw a steady growth in Karen's trust of her therapist. While there were a number of appointments "forgotten" or canceled, Karen used her sessions with profit. The ambivalence we saw in Karen's broken appointments could not be recognized by her and could not be brought into treatment. She did not dare acknowledge negative feelings toward her therapist at this point in treatment, even as she could not acknowledge the full strength of her negative feelings toward her parents.

Karen, as a needy child herself, welcomed the comfort and praise that came to her from the therapist. As an adolescent mother, she began to experience pride in her child and in herself as a mother. Every change in Nina was justly attributed to Karen by the therapist. And Karen, who had been the child in her family who could "never do anything right," began to blossom in the supportive, noncritical climate of this treatment which valued her as a young woman and as a mother. The therapist's professional caring for her as an adolescent in need probably satisfied deep longings in Karen for an understanding mother. She could speak of her private griefs with the therapist, of the anguish of her life at home, and, even knowing that neither she nor the therapist could change things at home, she took comfort from being heard and finding sympathy. Karen "understood" was on her way to becoming a mother who could in turn understand her child. The everyday griefs and disappointment of the baby could now touch her mother in a way that we had not seen earlier. She could now understand Nina's pain at the daily separations at the nursery and could find words of comfort and sympathy for Nina at the parting which caused the pain.

By the time Nina was 14 months old, Karen had become an empathic mother. We think the capacity to feel for her child emerged through the treatment in which she, both a mother and a child, came to know the qualities of empathy in her therapist.

CONSULTATION WITH THE NURSERY

Conferences with the director and staff of the nursery were an integral part of the therapeutic plan. With Karen's consent she and the therapist met frequently with the director and staff of the nursery for discussion of Nina's special needs and to work out a collaborative plan for facilitating all aspects of her development in the nursery. The therapist was able to make observations of Nina in the nursery which were discussed with the staff and with Karen.

As the only infant in a nursery that largely served a toddler group, Nina seemed lost and forlorn. There was no one person who "stood in" for mother, no one to whom Nina had an attachment. She was usually fed by "anyone handy" among the several volunteer aides. No written records were kept of her food intake or her general behavior during the nursery day. Older, aggressive children snatched toys from her or teased her while she looked on helplessly. In a nursery with eight to twelve scrappy and demanding toddlers, the forlorn complaints of the one baby were often not heard. When Nina cried as her mother left her in the morning, there was no one person to whom she could turn for solace. Some of the nursery aides found Nina's complaints annoying. Like Karen herself at the start of treatment, the aides could not acknowledge the legitimacy of a child's grief at separation from her mother.

In the course of collaborative work with the nursery many favorable changes took place. Karen's central importance for her baby was acknowledged, and the nursery staff made special efforts now to invite Karen to make frequent visits to the nursery as her school schedule permitted, and to support our plan in which Karen would feed Nina her lunch. One of the staff aides was assigned as Nina's primary caregiver in the nursery. While this plan never worked out ideally (as in many nurseries, there were shift changes and change of personnel), there was enough continuity, finally, in the relationship between Nina and one or two aides to give stability to a situation that had had none earlier.

The nursery staff became more attentive to Nina's nutritional needs and, within the limitations of an overworked staff, made efforts to monitor food intake and to give reports to Karen. The nursery's collaboration in the nutritional program made its own important contribution to Nina's steady weight gains.

ASSESSMENT OF NINA AT 14 MONTHS

At 14 months of age (seven months after treatment had begun), Nina had reached nutritional and psychological adequacy. Karen had summoned all of her resources to collaborate with the therapist in bringing about these important changes. Karen's own mood had brightened, she was enjoying her baby, she was becoming a competent mother. She now looked pretty and well-groomed. But our clinical judgment was "still a seriously depressed adolescent girl; in need of long sustained help from us."

FIGURE 1. Weight and Height Curves

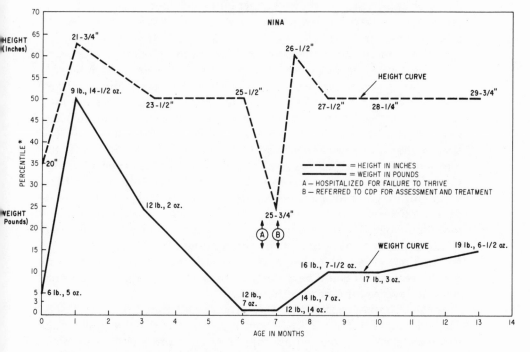

NOTE: * Birth percentile based on Colorado Intrauterine Growth Charts; other percentiles based on the Anthropometric Chart of Children's Medical Center, Boston.

Nina was a healthy, lively child whose weight had moved to and remained at between the 25th and 50th percentiles. The once-silent baby had become positively garrulous! On tape during her 14-month developmental assessment we see and hear her chattering in jargon with her mother, a jargon interspersed with intelligible words. She is "reading" a book to her mother at one point, naming pictures, "telling a story" with great expressiveness and a fine parody of English.

Impressive gains were seen in the 14-month testing. At 8 months Nina's MDI had been a respectable 110; at 14 months it was 133, equivalent to expectations for an 18-month-old. Our analysis of test results showed that the spurt in language development was largely responsible for these gains.

Nina's attachment to her mother had become strong and secure. In all the ways in which we could assess the quality of this attachment, Nina met our expectations for a 14-month-old child. In all of our observations she employed her mother as a secure base for exploration and moved confidently in her explorations while occasionally "touching base" with her mother through a glance or a smile or a vocal greeting or motor approach. She showed affection toward her mother in a natural and joyous way. She trusted her mother and confidently expected to be understood.

At the nursery she protested bitterly when her mother left her each morning. But when her mother spoke lovingly to her at the moments of separation and reminded her that she would be back, Nina could be consoled. She knew that her mother understood. And while the nursery situation had improved, with many accommodations to our suggestions and Karen's, it was not really possible for the small nursery staff to offer the kind of substitute mother care that Nina and other babies her age needed. Nina coped gamely with the less than ideal day care plan. She even learned to escape with agility from the battling older children and to assert her rights to property. But more than once during nursery visits the therapist saw Nina with a sad and resigned look upon her face after her mother left, sometimes sitting immobilized on the floor with huge tears rolling down her cheeks.

Karen herself spoke of her heartbreak at leaving Nina in the morning. She wished it could be different, but there were no better alternatives in daycare for a baby of Nina's age.

Nina's adaptive capabilities were now demonstrated in many forms. The old passive withdrawal and vacant staring had disappeared. Under moderate stress she reacted appropriately with protests or tears, then reconstituted herself with help and often without help. In problem-solving situations she persevered and took pleasure in finding the solutions. (Earlier, at 7 months, she would have given up with a faint cry and withdrawn.) The motor stereotypies had disappeared. There was good coordination of sensorimotor schemas.

In doll play she showed much tenderness and solicitude toward her dolls in feeding and dressing, a sign to us that she knew loving care from her own mother.

She was very much "a person," and gave positive signs of the differentiation of "self" and "other" in her behavior toward persons and objects. In informal observations we saw evidence that she had attained a high level of object permanence, roughly equivalent to the conceptual development of an 18-month-old child.

All this had been achieved by Karen's devotion and her use of our help. Yet Karen herself was still anorexic, and her depression, though moderately improved, was still present.

The Second Phase of Treatment: 15 to 25 Months

While Nina had attained nutritional and psychological adequacy by 14 months of age, our clinical assessment gave us clear indications that treatment of child and mother should continue. As long as Karen's depression and anorexia remained (even in moderate form), Nina—still so young—was regarded as being at risk. Karen herself remained in our view an endangered adolescent until such time as our work would bring some resolution of major psychological conflicts.

It is important to justify our reasons for continuing Karen's and Nina's treatment in the program. It might be argued fairly that our work on behalf of Nina had attained its goals. Would it not be more practical to arrange for treatment of Karen in another clinic specializing in work with adolescents? For Karen herself, there might be justification for such a plan, but for Karen as mother and for Nina, we could find strong arguments for their continuing in our program. We could predict that Karen's unresolved adolescent conflicts would surface in the course of her child's own development. If we were present throughout the period of early development, our own relationship with Karen would advantage us greatly in dealing with developmental problems as they emerged. And Karen, too, was our patient. The relationship of confidence which she had developed with her therapist put our clinic in the strongest position to help her examine her own problems and her relationship with Nina.

During this phase of treatment we saw that much of our early work was being sustained. The attachment between mother and child was strong and mutually rewarding. But attachment alone cannot provide solutions to all problems in parent-child relationships and child rearing. And very shortly, as we moved into this second phase of treatment, conflict emerged between Nina and her mother.

DEVELOPMENTAL CONFLICTS

At 15 months we began to get reports that Nina was becoming a cranky baby at bedtime and bath time. Karen complained of a new obstinacy in Nina. There were temper outbursts during the day. And Nina protested against going to sleep at night. Frequently she wakened at night.

As the therapist began to explore the areas of conflict between mother and baby, each inquiry brought uncertain answers. Did Nina waken with anxiety at night? No. She only seemed to want to play with her mother. How long did Nina nap during her day at the nursery? Karen did not know. (The aides at the nursery did not know, either.) We ourselves were not ready to give a complex meaning to the night wakening without practical information. After all, it was possible that Nina, bored during the long days at the nursery, slept for several hours in the morning and afternoon and was simply ready to start her day at three or four in the morning. But the constellation of problems—night wakening, temper tantrums, conflict with mother—suggested another line of inquiry to us. We had seen this constellation of problems in the second year when extraordinary demands were being made upon a child in one or another developmental area, and one of the most common areas of conflict was toilet training (Fraiberg 1950). The therapist began to make tactful inquiries.

Karen said that she had begun toilet training with Nina. Nina, she felt, was old enough to "understand" at 15 months. (We recall that Karen had been ready to begin toilet training when we first met Nina at 7 months, and had postponed doing so only on the suggestion of the therapist.) The therapist began to raise tactful questions about Nina's readiness for toilet training. She suggested too that some of the tantrums and the obstinacy Karen was now seeing in Nina might be a reaction to the beginning of toilet training and a sign that Nina was not yet ready. The therapist sketched for Karen the dilemma of the toddler who loves her mother and wants to please her mother but can't yet postpone an urge to urinate or defecate, or understand the mysterious process of using a potty chair or toilet.

Karen, ordinarily so compliant that we were pained for her, began to bristle. She tightened up visibly during these discussions with the therapist. A muted anger was in her voice. There were long silences. When the therapist touched upon Karen's own feelings, screened by silence, Karen of course denied them.

And Karen, for one of the rare times in her treatment, could make no use of the therapist's suggestions. She pursued toilet training with Nina with an energy and insistence that was rarely seen in her. She complained about Nina's obstinacy and her temper, and could not look at "reasons" or "causes." When the therapist asked Karen's help in understanding the problem, and invited concrete illustrations, Karen described a typical episode with Nina.

The weather was warm, so Karen was dressing Nina only in diapers. They were disposable ones, with little tabs to keep them closed, and Nina could, and did, pull them off. Then, without a diaper, she would urinate all over the floor. The therapist asked what would happen next. Karen said that she would tell Nina, "If you have to pee, tell me, and I'll put you on the pot." But Nina would *not* tell her mother, and even began playing with the urine as Karen tried to clean it up. Karen would become upset, and Nina would have a tantrum. Karen would put Nina in her crib and try to diaper her, but Nina would protest and throw the diaper out of the crib.

Although Karen had raised this as a difficult incident, she was not able to accept even a gentle questioning of her handling, and certainly would not hear advice on how to change it. Her reactions ranged from simple avoidance by changing the subject to a stubborn repeating of her plans, and finally, an unusually sullen denial of having any concerns at all about toilet training!

A THERAPEUTIC DILEMMA AND ITS RESOLUTION

It struck us, as we reviewed these sessions, that Karen was behaving as if someone were forcing *her* to use a potty! The experience of training her child to use a potty had touched off profound conflicts in Karen's own personality. Our therapeutic dilemma was obvious. There was no way in which our treatment could easily dredge up the repressed conflicts of a mother's early childhood and free her to use our guidance on behalf of the baby. However, there was another route that suggested itself to us. While Karen's original conflicts were not accessible to us, their derivatives in personality might be. What we saw in Karen's adolescent personality on the ego side were conflicts of "autonomy and submission," in Erikson's terms (Erikson 1950). Karen's own autonomy was threatened by our work around these issues, even as her child's autonomy was threatened by her mother's demands.

The therapist began this work by suggesting the understandable annoyance Karen might feel at being given advice. Karen denied anger at the therapist, but went on to say in an irritated tone, "People have been giving me advice ever since Nina was born. I think I'm the only one who can know what to do for my child." The therapist tried to connect their discussion of toilet training to Karen's fear that she was being told what to do, but Karen denied this. Despite the denial, the therapist moved into a description of a working relationship, to give Karen a sense of how *her* needs could be understood and how a problem could be discussed without her being told what she had to do.

The therapist said it could be valuable to have a person to talk to and sort out some of the many things happening so that Karen could make the best decisions for Nina and herself. At the same time, the therapist was sympathetic and supportive of Karen's possible needs and feelings. She commented that one would expect that Karen was at a point in *her* life where she would need more time for herself, and the more independent Nina was, the more easily Karen could find time for school-work and friends. The therapist also noted that one had only to spend a few delightful minutes with Nina to know that Karen had her own good ideas about how to do things for and with Nina. She also understood that Karen must get very tired of discussing toilet training. She added, however, that if Karen could share with the therapist what was happening, it would be of interest to her and might be of help to Karen.

The therapist's expression of sympathy for Karen's feelings and respect for her ideas was repeated over a number of weeks. During this time, Karen continued to report on toilet training, but the problems gradually decreased. She had instituted expectations about afternoon use of the potty, when she and Nina could be at home together, and she did not expect dry nights or dry days at the nursery. Gradually, Nina began asking for the potty, and toilet training proceeded without further incident. Concomitantly, the sleep problems and tantrums disappeared and Nina again enjoyed her bath.

While Karen had in fact been ignorant of her child's developmental needs and abilities, she was not able to use even gently presented, uncomplicated developmental information until her own needs and abilities were recognized, acknowledged, and respected. At this point, two things occurred: First, there was a new comprehension of her child's situation and a change in her behavior. This occurred even without an unraveling of the conflicts that had presumably contributed to making this situation especially problematic. Second, she began to move from these real but transient developmental issues to a presentation of the longtime family concerns raised much earlier in treatment.

At this point of treatment, Evelyn Atreya, who had been the first therapist for Karen and Nina, moved to another city and Deborah Cherniss became the primary therapist for the family.

Understandably, much time was spent in helping Karen to speak of the loss she felt when her first therapist had to leave her. It was as difficult for Karen to speak of loss as it was to speak of any form of emotional pain. Gradually the relationship was transferred to her new therapist. Nina too missed her first therapist and words were found to explain to the 2-year-old how sad her therapist had felt when she needed to go away, and how sad it was for Nina when someone she liked so much could not stay with her.

Maternal Depression and Family Issues: 25 to 30 Months

The focus of the work that now continued was closer to the work of the first period than that of the second. All the difficult family concerns which had been immediately apparent, but had never been central, now became main themes. As Karen described the people and relationships in her family, her depression again emerged as a major issue.

A CONTRASTING PICTURE OF CHILD AND MOTHER

At 2 years, Nina was a delightful and engaging child. Her fine development had continued in all areas. She had a wide range of affect, from joyful and exuberant to solemn and unsmiling; typically, she had an air of cheerful involvement in people and activities. Her play was nicely sustained, creative and entertaining to herself and onlookers. Her language was excellent, and she used both play and language to engage her mother and the therapist. Regardless of her mood or activity, Nina was *very* assertive and definite.

A striking contrast to her daughter's liveliness and involvement was Karen's depression. Initially, as Karen began to describe her family in greater detail than ever before, she was anxious but self-possessed and even articulate. Over the course of several sessions, however, a gradual change took place. She began staring off into space, seeming to fade away psychologically. When the therapist inquired about this, Karen talked about her lack of appetite, weight loss, insomnia, severe headaches, and dizziness. While some of these symptoms had been reported on and off throughout the treatment, they had not been occurring during visits. Following the very first months of treatment, Karen had become involved and quite active during meetings with the therapist. Now, she began to appear increasingly tired, sad, fragile, and waiflike. She would sink into a lethargic, almost immobile, posture and stare into the distance. Frequently, it seemed that both Nina and the therapist had to recall Karen from some sad reverie.

Still, Nina's assertiveness and her winsomeness could always rouse her mother's interest. Karen responded with pleasure to Nina's precocious games, and it often seemed that only Nina had the power to elicit a smile from her mother. Karen was able, however, to be firm when necessary, handling well what could become demanding or obstinate behavior. She also seemed to be able to act on Nina's behalf with her family, refusing to discipline Nina harshly, despite her family's criticisms of her for "spoiling Nina."

In general, Nina was a charming child who was developing exceptionally well. With support, Karen seemed to respond well to Nina's developmental needs. But Karen was describing real and distressing personal problems to the therapist. These centered on her family situation and Karen's longtime unhappiness with it. Although these troubles were not having a discernible negative effect on Nina, we felt concerned as to whether this would ultimately affect Karen's functioning.

We were worried about whether Karen could continue to protect Nina so successfully.

In an effort to understand more, a new emphasis in treatment was attempted. Although support and developmental guidance were still major areas of discussion, a more focused attention was now given to Karen's feelings about family, friends, and therapist.

SPECIFIC PROBLEMS

Karen talked haltingly about her concerns. She told us that she worried a good deal about what effect her family's constant chorus of criticism of her would have on Nina. She was afraid that Nina would learn from them to criticize, deprecate, or ignore her, as they did. Simultaneously, she began to express some resentment toward her parents for their lack of interest in her, her doings and plans, and, worst of all, their total lack of sympathy for her situation. They simply had no understanding, Karen felt, of what a burden it was for a high school student to try to raise and support a toddler. They minimized these difficulties as they had always minimized everything in regard to Karen—or so it seemed to her. It made her feel terribly insignificant—as if she weren't there—as if, Karen said, "I had just faded away." As Karen began reporting loss of weight and lack of sleep the therapist became increasingly concerned that this "fading" could become all too tangible.

Karen was immobilized and passive—in and out of sessions. Not only did these symptoms express complex conflicts, but the symptoms themselves added to Karen's physical and emotional suffering. Karen would remain chilled at night rather than ask her parents for more blankets. On the other hand, however, neither could she supply them for herself. It was clear that Karen was very unsure that she should really have *anything* for herself—comfort, friends, or even time alone. She found it impossible to plan anything. High school was ending and she was overwhelmed at the prospect of trying to sort through what she should do and how she could possibly work, go to school, and somehow take care of Nina. Many sad and helpless feelings from the past and the present and fears for the future were experienced by Karen and experienced, in good measure, as somatic symptoms. She also began to withdraw even more from others, to some degree including Nina. Despite descriptions of her parents' treatment of her, their insensitivity and the minimization of her needs and feelings, Karen rarely experienced any anger toward them. Instead, she vacillated between resignation and mild resentment, usually resolving the ambivalence with a shrug of helplessness, an averted gaze, and some somatic expression. All of these things made us feel that it was necessary to make some attempt to help Karen further.

KAREN'S TREATMENT: A SHIFT IN FOCUS AND STRUCTURE

Until this time all treatment sessions had included both Karen and Nina. Now, however, it seemed to us that a change might be useful. Given Nina's age and comprehension and her mother's very troubling symptoms with their attendant withdrawal, it seemed that both Karen and Nina might benefit from Karen's having individual sessions. While certainly Nina sometimes witnessed the family's derogatory treatment of her mother, the therapist wished to support Karen's protection of Nina in regard to them. It did not seem useful to have Nina a witness to her mother's upset and depression as she recounted these incidents and feelings. We also wanted to offer Karen a time of her own, both as an opportunity for discussion, not always possible with an active preschooler present, and as a way of demonstrating respect and concern for Karen's own needs and feelings.

Thus, as occasionally occurs in our work, the situation called for a modification of the usual joint parent-child sessions. For Karen and Nina, a structure used in similar situations seemed indicated: The regular joint sessions changed from weekly to biweekly, and additional weekly individual sessions were offered to Karen. This plan continued until treatment ended.

It should be emphasized that although Nina was seen less often, she was still very much in the center of the work. Important connections between Nina's behavior and external events continued to be made by Karen and the therapist. On the few occasions where there were difficulties, discussion of incidents quickly led to Karen's understanding and effective handling. Nina had a period of toileting accidents and was cranky and clinging. At one time, Karen would have been annoyed and frustrated and would have lacked any understanding of how to handle this. She would have had difficulty even in discussing this with the therapist. Now, in conjunction with the therapist, she could link recent separations in the family to the "accidents" Nina was having. She could see how these separations could make Nina fear losing her mother, and Karen could reassure Nina that this would not happen. In time, this way of thinking about Nina's behavior became very natural to Karen.

Instead of presenting problems, she began presenting solutions. With shy pride, Karen would describe not only a source of concern but the way in which she had dealt with it. Karen became increasingly able to control and to change external events to Nina's benefit. Karen was able to mobilize herself, and to be assertive and active on Nina's behalf. When she felt Nina was not treated properly, she was able to express anger on her behalf. This ability to express (and to experience) anger, and to act on Nina's behalf, remained in contrast to her own ability to experience anger and to act on her own behalf.

Any attempts, however gentle, to move Karen to some slight recognition of her own upset or negative feelings continued to result in an increase in somatic complaints. Karen was able to say to her therapist that she had been holding back feelings for so long that she simply did not know what they were any more. Affects momentarily there were quickly lost, and Karen would become mute and remote. Many times Karen reacted with extreme discomfort at the gentlest inquiries from the therapist. This happened when the therapist wondered with Karen if she sometimes disagreed with the therapist but could not feel comfortable saying so. Over a period of weeks, it became clear that Karen could not use even the most delicate and tactful of such suggestions, imbedded though they were in the general structure of support and guidance. Nonetheless, there were ways of structuring visits that proved very useful to Karen. Focusing on Nina and understanding the way events affected her behavior was the one way in which Karen could experience the relationship between her early experience and feelings and her present feelings and difficulties. She was not yet ready for sustained exploration, but she could benefit from the meaningful glimpses and could say so.

Seeing Nina in certain situations evoked memories for Karen which she could link to early feelings. As Karen watched her own mother begin to make many demands on Nina, Karen was able to remember the resentment and sadness she had experienced as a child. Karen was able to talk about Nina's assertiveness in contrast to her own passivity. She recognized her encouragement of Nina's assertiveness and began to think about why it was that she wanted Nina to be so assertive, and what being passive meant to her. Throughout this difficult time, Karen never missed an appointment, and it was evident that she continued to perceive the therapist as both committed to and concerned about her and her child.

The time served both diagnostic and therapeutic purposes. It reassured Karen that she was in control and that she would decide with us what was appropriate for us to do. In addition, out of this period there emerged the first real efforts that Karen had been able to make regarding plans for her future. It seemed to us that it would be very useful to continue to provide support and developmental guidance, to exploit the parallels that Karen found useful between Nina's experiences and her own, and to work with her as best we could toward an intelligent plan for her future and her future independence.

Situational Changes and Resolution: 30 to 38 Months

The last period in treatment was a time of important developmental growth for both Karen and Nina. Karen was finishing high school, and she was able to consider decisions about college, which she had previously avoided. Nina too was at a "graduating" point. She was now old enough to move into a preschool program for which, socially and intellectually, she was more than ready. Treatment concentrated on understanding and facilitating these changes for them both. For Karen, the decisions focused on going to college and moving out of her parents' home. This meant making an investment in her own future and separating from her family. For Nina, the move to a program designed for older children meant giving up babyhood. This too had meaning for Karen, who, like many parents, saw Nina's new school as symbolic of Nina's growing away from her. In general, this was a time of much external change. In addition to Nina and Karen both beginning new school "careers," they moved out of the home they had shared with Karen's family and, once settled in their new lives, terminated their treatment with us. The reactions to these changes were each addressed by a combination of developmental guidance, emotional support, practical help, and judicious acknowledgment of feelings.

MAJOR MOVES AND INTERVENTIONS

With the end of high school approaching, Karen had to decide whether and how she might go to college. Only during these sessions, spent in considering alternative schools and jobs, did it become clear to the therapist, and probably to Karen, that Karen was potentially a very capable student and that she had long cherished a dream of college. It also became very clear that Karen was setting up all kinds of obstacles to achieving her dream. Dreams were fine, but in fact, she was not applying for financial aid. The therapist engaged Karen in a discussion of what going to college meant to Karen and then discussed how her parents felt about her going to college. Karen said, "My parents think it's a big joke." Karen said that they never asked her about schoolwork and that they always belittled any of the courses in which she did well. The therapist said it sounded as if Karen's family had very different ideas about why one went to school and what courses were important. The therapist also acknowledged that in reality Karen had given a great deal of thought to school and had abilities and plans that she wanted to pursue. This straightforward discussion of the situation somehow enabled Karen to reconfirm her interest. Suddenly, the financial difficulties no longer seemed insurmountable, and Karen was able to apply for financial aid.

Karen's decision to go to college also led to her separation from her family. She had her choice of two schools, one close to her family and the other in a nearby community. By choosing the farther school, she created a rationale for moving out of her parents' home that did not necessitate her confronting either them or herself with any negative reasons for the move. The therapist discussed with Karen what she wanted and how she might proceed. This involved a careful examination of how Karen would present her plan to her parents, how they were likely to respond, and how Karen would handle their responses. Also, the therapist commented that leaving home involves, for many young people, a sense of the ending of a very important period in their lives. She said that this feeling might be even more heightened for Karen because at the same time, Nina was moving on to greater independence. This transition allowed the focus to shift to Nina, a focus with which Karen was more comfortable. In that framework, as they talked of what Karen wanted for Nina, despite the loss that *she* might feel, Karen was able to realize that the move from her parents' home meant to her that she would never have the attention, valuing, and love from her parents for which she had longed. The kind of parent she wished to be to Nina was a kind of parent her parents had never been able to be to her. When these feelings were experienced and talked about, some of the ambivalence which had been keeping Karen from actively planning for new living arrangements was sufficiently resolved for the move to take place.

Nina was directly and profoundly affected by moving. The relocation to a nearby community meant leaving both her grandparents' home, where she'd lived since birth, and the nursery where she'd spent the last eighteen months. She was the youngest of the children at her preschool center. In her typically active, coping style, Nina emulated the older children and quickly established herself with them in quite a sturdy fashion. Her reactions to all the changes that had occurred, however, were touchingly apparent in the play sessions.

Nina began trying to climb into the dolls' bed and into the dolls' high chair. At the same time, she also began climbing on the furniture in a dangerous way. When the therapist reflected that this seemed to give a very graphic picture of the feelings that Nina must have about being the baby and being the big girl, Karen immediately felt this was true. She connected it to the recent moves and spontaneously provided Nina with a lot of opportunities to be cuddled and babied by her, and to play with her. Karen managed beautifully to avoid infantilizing Nina in some detrimental way, yet provided the freedom for Nina to express her wishes and feelings. After a few weeks of an unusual amount of cuddling, Nina seemed comfortable and began again to enjoy the more typical imaginative doll play which had filled her time before. Much of this doll play expressed Nina's pleasure in being a good and loving mother, like her own.

NINA LEADS THE WAY: NEW INSIGHTS FOR KAREN

There were other ways in which the focus on Nina allowed Karen the direct freedom to experience some of her own feelings. Nina's energetic play was usually very charming, but on occasion she was quite capable of very demanding and irritating behavior. The therapist increasingly felt that Karen was really exceptionally patient and tolerant of Nina's unpleasant behavior—to a fault. When the therapist merely commented, finally, on Karen's surprising patience, Karen explained that if she acted or felt angry at Nina she felt very bad and guilty. One of the things the therapist and Karen learned as this was discussed was that in addition to Karen's own internal difficulties with anger, the therapist had unwittingly contributed to the situation. All of the tolerance for Karen and the understanding and patience toward both parent and child had been "taken over" by Karen as a model. It was as if she really thought she had not been "given permission" to be annoyed at her mischievious, assertive little girl. This became an important topic to be discussed and understood, and although basic shifts simply could not happen, our role in this could certainly be dramatically modified.

When Karen began to understand that a mother can love her child very much and still be angry with that child, there began to be perceptible changes in Karen. She became discernibly more relaxed and active and allowed more irritation and anger to show, both toward Nina directly and in speaking of her parents. Some of the entrenched defenses against anger shifted as, through gentle support and acknowledgment of her feelings, Karen could experience that having both positive and negative feelings toward Nina was expectable, allowable and—most important—not dangerous. The reassurance seemed to occur as she gradually experimented with experiencing and acknowledging more negative feelings and found they could be acted upon comfortably and appropriately. She learned that she did not need to fear either herself or Nina.

Karen became much more consistently active and involved, and she began to look more rested and relaxed. She began describing how she was trying to help Nina to express anger, letting Nina know that it was all right to be mad, to talk about it and then to make up. Simultaneously, she began telling the therapist with appropriate affect of *her* annoyance with *her* parents at their behavior around her college plans. With this acknowledgment, at last, of anger toward her parents, significant changes took place. Karen now began to separate from her parents emotionally and in reality.

This was, then, another change in a period of changes. There were moves from home and schools and there were changes in Karen's view of herself and in her ability to acknowledge her feelings and to act on her own behalf to meet her needs.

It was not an easy time for Nina. While her mother could envision all kinds of positive outcomes from these changes, for the most part Nina could only experience the loss of familiar places and people. It was very nice that Karen was perceptive of Nina's reactions and was able to understand and handle them in a sensitive and effective way. The situation became a new and stable pattern for Nina and Karen, one into which they comfortably settled after an initial, expectable period of stress.

As these changes were getting stabilized, the therapist began discussing with Karen how she thought they might use their sessions. Karen still had many of the same difficulties: She continued to suffer some somatic complaints, she was often passive, sometimes sad, and failed most often to experience the painful affect that her manner and behavior still reflected. She did not, however, experience these things as problems—or at least as significantly interfering. She had made important changes in her life, increasing her opportunities for satisfying relationships and a sense of self-worth, and she was a consistently sensitive and responsive mother to Nina. Of great importance and significance was the fact that she had maintained a very positive and rewarding relationship with a young man for some time. He was someone who valued her, treated her well, and made her feel important and cherished. It seemed to us reassuring and promising that she could enjoy this and that she did nothing either to spoil it or destroy it.

Nina was thriving in every way. Thus, when Karen did not feel that there were concerns and problems on which she wished to focus but instead could express some hesitant pleasure in the possibility of independence, the therapist introduced the idea of an ending point for their work.

TERMINATION

Long before the changes in Karen's and Nina's situation had been made, the therapist had suggested to Karen that she was not always going to need someone to help her and that the therapist was confident that Karen would sometime be able to do very well on her own. It was made clear to Karen that ending was a possibility to be considered together, when the situation was stable. When this occurred Karen was ready, if not eager, to terminate. The time at which they would end was mutually agreed to. Karen and the therapist reviewed the work they had done and reaffirmed Karen's continued competence as a mother.

The therapist spoke of the work as a confirmation of Karen's own very good ideas and knowledge, pointing out that while Karen at times had needed some help in determining what was best for Nina, she had mostly needed support in order to do what she herself had felt was best. To this, Karen responded that long ago, in their initial meetings, the therapist had been the first to make Karen feel that she had the right and the capacity to be Nina's mother.

Karen said that even in the first months of treatment, "I never felt I was a bad mother when I came *here*. It was really nice to come and know that I was doing *something* right. It was very reassuring. People here knew I couldn't do everything right but that I certainly tried." The therapist said that she knew that it had been hard for Karen because Karen had not had support at home—and every mother needs that. Karen then said that during the past year she guessed she should have known that things were all right with Nina just by looking at her, but this was very hard, being with her family, and again, she needed to know she wasn't doing things wrong. Karen now felt confident about herself, and while shyly sad about termination, she was able to say that "ending is taking a step forward for myself."

FOLLOW-UP

Eight months after termination, Karen called the therapist and wanted additional information about financial resources they had previously discussed. At that time, the school situation for both of them was still stable, and Karen reported that she and Nina were living with a good friend, one of several who supported her endeavors. From her descriptions, it sounded as though Karen had found a new "family," in which both she and Nina were valued and nutured.

Discussion

AN OVERVIEW OF TREATMENT

When Karen first came to the Child Development Project, she was a passive, timid girl, uncertain of either her rights or her ability to mother her child. Two-and-a-half years later, when treatment ended, she had become a competent and confident parent. Nina, a joyless, wary, starving infant, had become an active, assertive, and delightful child, who was thriving in every area of development. To some extent, natural developmental processes were at work: Karen at 18½ had greater emotional maturity and a larger fund of interpersonal experience than she had had at 16; and at 3 years, Nina certainly had many more skills than she had had at 7 months. However, given the many residual effects associated with failure to thrive, as well as the specific family and economic stresses for this mother and child, more than maturation and the passage of time had been necessary to ameliorate the serious problems they presented.

The therapist responded to these problems in a variety of ways. In the first part of treatment, both difficulties and strengths were identified, and treatment focused on the development of a trusting relationship and the support of Karen's maternal abilities. As treatment progressed and the failure to thrive syndrome was no longer a concern, the focus shifted to developmental issues, such as toilet training. The most important element in this next treatment period was the therapist's recognition, acknowledgment, and respect for Karen's needs, wishes, and feelings.

As Nina's situation and the mother-child relationship became increasingly stable and secure, Karen's own depression became a major area of concern. Her physical and emotional debilitation and immobilization were interfering with her functioning and were making her less accessible to Nina. Because of this, the structure of treatment changed. Individual sessions for Karen were now added to the joint sessions with Nina, and in the individual sessions the therapist attempted to focus more directly with Karen on her conflicts and her strong defenses against them.

The intensification of somatic symptoms which had suggested this approach worsened, and the therapist decided to return essentially to the earlier focus, retaining what seemed to be a useful structure for the sessions. Individual sessions for Karen were continued, along with the joint sessions with Nina, and the therapist provided continued solid support. Karen's more defended feelings were dealt with essentially through her identification with Nina. There were also some shifts in her ability to deal with anger when Karen's overly "patient" responses to Nina were commented upon and then explored with her. Finally, in a period of many important situational changes, treatment concentrated on Nina's and Karen's needs and on alternatives for meeting them, as well as on support and tactful acknowledgment of Karen's feelings as she made decisions and took actions which had special and poignant meaning for her.

DEVELOPMENTAL GUIDANCE

The various methods of treatment used by the therapist in work with Nina and her mother typify developmental guidance in our work. As in any therapeutic work, the treatment alliance is fundamental, but in developmental guidance this aspect is central. In addition to the trust based on the therapist's constancy and reliability, the alliance is founded in large part on a mutual concern for the child. The therapist allies himself with the parent's abilities and investment in the child, even though he may often have to search out and elicit such strengths. There is a consistent, strong recognition of even the most tenuous connections between parent and child and the steadfast support of these. The effect is to considerably enhance those connections and gradually to enlarge the positive areas of connectedness.

The parents are perceived and explicitly treated as indispensable partners in the treatment process, and they understand the view that, of course, parents want what is best for their child. Demonstrating interest in and respect for their ideas and skills in interacting with their child, the therapist communicates his firm belief that the parents have a knowledge of and relationship to the child that others cannot have. Even the most competent helpers (nursery staff, family, or therapist) can only contribute to making that very special relationship more satisfying and pleasurable—they cannot replace it. As was true for Karen, many parents are able to articulate later in treatment how crucial for all subsequent work is the initial firm recognition and support of their own investment in their babies.

As trust in the treatment relationship develops, the therapist's commitment and expertise work together to facilitate the understanding and handling of problems. The parents know the therapist is not critical of them; he respects them, is interested in them, and is concerned about their well-being as well as their baby's. The therapist's questions and comments make them confident of his knowledge and understanding of infants and parents. This combination of respect, concern, and knowledge makes it possible for the therapist occasionally to provide normative expectations for development as well as suggestions for the smoother negotiation of developmental tasks.

Rarely does the therapist give direct advice. Instead, he helps the parents articulate their questions, observations, and ideas and then works together with them to find solutions to their shared concerns. Often this will take the form of discussion about the ways in which the parents have already attempted to handle the situations and about what else they might try to do. This is done in the context of their own needs and feelings. For Karen and Nina toilet training could not proceed smoothly without recognition of Karen's concern with independence; for other teenage parents on welfare, feeding the baby may be difficult because of their own real hunger. Without recognition of such important elements, discussion of solutions has little chance of success.

In addition to information and discussion of the meaning of behavior and alternatives to handling it, the therapist also provides a more objective basis than a parent may have for viewing the child. He can help separate serious concerns from transient problems. The therapist can become a repository of the past, especially as the contacts continue and a mutual history is built, putting into a broad context the child's developmental regressions, plateaus, and progress.

Another major aspect of developmental guidance is emotional support and empathy. The therapist provides this both at times of crisis and of pleasure. When problems arise suddenly or persist drainingly, or when family and friends react critically and disparagingly to the child or parent, the therapist can draw not only upon belief in but knowledge of the parent's commitment to the child. Support is offered by the therapist's explicit faith in the parents, despite their fears of wrongdoing or failure. This was particularly important for Karen. Sharing the joys of the child's progress, pointing out newly observed achievements, and appreciating parental triumphs is another way of providing emotional support. An important dimension is added to this when it is possible to link the child's good progress to good things the parent has done.

Practical help is often an integral part of the work with young children and their parents. Having arrived at a joint decision with the parents about the child's or parents' needs, the therapist must then help the parents find the most appropriate resources. For Karen and Nina, this was most important in terms of schools and housing. For many lower-income families, medical, legal, and financial aid are often necessary. Even financially comfortable families may need help in finding good services or in meeting a handicapped child's special needs. Recognition of these practical needs and help in meeting them, whether through discussion with the parent, exploration of community resources, or dealing with other agencies, is part of developmental guidance.

Finally, the therapist collects ongoing observations and processes them for continual evaluation of the situation. Throughout the work the therapist is assessing what the parents can give to the child and what their psychological availability is to treatment. The therapist not only supports and extends the parents' strengths and resources, but also explores those areas which seem to be sources of difficulty. If it becomes apparent that the difficulties may greatly interfere with the work and by extension, the child's well-being, the work is modified. While for Karen this was not indicated, for some parents interpretive treatment may be incorporated with developmental guidance, or referral to another agency may be made for treatment focused primarily on the parent, rather than on the child, while our work continues.

CONCLUSIONS

The work with Nina and Karen demonstrates the value of developmental guidance. For them, two aspects of this treatment mode seemed vital. First, much of the work was built on strengthening the attachment between them and supporting Karen's sense of her rights and capacities to mother Nina. Second, for this young girl who felt generally helpless and worthless, the therapist became someone who believed in her importance, competence, and right to be cared for and respected. With this encouragement, with help in finding resources and with some developmental information, advice, and support, Karen was able to act in ways that had important positive effects for both herself and Nina.

Obviously, some aspects of Karen's conflicts and depression remained. At the same time, the work based on support and respect had contributed to a strong, positive mother-child relationship. While still troubled by intrapsychic and intrapersonal conflicts, Karen was able to protect Nina, and Nina, in turn, gave her mother both the love for which she longed and which lightened her depression, and irrefutable evidence of Karen's success as a parent. Developmental guidance did not provide a remedy for all of the serious problems that had existed for Nina and Karen. It did, however, provide a foundation of trust and confidence which had vital effects and which would serve them well in their future.

BIBLIOGRAPHY

Erikson, E. 1950. *Childhood and Society.* New York: Norton, pp. 364–365.
Evans, S. L., Reinhart, J. B., and Suscop, R. A. 1972. "Failure to Thrive: A Study of 45 Children and Their Families." *Journal of the American Academy of Child Psychiatry* 2:440–457.
Fraiberg, S. 1950. "On the Sleep Disturbances of Early Childhood." In Eissler, R. S., et al., eds. *The Psychoanalytic Study of The Child,* vol. 5. New York: International Universities Press, pp. 285–309.
Fraiberg, S., and Bennett, J. 1979. "Failure to Thrive: Treatment in an Infant Mental Health Program." (Unpublished)
———. 1978. "Intervention and Failure to Thrive: A Psychiatric Outpatient Treatment Program." *Birth and the Family Journal* 5:4.
Freud, A. 1946. *The Ego and the Mechanisms of Defense.* New York: International Universities Press, pp. 149–180.

Glaser, J. H., Heagarty, M. C., Dexter, M. B., and Pirchik, E. C. 1968. "Physical and Psychological Development of Children with Early FTT." *Journal of Pediatrics* 73:690–698.

Leonard, M. F., Rhymes, M. P., and Solnit, A. J. 1966. "FTT in Infants." *American Journal of Diseases of Children* 3:600–612.

Shaheen, E., Alexander, D., Trukowsky, M., and Barbaro, G. J. 1968. "FTT—A Retrospective Profile." *Clinical Pediatrics* 7:255–261

Whitten, C. F., Pettit, M. G., and Fischoff, J. 1969. "Evidence that Growth Failure from Maternal Deprivation Is Secondary to Undereating." *Journal of the American Medical Association* 209:1675–1682.

VI

Robbie: Coping with Trauma in the Neonatal Period

CAROLYN R. ARADINE
VIVIAN SHAPIRO
HOWARD UMAN

THIS CHAPTER describes the developmental guidance and supportive interventions provided to one critically ill premature infant and his parents throughout the first year of the child's life. This infant also experienced severe respiratory obstruction which necessitated a long-term tracheostomy, adding a potential handicap to his development of language and social interactions. The work described was done collaboratively by a pediatric nurse who worked as the family's primary Child Development Project therapist with members of the health care system. The chapter illustrates the use of developmental guidance in a medically high-risk situation.

Background

The infant who is born early has many immature body systems. Sophisticated medical measures are now available to assist such infants. Their care, however, requires separation of the baby from the parents. Even though the parents may visit the baby daily, they may be restricted in many ways from interacting with him, both because of his immaturity and of his need for specialized medical equipment and treatments. Despite the value of these treatments, such separations constitute a crisis for both the infant and the parents—but especially the latter. Early contact of the kind that promotes infant attachment to parents and parental attachment to the infant may be very limited.

The respiratory system of an immature infant often requires assisted ventilation until the baby is capable of sustaining his own respiration. Various assistive measures may be used. Endotracheal intubation with assisted ventilation by a respirator may be necessary. One of the hazards of such endotracheal intubation is damage to the vocal cords, larynx, or trachea. If damage is severe, scarring and stenosis (narrowing) of the trachea or associated structures may result. In the presence of severe narrowing, normal respiration is severely compromised. Tracheostomy, the placement of an artificial airway into the trachea below the narrowing, may become essential to sustain life.

The presence of a respiratory obstruction necessitating a tracheostomy, especially if it is necessary for a prolonged period, may pose a severe developmental handicap to the infant, especially in the areas of language development and social interaction. In addition, there are severe medical risks, including a high incidence of infections, respiratory arrest, and death (Aberdeen and Downes 1974; Freeland et al. 1974; Fearon and Ellis 1971; Fearon and Cotton 1974; Holinger et al. 1976; McGovern et al. 1971; Parkin et al. 1976). Prolonged use of the tracheostomy with infants is a relatively new medical practice. Medical experience and research are still limited. Such infants may be hospitalized for extended periods, but their home care is a new and frightening process to both parents and professionals, whose questions about how best to provide care to these children remain unanswered. There has been little research on the development and home care of these infants (Aradine 1978).

Long-term hospitalization of sick infants in itself poses many difficulties for infants and parents. Attachment may be impeded. Economic need may be severe. Frequent visiting by parents may be very difficult. The continuing needs of all family members must be carefully balanced. The resulting stress and strain are accompanied by worry.

Simultaneously the parents are experiencing their own psychological crises, and some emotional adjustment is necessary. They may at the same time be faced with painful and difficult decisions related to the care of their newborn infant, whose life may be recurrently threatened. Urgent questions about their relationship to the baby face the parents. How close should they let themselves feel to the infant? Mothers who have experienced the closeness of carrying the fetus through the pregnancy may feel this question very poignantly. Their desire to be close to the infant and on the other hand their grief over the baby's condition may be especially difficult to bear, even though it is normal for such feelings to occur. They may feel they have failed as parents. They may also find themselves experiencing differing feelings toward the baby and his situation. They may or may not have the resources to deal with the crisis by themselves.

In the following case we address these multiple concerns for a sick premature infant and his parents. We describe the supportive and developmental guidance provided for the family.

Robbie and His Parents

Robbie was born very prematurely, at twenty-seven-weeks gestation; he weighed 2 pounds 5 ounces. The pregnancy had been complicated by recurrent bleeding. Statistically, his risk of mortality at birth had been greater than 50 percent. He was hospitalized in a busy intensive-care nursery, surrounded by a vast array of complex medical equipment, bright lights, and the constant movement of many staff members caring for many very ill infants.

Following a stable first week, Robbie experienced multiple medical problems: progressive respiratory distress, apnea, bradycardia, anemia, acidosis, sepsis, and a patent ductus arteriosus. He required extensive treatment. Fluids and nourishment were administered through tubes; intravenous tubes entered his scalp veins, and a nasogastric tube was passed through his nose to his stomach. For seven days his eyes were patched while he lay in the isolette under bright lights, receiving phototherapy to lower his elevated bilirubin. Cardiac surgery was necessary at age 1 month to close the patent ductus. Respiratory distress and apnea progressed and required endotracheal assisted ventilation for two-and-a-half months. The endotracheal tube passed through his mouth into his trachea and was connected to the constantly pulsating respirator. Monitor leads to check respiration, temperature, and heart rate were attached to his chest. Medications were required to treat his electrolyte imbalances and infection. Robbie could be touched in the isolette but not yet held. It was difficult for his parents or others to see the "real baby" in the midst of all this equipment. This was not the baby the Richardses had dreamed of bearing. In addition to these difficulties, Robbie's course had been further complicated by a possible intracranial bleed and a respiratory arrest requiring resuscitation. Robbie's early weeks were a constant series of ups and downs. There were many points at which his parents feared he might die.

Mr. and Mrs. Richards were a handsome, dark-haired young couple. They were sensitive, well educated, and emotionally healthy. Faithfully, they visited the baby daily. In their deep grief, however, they found it impossible to call the baby by name, to put their feelings into words for one another, to share their deep sadness and fears, or to explain the baby's condition to their school-age daughter.

The First Child Development Project Visit

When the baby was 6 weeks old, Mrs. Richards approached the Child Development Project and asked for help. She phrased the dilemma eloquently: "I don't know how close to let myself get to the baby. There have been so many ups and downs. There is a great risk that he will not live; he may be brain-damaged. If he does live, he may need a tracheostomy to help him breathe. If so, he will not be able to vocalize or cry. He will probably need to stay in the hospital. How could you take care of a baby at home who can't cry, who might need you in the middle of the night and whom you might not be able to hear?"

The baby was receiving excellent medical care. The parents felt, however, that they were obtaining inadequate information and inconsistent support from hospital staff. Each month there was a new rotation of doctors; differing explanations added to the parents' confusion. There were many different nurses caring for Robbie. The staff encouraged Mrs. Richards to participate in the baby's care, but there was no one person who could help her assess the situation and her feelings.

The first visit, made with Vivian Shapiro, a member of the Child Development Project intake committee, illustrates our approach and describes the family's difficulties. Mrs. Richards expressed grief, sadness, and worry with tears and words. Mrs. Shapiro listened sympathetically. She wholeheartedly supported Mrs. Richards's desire to request an appointment to talk to a senior physician about her baby's progress. She helped Mrs. Richards clarify her feelings, experiences, and questions. Mrs. Richards spoke of the terrible difficulty of not having the baby at home, of being uncertain about the future, of having feelings of love and attachment toward the baby and not yet being able to hold or care for him. Mrs. Shapiro pointed out that parents often find it difficult to talk to each other about their feelings and grief because each handles it at his or her own pace, and frequently these are not the same.

Mrs. Shapiro then asked Mrs. Richards to tell her about the baby and her visits to see him. Mrs. Richards could only describe the machinery: the isolette, the many tubes, the respirator, and monitoring devices. Focusing on the baby, Mrs. Shapiro asked, "How do you comfort the baby?" With surprise at the question, Mrs. Richards brightened and replied, "It is remarkable. You can see him crying even though you can't hear the sound. There are his facial expressions and his movement." Mrs. Richards described how she could put her hands through the isolette and pat the baby's bottom and he quieted. With a small laugh she added, "I know that he probably does this for all the nurses too. It's not just for me." Mrs. Shapiro told her that although this was true, it was important that she was doing this, that she came to see the baby, that he felt her handling him, and that she had the pleasure of comforting him. Mrs. Richards became calmer and said, "I want to tell Ann that she has a baby brother." They talked about what to tell Ann and what Ann might be worried about. Mrs. Richards was sad but relieved as the visit ended. She thanked Mrs. Shapiro for the opportunity to talk about what had been happening. Mrs. Shapiro offered her the continued help of the Child Development Project, which Mrs. Richards gratefully accepted. She introduced me, the therapist,* and I then began to meet with Mrs. Richards weekly to help her face the difficulties, whatever the baby's course would be.

The Early Work

During the first two months of work, I met with Mrs. Richards at the office or at the hospital weekly. I began by focusing on Mrs. Richards's own emotional needs in response to the baby's continued uncertain course and the difficulties she was encountering in dealing with the hospital system. Developmental guidance about the needs and characteristics of premature infants was intertwined with emotional support and clarification of information received about the baby's health status. The developmental guidance also included attention to the needs of the Richards's older daughter, Ann, and the questions and worries she might have about the baby. Mrs. Richards discussed with me how to help Ann understand the baby's condition.

Robbie developed pneumonia. It was another setback, and his parents again feared he might die. Mrs. Richards had many questions

---

*Carolyn Aradine was the therapist and is subsequently referred to as "I" in the text.

about his medical status, but hesitated to "bother the doctors." Instead, she sought resource materials in the library. Simultaneously, the parents worried about the competence of yet another new rotation of physicians. They wanted to talk with the senior staff physician who had met with them once earlier, but hesitated to request this. They did not want to antagonize the staff and seemed to fear that asking questions or "special favors" might do so.

I listened with sympathy to Mrs. Richards's concerns. I provided a background of general information and responded to her questions about pneumonia. I then encouraged her to discuss the specific questions about Robbie with the physicians providing his care. It was important to hear the specific answers about his condition from those caring for him. To help her do so more easily, I helped Mrs. Richards formulate the specific questions, supported her right to ask these questions, and encouraged the Richardses to make an appointment to talk over their concerns about the baby with the physician of their choice. Upon receiving this support and guidance, Mrs. Richards contacted the physician. He met with both parents and agreed to follow the baby and periodically talk with them. They felt much relieved.

At the same visit, Mrs. Richards introduced the baby to me by a photograph. She then spoke of another concern. She wanted to touch the baby, but he squirmed in response. She was afraid that Robbie was learning that touch only brought painful procedures. She was well read in infant development and wished the nurses would provide more stimulation that was unrelated to procedures. As we talked, I helped Mrs. Richards identify ways she could provide comforting touch to the baby. I suggested she also talk soothingly to him, providing vocal stimulation as well.

Robbie gradually improved, and recovered from his pneumonia. His parents were able to hold him for the first time when he was 2 months old. During a visit with me to see Robbie in the intensive-care nursery a few days later, Mrs. Richards saw her baby in the alert and awake state for the first time. I observed as Mrs. Richards held her infant and as she talked with staff members about his progress and condition. In spite of all the difficulties, Mrs. Richards was very comfortable holding her infant and in tune with his signals. Reciprocal attachment between mother and infant seemed to be progressing well. Mrs. Richards held Robbie and rocked him gently, looking down tenderly at him. His eyes sought her face and studied it. Their eyes met frequently. Robbie wiggled and squirmed, mother gently soothed, patted, rocked, and comforted him, quietly responsive to each signal. As I observed, I pointed out to Mrs. Richards the baby's developing capabilities to see, feel, hear, be comforted by, and seek mother's attention.

During the visit, I also observed Mrs. Richards's interactions with

Robbie's nurse and his physicians. She was attentive to the detailed discussions with these staff members while simultaneously holding and responding to Robbie. She asked her questions with ease. I subsequently reviewed these discussions with Mrs. Richards and answered the few questions she had.

A significant milestone in the process by which the Richardses claimed this baby as their own occurred about this time. The Richardses had chosen to name the baby after father and grandfather; they would use his middle name, Robbie, to avoid confusion with father. Initially, however, they had used no name, but had referred to their son as "baby," "boy," or "he." Now, after two months, they began to call him Robbie. They requested the hospital staff to do the same, although they actually feared that this might cause confusion and somehow jeopardize his care.

At age 2½ months, new difficulties arose. Extubation was attempted, but respiratory distress recurred. Subglottic stenosis, severe swelling and narrowing of the subglottic area of the trachea, was identified. Surgery to perform a tracheostomy was advised and performed. Robbie was then able to be weaned from the respirator and to breathe unassisted through the tracheostomy tube. His condition improved. He appeared now to be a much more comfortable baby and was moved to a crib. Fewer tubes and less equipment were now needed. Although no one could predict how long he might require the tracheostomy (and estimates varied from a few weeks to twenty years!), the Richardses began to look toward a more hopeful future and to anticipate Robbie's coming home. They began to learn the measures his care would require.

Mrs. Richards continued to speak of worries about Robbie's medical condition, care, and development. Would she be able to treat him like a "normal baby"? She worried about his silence, imposed by the tracheostomy; he was unable to vocalize or cry aloud. What would that mean about his future speech? Although there was little information available with which to provide answers, I continued to listen, to point out Robbie's abilities, and to look with Mrs. Richards at the ways in which the baby did communicate with her by means other than voice (eyes, movements). I encouraged the parents in their "pact" always to hold Robbie when they visited and to talk to him as they did so. I supported their need to continue to gain the necessary medical information. When Mrs. Richards noted that she and her husband heard different things when the doctors talked to them, I reassured them that this was a common experience, but encouraged them to meet together with the doctors whenever possible to limit discrepancies in the information received. The Richardses also sought written information about infant development, prematurity, and the effects of hospitalization. In addition to reviewing questions raised by their reading, I provided selected materials I felt would be helpful to Mrs. Richards and subsequently discussed these with her.

A NEW CRISIS: TRANSFER

At age 3 months a new crisis loomed. Robbie no longer required intensive neonatal care. Transfer to a constant-observation nursery on another unit was proposed. Mrs. Richards became gravely concerned. Again there would be different doctors and nurses and new ways of doing things. Would Robbie receive equally good care? To whom would the parents turn for help and answers to their questions? I reassured Mrs. Richards of my continued availability and discussed the information about the new unit that had been provided in anticipation by staff members.

Despite preparation, the transfer three weeks later was an extremely painful time for the parents. I met Mr. and Mrs. Richards at the hospital soon after the transfer. Mrs. Richards poured out a torrent of worries. It seemed to her that there had been one crisis after another, including changes and lapses in Robbie's care. Communication from the staff members to them seemed curt and uninformative. Staff members repeatedly asked the parents how the intensive-care nursery had done things; the parents heard these questions as expressions of staff insecurity and inexperience. They wondered if there was any communication between units. They could not identify which doctor was responsible for Robbie. They were frightened.

The Richardses again felt distrustful of the hospital system and devised their own strategies to meet the crisis. Mrs. Richards felt that the staff had to prove their ability to care for Robbie. The Richardses began to visit the hospital many times each day, often unannounced and at unusual hours, to "check up on Robbie's care." They brought their legitimate complaints to the nursing director and to Robbie's doctor in the intensive-care nursery. They turned to me for guidance and emotional support.

As I listened sympathetically, Mrs. Richards, near tears, poured out her worries. I then met Mr. Richards for the first time and listened as well to his concerns. I affirmed the parents' decision to appeal to hospital staff members for assistance and encouraged them to meet with these people to discuss their concerns. These meetings resolved many of the difficulties. A primary nurse* was assigned to provide and co-

---

*Primary nurse means one registered nurse assigned to provide care to a particular baby whenever she is working. She plans care, coordinates that care with nurses who assist her on other shifts, and is the major nursing person to discuss the baby's care with the parents.

ordinate Robbie's care. This intervention clearly facilitated meeting both the baby's and the parents' needs.

At this point it became evident that collaboration among the parents, the Child Development Project therapist, and hospital staff members was imperative. With the parents' permission, I communicated directly with the primary nurse as well as with them. Collaborative plans were made for Robbie's nursing care, promotion of his development, and the planning for his discharge. Unfortunately, we were unable to establish the same primary responsibility and coordinated planning with Robbie's physicians. Rotations of pediatricians and specialists continued without any one person assuming responsibility for medical coordination and communication with the parents.

CONTINUED HOSPITALIZATION

Robbie remained hospitalized for another four months. Every seven to fourteen days he underwent general anesthesia for direct laryngoscopy and dilation of the stenosis. Such intrusive procedures are stressful. Robbie tolerated the procedures well, but his weight gain was slow. His development progressed at a rate consistent with his age corrected for prematurity. The therapist, nurses, physical therapist, and parents designed and instituted interventions to promote his developing abilities. His parents obtained tiny, lightweight rattles and squeaky animals which could be handled by Robbie. A mobile with music box provided visual and sound stimuli. Robbie was placed in varied positions, including prone and supported sit, to foster head control. His parents and nurses cuddled him, held him in the ventral position, made frequent eye contact, and talked with Robbie to foster human relationships. He was held for feedings.

Both Mr. and Mrs. Richards were daily visitors and active participants in Robbie's care. Both learned his total care regimen, including all aspects of tracheostomy care and postural drainage as well as his routine infant care. The parents arranged their schedules to spend different periods of the day with Robbie, thus providing more direct parental attention and care. Continuity of his care was maintained by his primary nurse and a small number of assisting nurses. These nurses also provided support and thorough instructions to his parents.

During Robbie's continued hospitalization, I met weekly with Mrs. Richards. Visits alternated between office visits with mother alone and hospital visits with mother, Robbie, and staff members. There continued to be three major components of the work: emotional support for Mrs. Richards; developmental guidance; and facilitation of communication with the hospital staff. To these, a fourth component was added: planning for Robbie's eventual discharge. I began to anticipate home care with Mrs. Richards. What would be her own emotional responses to the new responsibilities of Robbie's care? What changes and needs would the family experience?

Developmental guidance was a major facet of the work at this time. Mrs. Richards worried that long-term hospitalization could be a major obstacle to her baby's development. At each visit, Mrs. Richards shared her observations and questions about Robbie's development with me. During hospital visits, we observed Robbie's abilities together. We sought to understand his cues, to pace interactions, to play sensitively with him, to provide toys and opportunities that would promote his developing abilities, and to observe his developing attachment to his mother. As I watched mother and baby throughout these interactions, I pointed out the present and emerging aspects of Robbie's abilities (his beginning smile, his particular comfort in mother's arms, his hands beginning to reach and come to midline, his expressive face and attentive gaze). Mrs. Richards responded readily to these observations and to my descriptions of things she was already doing to promote his development. My reviewing these observations with Mrs. Richards seemed to be an important source of support. It validated for Mrs. Richards the value and results of her many efforts to help Robbie. Most important, it helped Mrs. Richards to recognize the behaviors that indicated Robbie's increasing preference for mother. These rewards from Robbie encouraged Mrs. Richards as she provided his daily care.

When Mrs. Richards conferred with me about what toys Robbie might find useful, I responded in two ways. I concurred with Mrs. Richards's judgment and encouraged her to secure the toys she had suggested might be useful. Second, I showed her some additional toys that Robbie could enjoy and that were small and lightweight enough for him to handle. By the following week's visit, many of the toys discussed had been provided for Robbie by his parents.

Developmental observations guided my recommendations to Mrs. Richards. Robbie's prematurity at birth required that guidance be given in accord with gestational rather than chronological age. His long hospitalization and complications further delayed some areas of development. The usual infant guidelines were only helpful in providing the sequence in which abilities emerge. Specific activities had to be guided by observations of his emerging abilities. His progress was often inconsistent, advancing at varied rates in different areas of development. For these reasons, Mrs. Richards found the ongoing developmental guidance especially supportive.

Language development was of particular concern because of the tracheostomy. Although Robbie cried, his cries were silent; he was not yet able to make any vocal sounds. However, he was alert, attentive, and himself very much interested in sounds. He attended and turned to sounds such as the spoken voice, his music box, other toys that made noise, and environmental sounds. Guidance was directed toward encouraging Mrs. Richards to talk with Robbie as she cared for and played with him, even though she was deprived of the vocal response which would have reinforced her efforts. I acknowledged the difficulty of the task and helped Mrs. Richards observe Robbie's visual and motor responses to her voice. Together we discussed the discomfort we both felt because there was little information and no certainty about Robbie's future speech. I explained, however, that hearing conversational language and identifying Robbie's behavioral responses and signals were very important contributions to his future language development.

The physiological organization of an infant is promoted by consistency in those giving him care. (Burns et al. 1972.) Combined with sensitive responsiveness to the infant's signals, continuity is a critical factor in infant development. Consistent caretakers are able to read an infant's cues more readily and to pace their responses to his needs. The foundation is thus laid for enabling an infant to distinguish and trust the special people in his world. Robbie's parents and his nurses tried to provide as much consistency as possible throughout his hospitalization. Although within the hospital structure it was not possible to provide a single continuous caregiver, limiting the number of people would facilitate Robbie's development and growing attachment to his parents. His parents came daily to care for him. I stressed the importance of continuity and observed Robbie's developing states, changing patterns, and preference for his parents. I observed Robbie's first smiles and reassured Mrs. Richards that they were appearing at the appropriate gestational age. I emphasized that Robbie's turning to his mother's voice and beginning to watch her arrival and departure were signs of attachment and beginning differentiation of mother.

Continued emotional support was another essential ingredient of the work with Mrs. Richards. In weekly meetings with me, she had the opportunity to express the joys and sadness, the strains, the worries, the doubts, and the anger she experienced during Robbie's extended hospitalization. It was sad waiting so long to bring her baby home. It was frustrating not to be able to anticipate and plan exactly when he could be discharged. It was difficult to arrange schedules so someone could be at the hospital with Robbie when he was awake. As he grew older and his schedule changed, the Richardses had to readjust their schedules. The parents' and nurses' plans sometimes differed, resulting in tensions and miscommunications. Did the baby "belong" to the hospital or to the parents? Mrs. Richards felt pressured to provide all of Robbie's care exactly and correctly. She knew that his discharge was in part dependent upon her ability to do so. More than that, she worried whether she would be able to do all Robbie needed when he came home.

In addition, Mr. and Mrs. Richards and Ann had needs of their own to be met. They needed a respite from the demanding pace of the long hospitalization. Mrs. Richards had not been able to complete her own educational program as planned. Mr. Richards was extremely busy. He was also concerned that they find time to visit his mother who was ill but lived far away. I listened with sympathy and helped them to clarify and so to resolve many practical difficulties and conflicts between their own and Robbie's needs.

Communications with the nursing staff were generally much improved. The primary nurse played the central role in keeping communications open and coordinating them. She tried to promote and clarify communications among the physicians involved and between the rotating medical staff and the parents. I encouraged Mrs. Richards to ask her questions and express her doubts to the staff. At times I helped her formulate the questions. At other times I clarified what seemed to be conflicting or incomplete information.

PENDING DISCHARGE

The prospects and plans for Robbie's discharge had always been vague. Discharge was to be linked to a "magic weight" of 10 pounds, a figure with no special rationale other than its signifying Robbie's becoming "bigger and more stable." His parents had learned the measures necessary to his care and proceeded to perform them at the hospital. However, the physicians were still hesitant about discharge; they had "never before let such a small child with a tracheostomy go home." The parents resigned themselves to a continuing hospitalization and made their other family and vacation plans accordingly. Mrs. Richards expressed her sadness and uncertainty to me. Simultaneously she continued to pursue plans to get the needed equipment and supplies ready at home for Robbie's eventual arrival.

With a new rotation of medical personnel, the plans for discharge appeared to change abruptly; Robbie might be going home soon, it seemed. Communications from the hospital conflicted. The parents were not consulted about the potential date for Robbie's discharge. As they attempted to sort out explanations for the change, they felt confused, angry, and disappointed. There was conflicting pressure on them, from the hospital and from their own need for a vacation before assuming Robbie's full care at home.

During meetings with me, Mrs. Richards's discomfort and ambivalence about Robbie's situation and the pressures she felt began to be expressed. There were multiple complaints about Robbie's care and the poor communications from the staff. She displayed little affect, however.

The Richardses needed relief and some time for themselves. They left, abruptly, on their scheduled two-week vacation. The minimal communication of their plans to the hospital staff seemed uncharacteristic of these dedicated, highly invested parents. I understood, however, that the Richardses were responding to stress from the uncertainty and helplessness they were feeling about Robbie's pending discharge. In part, their mode of leaving expressed a defensive withdrawal and ambivalence which they could not yet articulate. Simultaneously, other family responsibilities added to their concern and drew them away.

Upon their return home, the Richardses were greeted by Robbie's smiling at them. The nurses observed that he had missed them during their absence. He had smiled less, eaten less well. Mrs. Richards too confided to me that she had been full of worry while away from Robbie. She had not known how he was doing each day and had not been able to call regularly for progress reports.

The focus of the work now shifted directly to Robbie's coming discharge. The Richardses resumed preparation for home care under the guidance of the primary nurse. Soon they had mastered tracheostomy tube changes, the final hurdle. The equipment for home use arrived. With encouragement from the examples of two other families who were managing well in tracheostomy home care with their toddlers, Mrs. Richards began to believe that Robbie would grow up. She was beginning to distinguish her now-thriving infant from the baby who had survived so precariously in the intensive-care unit six months earlier.

During this period, my position allowed me to provide continuity between hospital and home—a critical link. My continuing emotional support and developmental guidance with Mrs. Richards centered on two areas: (1) anticipating the needs, adjustments, and feelings the family might experience when Robbie came home, and (2) collaborative discharge planning with the hospital staff. Subsequently, I would also continue the work with them at home.

At Mrs. Richards's request, I now made a home visit. Mrs. Richards expressed multiple worries about caring for Robbie at home. How would she manage the equipment? Would Robbie get sick again? How could she prevent it? Would he have breathing problems? How could they best arrange their compact home to accommodate the furniture and equipment needed? I understood Mrs. Richards's worries and provided information when this was relevant. Together Mrs. Richards and I moved from room to room discussing arrangements for Robbie's care and equipment. Mrs. Richards had prepared well. She needed reassurance to this effect. I supported her excellent planning and reassured her about the adequacy of the provisions she had made. I then helped her focus on how she would feel when Robbie came home. What changes did she anticipate would be necessary for the family? What hopes and disappointments did she have? Mrs. Richards's underlying worry gradually came to the surface: How different or how like a normal baby would Robbie be?

Over the subsequent visits during the month before his discharge, Mrs. Richards and I continued to pursue this question and plans for Robbie's home care. Worries about Robbie's development were explored. Finally the discharge date was set. Mrs. Richards was solemn and sad. Slowly, she shared the "bad news" with me; she had just also been told that the tracheostomy would be "permanent." Angrily and in tears, Mrs. Richards poured out sadness and worry about the future for Robbie and for herself. It seemed now that she would never be able to treat him as a "normal kid." Would he be able to run and play? Would he be developmentally delayed? Would he talk? They would be tied down! Would there be anyone who could help them care for the baby? Mrs. Richards's expression of profound feeling was followed by her regaining composure and resuming the making of more precise plans for the baby's discharge. Subsequently a conference with the physicians was arranged, which clarified Robbie's medical situation and again instilled some hope. He would need the tracheostomy for an indefinite period of time; no one could predict how many years it would take until the scarred area grew enough to allow normal respiration. But future surgical repair was a distant possibility. The Richardses felt some relief, but there was continued uncertainty which no one could remove about what Robbie's future would hold.

Throughout the last month before discharge, collaborative planning with the hospital staff facilitated the coordination of available community resources. The public health nurse and respiratory therapist would make home visits. I would continue weekly contact to provide emotional support and developmental guidance. I was also the one consistent professional link between the hospital and Robbie's home care.

Medical coordination and planning, however, were fragmented. No one assumed responsibility for Robbie's present or future medical care. He was scheduled for return visits to ENT, eye, and premie follow-up clinics as his physicians planned. The Richardses contacted their family pediatrician, who agreed to provide Robbie's general pediatric care, but chose not to see Robbie or his parents prior to discharge. The significance of the transition from hospital to home care was not recognized by the medical team, who saw Robbie's problems as resolving themselves. The parents' anxiety in response to this tremendous adjustment was not acknowledged by the physicians.

Just prior to Robbie's discharge, Dr. Howard Uman, who was then pediatric chief resident at the hospital, joined the Child Development Project staff. At my request he agreed to serve as pediatric consultant and to provide medical continuity for the family within the hospital system. The Richardses welcomed and eagerly accepted his assistance. His participation relieved them of many of their worries about future difficulties with new and different hospital staff members who might not be familiar with their child and his medical history.

DISCHARGE

Discharge planning and preparation were completed. The discharge date was established. Mr. and Mrs. Richards took a brief vacation in order to obtain a bit of respite from all family responsibilities. At age 7 months Robbie arrived home to the secure care of his parents.

The actual transition to home was easier than the parents had anticipated. Robbie adjusted readily to his new environment. Mr. and Mrs. Richards were both home for the first few days. They were themselves surprised by the ease of the transition and their own adjustment. Their primary worry was the ever-present possibility of Robbie's developing respiratory difficulties. How would they hear him if he needed them? Nights were the time of greatest worry. Initially they got up every hour to check him. Gradually they realized that they could hear the movements by which Robbie signaled distress. By the end of Robbie's first week at home, the Richardses had assumed a more normal regimen, checking him at regular intervals, when indicated by his signals and when he seemed to have increased secretions.

I remained in close touch with the family during this transition period. I talked with Mrs. Richards on the day Robbie arrived home. I made a home visit a few days later during Mrs. Richard's first full day alone with the baby. The family managed well and did not need extra help but were greatly reassured by the availability of help and support should a difficulty or questions arise.

Follow-up at Home

Throughout the rest of Robbie's first year (7 to 12 months), I met weekly with Mrs. Richards and Robbie at home. Mr. Richards joined us for some visits. I continued to provide support and to supply appropriate developmental guidance to promote Robbie's growing abilities. The parents' feelings and concerns about his care and development and the restrictions this imposed on their lives were discussed. Periodic video-tapes of Robbie with his mother were made. Selected Bayley items were administered to demonstrate his abilities. Review of these obser-vations enabled me to analyze Robbie's developmental abilities and progress. I reviewed the tapes with Robbie's parents. Together we dis-cussed his abilities and considered various ways in which Robbie's de-velopment could be facilitated by his parents.

Robbie progressed well at home, moving ahead steadily in all areas. His parents provided his care competently. Father participated actively when home. Robbie's extensive regimen of care was time-consuming. Tracheostomy care, suctioning, postural drainage, feeding, diapering, and dressing frequently filled the greater part of each waking period. Mrs. Richards used every available moment to provide play and devel-opmental stimulation but often felt a happy play time with her baby was missing.

In providing Robbie's twenty-four-hour care, Mrs. Richards was es-sentially homebound. Because of his severe prematurity, Robbie's short periods of wakefulness were like those of a younger baby. These limited Mrs. Richards's activities. Visiting by friends and family was initially curtailed for fear of exposing Robbie to infections. Those who did visit came infrequently. My visits and discussion of the family's isolation helped to counteract some of the loneliness and helped Mrs. Richards discover ways to become less isolated. Mr. Richards cared for Robbie for periods during the week, which allowed his wife to get out to shop, do family errands, and occasionally see friends. Visits with Robbie to see grandmother who lived nearby were introduced.

Continuing developmental guidance evolved parallel to Robbie's progressing developmental abilities. At each visit, Mrs. Richards and I watched and interacted with Robbie and discussed our observations. Opportunities that allowed gross and fine motor skills to be developed were discussed. Recommendations made by the physical therapist were encouraged to promote Robbie's motor skills. Social games, which in-cluded talking to Robbie while providing care, peek-a-boo, and songs were encouraged. Together mother and I observed Robbie so that we could continue to read his signals and put these into words with him. Mrs. Richards raised questions and observations that concerned her, and I offered the appropriate developmental information. As Mrs. Richards recognized more of her son's capabilities, she was able to put into words her comparisons of a "sick" and "healthy" baby and move toward viewing Robbie as a "normal child."

Several areas of concern in development received particular empha-sis. At 8 months of age, Robbie was exquisitely sensitive to strangers and to separation. He watched strangers with a sustained wary gaze.

He followed his parents' comings and goings with intense, sad eyes. These were age-appropriate behaviors, but his responses were exaggerated. Mrs. Richards recalled how Robbie had watched her through the window between his crib and the hallway when she arrived and left the hospital. His gazes were a difficult reminder of how painful those early separations had been for her. These repetitions raised again the unanswered questions of what effect Robbie's difficult beginning would have on his future development. Although I could provide no definitive answer, I sympathized with Mrs. Richards's worries and listened to her feelings. Guidance was offered about practical ways to make everyday separations and strangers' visits less stressful for the baby (e.g., keeping in visual and auditory touch with mother and putting what was occurring into words).

Despite his intense visual interest and investment in his environment and his expressive facial gestures, Robbie did not frequently seek or maintain eye-to-eye contact with people. This too raised serious questions about his early experiences. He had had contact with many people. An intimate relationship with his parents had not been available around the clock until he was 7 months old. A videotape of Robbie with mother at home highlighted this aspect of communication and interaction for both the parents and for me. As the parents watched the tape, both commented upon his infrequent direct eye contact. I then addressed the sadness this caused the parents and the difficulties they felt in reading his signals. The Richardses and I made conscious efforts to gain and maintain eye contact with Robbie when interacting during play and care.

The development of speech was another major area of concern. Although both the Richardses and I had been told that "children with tracheostomies eventually do talk," there was no research or literature that could be located to provide any reassurance or guidelines. Robbie was silent. He could not yet produce vocal sounds or cry aloud. Again I addressed the parents' feelings. I provided ongoing encouragement to the parents as they attempted to keep talking to Robbie in the absence of vocal feedback. I encouraged games by which he could learn to make other sounds (such as clicking the tongue and lips). Robbie learned these readily, and reciprocal games developed.

The developmental guidance was combined with support and attention to the feelings of the parents. I attempted to keep a focus as well on the meaning the experience might have to the baby himself. The visits focused more careful attention upon development than one would normally do with a child and identified areas that required intervention. This was perhaps stressful for the parents. These visits, however, also served important positive functions for the parents by validating their observations on Robbie's developmental progress. Mrs.

Richards found it difficult to see the baby's progress when she was with him constantly. My periodic visits and the short videotapes which could be later reviewed confirmed progress and encouraged the parents.

CLINIC VISITS

Periodic contacts with the hospital continued to be a prominent part of life for Robbie and his parents. The stresses imposed by his early birth and multiple hospital experiences were reawakened by every visit back to the hospital. Difficulties of communication with hospital personnel recurred. These issues were discussed both with me during home visits and with Dr. Uman during clinic visits.

Robbie's four-volume chart did not readily communicate his history, care, and needs to new staff. Physicians unfamiliar with Robbie's care gave advice that contradicted previous advice and the parents' own observations and experience. The parents rarely saw familiar doctors. The clinic visits entailed long waiting periods. The hurried atmosphere did not lend itself to inviting or hearing the parents' questions. Developmental guidance and emotional concerns were ignored or avoided. Clinic staff did not have definitive answers to the uncertain issues of the duration of Robbie's tracheostomy and the development of speech; they did not address the parents' questions. The clinic visits were also often accompanied by "social visits" back to the nurseries. These reawakened the painful memories of Robbie's birth and hospitalization.

Dr. Uman accompanied the family to clinic visits as their pediatric consultant. He assisted the parents in formulating their own questions before the actual visits with the consultants. He improved communications by presenting a clear, concise summary of Robbie's history, current situation, and the objectives for his care. He spoke about Robbie to the physicians involved and helped them focus on the specific issues for the visit. Much conflicting advice was thus avoided. He reviewed the visits with the parents, explaining findings, procedures, and prognosis. Both he and I shared the uncertainties with the parents and addressed the "unanswerable" problems, always being attentive to the developmental and emotional implications of these problems, whose impact on their lives was bound to continue. Both of us remained available so that the Richardses could raise questions at their own pace. We encouraged them to talk of their feelings. As they did so, they gained new understanding.

READMISSION FOR EVALUATION

As Robbie approached his first birthday, his parents' anxiety heightened markedly. They had been told that Robbie would need to have another laryngoscopy when he was about a year old. The prospect of readmission to the hospital brought to their minds a resurgence of the medical uncertainties. The preceding months had brought them a measure of security, for he had remained healthy and had made steady developmental strides. When his tracheostomy had been occluded briefly he had been heard to vocalize—a fleeting taste of what had been so long awaited. It was permission to hope for the almost unthinkable—that Robbie could become completely normal and speak.

During visits with both Dr. Uman and myself, the family began to comtemplate this new crisis. All of us prepared ourselves to encounter the impersonality and inertia of the hospital system and sought ways in advance to ease the difficulties that could arise. The parents began this process by questioning the need for laryngoscopy at this time. Would it change Robbie's management? Would separation from them be harmful to him? What were the risks of the procedure as well as of the anesthesia?

The ENT clinic was unable to respond fully to these questions. Readmission and reexamination were justified as being the "standard approach" and were discussed in a positive tone that implied, if it did not actually promise, good results. Further worries on the part of Robbie's parents were simply dismissed. The question of there being possible bad news was never approached.

The parents responded by shoring up their defenses and opted to admit Robbie as soon as possible, "so there would be less time to think about it." Dr. Uman listened, put into words for them that he "knew this would be hard," and then offered to go over with them what the procedure would actually entail. The parents accepted his offer, and he then reviewed in detail Robbie's medical difficulties and the risks of these "routine" procedures. It was not the first time that the information had been presented, but the review was important. We discussed the distortions and changes in the parents' perspectives which might have occurred since the earlier discussions. The need for Robbie to return to the hospital was established.

Readmission occurred just before Robbie's first birthday. It began with delays in the admissions department, but Mrs. Richards had learned to negotiate the system successfully. She suggested using this time constructively to get the needed laboratory studies and x-rays. The infant unit was friendly and familiar; the Richardses were greeted warmly by the nursing staff, who had reserved Robbie's old bed for him. His primary nurse once again provided his care.

Some of the pain of the past was revived for the parents as staff members persisted in addressing the baby by his first name rather than "Robbie." Reviewing his history added further pain. Both Dr. Uman and I visited Mrs. Richards and Robbie on the afternoon of admission. We were greeted with her concerns about getting Robbie's history accurately and her confusion about certain significant events. As we waited in anticipation of the following day's procedure, the topics of Robbie's cardiac surgery, his respiratory arrest, and his dependency on his parents were raised and explored.

The laryngoscopy was accomplished the next morning with only minor delays. Robbie tolerated the procedure well. His parents waited, but the specialists did not return to the unit with the long-awaited news of the results of the procedure. Later in the afternoon, Mr. Richards spoke with a doctor briefly on the telephone, but the promised face-to-face discussion with the ENT specialists never materialized. Robbie was discharged. His parents left, still unclear about the results of his reevaluation.

Mrs. Richards called and told me about these difficulties. Dr. Uman spoke with the ENT physician and then discussed the results with the parents. He was the bearer of difficult news. There was concern about a tracheal diverticulum forming from pressure of the tracheostomy tube. The narrowed area of the airway had not grown. The vocal cords had not been assessed. He offered his concern and support, yet two factors made this most difficult to transmit: the information itself was painful, and the telephone did not allow full assessment of Mrs. Richards's response. There must have been tears as she listened.

POST-READMISSION

The readmission was another turning point. It had raised new difficulties as well as heightening awareness of the painful past. To help the parents, Dr. Uman and I joined in a home visit with both Mr. and Mrs. Richards soon after the discharge. The meeting brought a review of the first year as well as a discussion of Robbie's current medical and developmental status.

Feelings and questions surfaced anew and were discussed. The Richardses now understood the hospital system and could clearly see the confusion and crossed communications that had occurred. They were disturbed by the deficiencies of the system that made it so difficult to meet both their own and Robbie's needs. They knew that Dr. Uman would soon be leaving and worried that discussion of difficult medical issues would lapse again. I reviewed the parents' concerns with them. I identified their need to have a complete written summary of Robbie's history to help them remember the details of his story without confusion and to allow them to present the facts readily to consultants who would see Robbie in the future. The summary of Robbie's growth and development was provided by the therapist. I agreed with the family in their decision to seek the care of an ENT specialist on a private basis. The initial visit with this specialist brought reassurance. The parents could now rely on him to know them and their baby and to provide continuing care and consistent recommendations. The Richardses were assured that I would continue to work with them.

CONTINUING WORK

This detailed story of our work with Robbie ends at the beginning of his second year of life. The work, however, continued. Further developmental and health guidance were provided as new phases of Robbie's growth occurred. The parents found that hospital visits and developmental questions were recurrent painful reminders of the difficult first year. Attention to issues of affect and communication became increasingly important in the continued work as Robbie still had little capacity to communicate vocally.

Despite the difficulties of the first year, Robbie and his family made outstanding progress. Robbie became a healthy, active toddler. He had no new medical complications and few illnesses. Hospitalizations were limited to those necessary for reevaluation by laryngoscopy, usually every six months. Although he still had severe subglottic stenosis requiring the tracheostomy, Robbie was an active, happy child. He visited friends, family, and other children with his parents and played happily indoors and outdoors. He made enormous developmental progress, although his development remained slightly delayed. He was developing receptive comprehension of language, and he communicated nonverbally with eloquent body language, pointing persistently, throwing things to signal anger, bouncing and dancing when happy, and smiling broadly to engage others socially. He began to vocalize around the tracheostomy tube. He was securely attached to his parents and sister and was clearly very precious to his parents. Mr. and Mrs. Richards both did exceedingly well in providing his total care. They were resourceful and creative in promoting his well-being. They could now enjoy the fruits of their efforts in Robbie's excellent progress. At the request of the hospital staff they talked with other parents going through the same difficulty with their children and provided information about how they had managed Robbie's care at home.

Summary

Robbie's story vividly portrays the difficulties imposed on a family by illness, developmental handicaps, and long and repeated hospitalizations. This case illustrates our use of developmental guidance. In particular, the Richardses' story demonstrates the interlocking aspects of the child's health, developmental, and emotional needs and the parents' needs for emotional support and guidance through the ongoing and recurrent questions posed by their child's condition. Our work, which combined psychotherapeutic and developmental knowledge and skills in health care, was effective in helping both the infant and the parents deal successfully with multiple crises.

In addition, consistent daily care from a small group of nurses and from his parents fostered Robbie's attachment, development, and internal organization. Recognition of and attention to the parents' questions and emotional needs and the provision of support and guidance helped them to face the uncertainties of Robbie's future, put into perspective the painful memories that resurfaced at each point of crisis, learn and provide Robbie's tracheostomy care competently, and cope with the frustrations and discontinuities of the health care system. As therapist, I provided a consistent resource to whom the family could turn whenever they needed help. Dr. Uman, the pediatric consultant, and I provided continuity within the complex system of medical specialty services. Occasionally, at the family's request, we intervened directly into the system on Robbie's behalf. Throughout all of the work we supported the parents' right to make decisions about their baby, to provide his care, and to work with their health resources.

This case also emphasizes the need for integration of psychotherapeutic and pediatric interventions in comprehensive care. It reiterates the need for ongoing developmental guidance for infants who are developmentally handicapped or affected by early illness and for their parents. This may be accomplished in many different ways by various combinations of professionals. Robbie's case illustrates one way, but is not intended to provide a model for *the* way to deliver all such comprehensive care. The principles, however, may be generalized for infants and their families facing and enduring neonatal complications.

BIBLIOGRAPHY

Aberdeen, E., and Downes, J. 1974. "Artificial Airways in Children." *Surgical Clinics of North America 54(5)*:1155–1170.

Ainsworth, M. 1973. "The Development of Mother-Infant Attachment," in Caldwell, B., and Riccuiti, H., eds. *Review of Child Development Research III.* Chicago: University of Chicago Press, pp. 1–94.

Aradine, C. 1978. "Development of Toddlers with Long-term Tracheostomies." Ph.D. thesis, University of Michigan.

Aradine, C. 1980. "Home Care for Young Children with Long-Term Tracheostomies," *American Journal of Maternal Child Nursing 5*:121–125.

Bell, S., and Ainsworth, M. 1972. "Infant Crying and Maternal Responsiveness." *Child Development 43(4)*:1171–1190.

Burns, P., Sander, L., Stechler, G., and Julia, N. 1972. "Distress in Feeding: Short-term Effects of Caretaker Environment of the First 10 Days." *American Academy of Child Psychiatry Journal 11*:427–439.

DeMonterice, D., and Filston, H. "Home Care of Infants with Tracheostomies." (Unpublished)

Fearon, B., and Cotton, R. 1974. "Surgical Correction of Subglottic Stenosis of the Larynx in Infants and Children: Progress Report." *Annals of Otology 83*:428–431.

Fearon, B., and Ellis, O. 1971. "The Management of Long-term Airway Problems in Infants and Children." *Annals of Otology 80*:669–677.

Freeland, A. P., Wright, J. L. W., and Ardan, G. H. 1974. "Developmental Influences of Infant Tracheostomy." *Journal of Laryngology and Otology 88(10)*:927–936.

Holinger, P., Kutnick, S., Schild, J., and Hollinger, L. 1976. "Subglottic Stenosis in Infants and Children." *Annals of Otology 85*:591–599.

Kaler, John, and Kaler, Hilary. 1974. "Michael Had a Tracheostomy." *American Journal of Nursing 74(5)*:852–855.

McGovern, F. H., Fitzhugh, G. S., and Edgemon, L. J. 1971. "The Hazards of Endotracheal Intubation." *Annals of Otology 80*:556–564.

Parkin, J., Stevens, M., and Jung, A. 1976. "Acquired and Congenital Subglottic Stenosis in the Infant." *Annals of Otology 85*:573–581.

VII

Ghosts in the Nursery: A Psychoanalytic Approach to the Problems of Impaired Infant-Mother Relationships

SELMA FRAIBERG

EDNA ADELSON

VIVIAN SHAPIRO

IN EVERY NURSERY there are ghosts. They are the visitors from the unremembered past of the parents, the uninvited guests at the christening. Under favorable circumstances, these unfriendly and unbidden spirits are banished from the nursery and return to their subterranean dwelling place. The baby makes his own imperative claim upon parental love and, in strict analogy with the fairy tales, the bonds of love protect the child and his parents against the intruders, the malevolent ghosts.

This is not to say that ghosts cannot invent mischief from their burial places. Even among families where the love bonds are stable and strong, the intruders from the parental past may break through the magic circle in an unguarded moment, and a parent and his child may find themselves reenacting a moment or a scene from another time with another set of characters. Such events are unremarkable in the family theater, and neither the child nor his parents nor their bond is necessarily imperiled by a brief intrusion. It is not usually necessary for the parents to call upon us for clinical services.

In still other families there may be more troublesome events in the nursery caused by intruders from the past. There are, it appears, a number of transient ghosts who take up residence in the nursery on a selective basis. They appear to do their mischief according to a historical or topical agenda, specializing in such areas as feeding, sleep, toilet training or discipline, depending upon the vulnerabilities of the parental past. Under these circumstances, even when the bonds between parents and child are strong, the parents may feel helpless before the invasion and may seek professional guidance. In our own work, we have found that these parents will form a strong alliance with us to banish the intruders from the nursery. It is not difficult to find the educational or therapeutic means for dealing with the transient invaders.

But how shall we explain another group of families who appear to be possessed by their ghosts? The intruders from the past have taken up residence in the nursery, claiming tradition and rights of ownership. They have been present at the christening for two or more generations. While no one has issued an invitation, the ghosts take up residence and conduct the rehearsal of the family tragedy from a tattered script.

In our infant mental health program we have seen many of these families and their babies. The baby is already in peril by the time we meet him, showing the early signs of emotional starvation, or grave symptoms, or developmental impairment. In each of these cases the baby has become a silent actor in a family tragedy. The baby in these families is burdened by the oppressive past of his parents from the moment he enters the world. The parent, it seems, is condemned to repeat the tragedy of his own childhood with his own baby in terrible and exacting detail.

These parents may not come to us for professional guidance. Ghosts who have established their residence privileges for three or more generations may not, in fact, be identified as representatives of the parental past. There may be no readiness on the part of the parents to form an alliance with us to protect the baby. More likely it is we, and not the ghosts, who will appear as the intruders.

Those of us who have a professional interest in ghosts in the nursery do not yet understand the complexities and the paradoxes in the ghost story. What is it that determines whether the conflicted past of the parent will be repeated with his child? Is morbidity in the parental history the prime determinant? This strikes us as too simple. Certainly we all know families in which a parental history of tragedy, cruelty, and sorrow have *not* been inflicted upon the children. The ghosts do not flood the nursery or erode the love bonds.

Then, too, we must reflect that if history predicted with fidelity, the human family itself would long ago have been drowned in its own oppressive past. The race improves. And this may be because the largest number of men and women who have known suffering find renewal and the healing of childhood pain in the experience of bringing a child into the world. In the simplest terms—we have heard it often from parents—the parent says, "I want something better for my child than I have had." And he brings something better to his child. We have all known young parents who have suffered poverty, brutality, death, desertion, and sometimes the full gamut of childhood horrors, who do not inflict their pain upon their children. History is not destiny, then, and whether parenthood becomes flooded with griefs and injuries or whether it becomes a time of renewal cannot be predicted from the narrative of the parental past. There must be other factors in the psychological experience of that past which determine repetition in the present.

In therapeutic work with families on behalf of their babies we are all the beneficiaries of Freud's discoveries before the dawn of this century. The ghosts, we know, represent the repetition of the past in the present. We are also the beneficiaries of the method Freud developed for recovering the events of the past and undoing the morbid effects of the past in the present. The babies themselves, who are often afflicted by the diseases of the parental past, have been the last to be the beneficiaries of the great discoveries of psychoanalysis and developmental psychology. These patients, who cannot talk, have had to await articulate spokesmen.

During the past three decades a number of psychoanalysts and developmental psychologists have been speaking for the babies. What the babies have been telling us is sobering news, indeed. This story you already know, and I will not attempt to summarize the vast literature that has emerged from our studies of infancy.

In our own work at the Child Development Project we have become well acquainted with the ghosts in the nursery. The brief intruders, which we have described, or the unwelcome ghosts who take up temporary residence, do not present extraordinary problems to the clinician. The parents themselves become our allies in banishing the ghosts. It is the third group, the ghosts who invade the nursery and take up residence, who present the gravest therapeutic problems for us.

How is it that the ghosts of the parental past can invade the nursery with such insistency and ownership, claiming their rights above the baby's own rights? This question is at the center of our work. The answers are emerging for us and in the closing section of this chapter we will return to the question and offer a hypothesis derived from clinical experience.

In this chapter we will describe our clinical study and our treatment through two of the many imperiled babies who have come to us. As our work progressed, our families and their babies opened doors to us which illuminated the past and the present. Our psychoanalytic knowledge opened pathways into understanding the repetition of the past in the present. The methods of treatment we developed brought together psychoanalysis, developmental psychology, and social work in ways that will be illustrated. The rewards for the babies, for the families, and for us have been very large.

In this collaborative work, Edna Adelson, staff psychologist, was the therapist for Jane and her family, Vivian Shapiro, staff social worker, was therapist for Greg and his family, and Selma Fraiberg served as case supervisor and psychoanalytic consultant.

Jane   .

Jane, who came to us at 5½ months, was the first baby referred to our new infant mental health project. Her mother, Mrs. March, had appeared at an adoption agency some weeks earlier. She wanted to surrender her baby for adoption, but adoption plans could not proceed because Mr. March would not give his consent. Jane's mother was described as "a rejecting mother."

Now, of course nobody loves a rejecting mother, in our community or any other, and Jane and her family might at this point have disappeared into the anonymity of a metropolitan community, perhaps to surface once again when tragedy struck. But chance brought the family to one of the psychiatric clinics of our university. The psychiatric evaluation of Mrs. March revealed a severe depression, an attempted suicide through aspirin, a woman so tormented that she could barely go about the ordinary tasks of living. The "rejecting mother" was now seen as a depressed mother. Psychiatric treatment was recommended at a clinical staffing. And then one of the clinical team members said, "But what about the baby?" Our new project had been announced and scheduled for opening the following day. There was a phone call to us, and we agreed to provide immediate evaluation of the baby and to consider treatment.

EARLY OBSERVATIONS

From the time Jane was first seen by us we had reason for grave concern. At 5½ months she bore all the stigmata of the child who has spent the greater part of her life in a crib with little more than obligatory care. She was adequately nourished and physically cared for, but the back of her head was bald. She showed little interest in her surround; she was listless, too quiet. She seemed to have only a tenuous connection with her mother. She rarely smiled. She did not spontaneously approach her mother through eye contact or gestures of reach. There were few spontaneous vocalizations. In moments of discomfort or anxiety she did not turn to her mother. In our developmental testing she failed nearly all the personal-social items on the Bayley scale. The test could not be completed. Jane was badly frightened by the unexpected sound of the test bell. After only a few more items her threshold of tolerance was shattered, and she collapsed into prolonged screaming.

The mother herself seemed locked in some private terror, remote, removed, yet giving us rare glimpses of a capacity for caring. For weeks we held onto one tiny vignette captured on videotape, in which the baby made an awkward reach for her mother and the mother's hand spontaneously reached toward the baby. The hands never met each other, but the gesture symbolized for the therapists a reaching out toward each other, and we clung to this symbolic hope.

There is a moment at the beginning of every case when something is revealed that speaks for the essence of the conflict. This moment appeared in the second session of the work when Mrs. Adelson invited Jane and her mother to our office. By chance it was a moment captured on videotape, because we were taping the developmental testing session as we customarily do. Jane and her mother, Mrs. Adelson, and Mrs. Evelyn Atreya, as tester, were present.

Jane begins to cry. It is a hoarse, eerie cry in a baby. Mrs. Atreya discontinues the testing. On tape we see the baby in her mother's arms screaming hopelessly; she does not turn to her mother for comfort. The mother looks distant, self-absorbed. She makes an absent gesture to comfort the baby, then gives up. She looks away. The screaming continues for five dreadful minutes on tape. In the background we hear Mrs. Adelson's voice, gently encouraging the mother: "What do you do to comfort Jane when she cries like this?" Mrs. March murmurs something inaudible. Mrs. Adelson and Mrs. Atreya are struggling with their own feelings. They are restraining their own wishes to pick up the baby and hold her, to murmur comforting things to her. If they should yield to their own wishes, they would do the one thing they feel must not be done. For Mrs. March would then see that another woman could comfort the baby, and she would be confirmed in her own conviction that she was a bad mother. It is a dreadful five minutes for the baby, the mother, and the two clinicians. Mrs. Adelson maintains composure, speaks sympathetically to Mrs. March. Finally, the visit comes to an end when Mrs. Adelson suggests that the baby is fatigued and probably would welcome her own home and her crib; and mother and baby are helped to close the visit with plans for a third visit very soon.

As we watched this tape later in a staff session, we said to each other incredulously, "It's as if this mother doesn't *hear* her baby's cries!" This led us to the key diagnostic question, *"Why doesn't this mother hear her baby's cries?"*

THE MOTHER'S STORY

Mrs. March was herself an abandoned child. Her mother suffered a postpartum psychosis shortly after the birth of Mrs. March. In an attempted suicide, she had injured herself and was horribly mutilated for life. She had then spent nearly all of the rest of her life in a hospital and was barely known to her children. For five years Mrs. March was cared for by an aunt. When the aunt could no longer care for her she was shifted to the house of the maternal grandmother, where she received grudging care from the burdened, impoverished old woman. Mrs. March's father was in and out of the family picture. We did not hear much about him until later in the treatment.

It was a story of bleak rural poverty, sinister family secrets, psychosis, crime, a tradition of promiscuity in the women, of filth and disorder in the home, and of police and protective agencies in the background making futile uplifting gestures. Mrs. March was the cast-out child of a cast-out family.

In late adolescence, Mrs. March met and married her husband, who came from poverty and family disorder not unlike her own. But he wanted something better for himself than his family had had. He became the first member of his family to fight his way out of the cycle of futility, to find steady work, to establish a decent home. When these two neglected and solitary young people found each other, there was mutual agreement that they wanted something better than what they had known. But now, after several years of effort, the downward spiral had begun.

There was a very high likelihood that Jane was not her father's child. Mrs. March had had a brief affair with another man. Her guilt over the affair, her doubts about Jane's paternity, became an obsessive theme in her story. In a kind of litany of griefs that we were to hear over and over again, there was one theme: "People stared at Jane," she thought. "They stared at her and knew that her father was not her father. They knew that her mother had ruined her life."

Mr. March, who began to appear to us as the stronger parent, was not obsessed with Jane's paternity. He was convinced that he was Jane's father. And anyway, he loved Jane and he wanted her. His wife's obsession with paternity brought about shouting quarrels in the home. "Forget it!" said Mr. March. "Stop talking about it! And take care of Jane!"

In the families of both mother and father illegitimacy carried no stigma. In the case of Mrs. March's clan, the promiscuity of their women over at least three or four generations cast doubt over the paternity of many of the children. Why was Mrs. March obsessed? Why the sense of tormenting sin? This pervasive, consuming sense of sin we thought belonged to childhood, to buried sins, quite possibly crimes of the imagination. On several occasions in reading the clinical reports, we had the strong impression that Jane was the sinful child of an incestuous fantasy. But if we were right, we thought to ourselves, how could we possibly reach this in our once-a-week psychotherapy?

TREATMENT: THE EMERGENCY PHASE

How shall we begin? We should remember that Jane and Mrs. March were our first patients. We did not have treatment models available to us. In fact, it was our task in this first infant mental health project to develop methods in the course of the work. It made sense, of course, to begin with a familiar model, in which our resident in psychiatry, Dr. Zinn, worked with the mother in weekly or twice-weekly psychotherapy, and the psychologist, Mrs. Adelson, provided support and developmental guidance on behalf of the baby through home visits. But within the first sessions, we saw that Mrs. March was taking flight from Dr. Zinn and psychiatric treatment. The situation in which she was alone with a man brought forth a phobic dread, and she was reduced to nearly inarticulate hours or to speaking of trivial concerns. All efforts to reach Mrs. March, or to touch upon her anxieties or discomfort in this relationship, led to an impasse. One theme was uttered over and over again. She did not trust men. But also, we caught glimpses in her oblique communications of a terrible secret that she would never reveal to anyone. She broke appointments more frequently than she kept them. With much difficulty, Dr. Zinn sustained a relationship with her. It was nearly a year before we finally heard the secret and understood the phobic dread that led to this formidable resistance.

There are no generalizations to be drawn from this experience. We have been asked sometimes if women therapists are more advantaged in working with mothers who have suffered severe maternal deprivation themselves. Our answer, after nearly eight years of work, is, "Not necessarily; sometimes not at all." We have examples in our work in which the male therapist was specially advantaged in working with mothers. We tend to assign cases without overconcern about the sex of the therapist. Mrs. March must be regarded as an exceptional case.

But now we were faced with a therapeutic dilemma. Mrs. Adelson's work was to center in the infant-mother relationship through home visits. Mrs. March needed her own therapist, Dr. Zinn, but a morbid dread of men, aroused in the transference, prevented her from using the psychiatric help available to her. With much time and patient work in the psychiatric treatment, we would hope to uncover the secret that reduced her to silence and flight in the transference to Dr. Zinn.

But the baby was in great peril. And the baby could not wait for the resolution of the mother's neurosis.

Mrs. Adelson, we soon saw, did not arouse the same morbid anxieties in Mrs. March, but her role as the baby-mother therapist, the home-based psychologist, did not lend itself easily to uncovering the conflictual elements in the mother's relationship to the child and the treatment of the mother's depression.

Since we had no alternative, we decided we would use the home visits for our emergency treatment.

What emerged, then, was a form of "psychotherapy in the kitchen," so to speak, which will strike you as both familiar in its methods and unfamiliar in its setting. The method, a variant of psychoanalytic psychotherapy, made use of transference, the repetition of the past in the present, and interpretation. Equally important, the method included continuous developmental observations of the baby and a tactful, nondidactic education of the mother in the recognition of her baby's needs and her signals.

The setting was the family kitchen or the living room. The patient who couldn't talk was always present at the interviews—if she wasn't napping. The patient who could talk went about her domestic tasks or diapered or fed the baby. The therapist's eyes and ears were attuned to both the nonverbal communciations of the baby and the substance of the mother's verbal and nonverbal communications. Everything that transpired between mother and baby was in the purview of the therapist and in the center of the therapy. The dialogue between the mother and the therapist centered upon present concerns and moved back and forth between the past and the present, between this mother and child and another child and her family in the mother's past. The method proved itself and led us, in later cases, to explore the possibilities of the single therapist in the home-based treatment.

We shall now try to summarize the treatment of Jane and her mother and examine the methods that were employed.

In the early hours of treatment, Mrs. March's own story emerged haltingly, narrated in a distant, sad voice. It was the story we sketched earlier. As the mother told her story, Jane, our second patient, sat propped on the couch or lay stretched out on a blanket, and the sad and distant face of the mother was mirrored in the sad and distant face of the baby. It was a room crowded with ghosts. The mother's story of abandonment and neglect was now being psychologically reenacted with her own baby.

The problem, in the emergency phase of the treatment, was to get the ghosts out of the baby's nursery. To do this we would need to help the mother to see the repetition of the past in the present, which we all know how to do in an office that is properly furnished with a desk and a chair or a couch, but which we had not yet learned to do in a family living room or a kitchen. The therapeutic principles would need to be the same, we decided. But in this emergency phase of the treatment, on behalf of a baby, we would have to find a path into the conflictual elements of the mother's neurosis which had direct bearing upon her capacity to mother. The baby would need to be at the center of treatment for the emergency period.

We began, as we said, with the question to ourselves: "Why can't this mother hear her baby's cries?"

The answer to the clinical question is already suggested in the mother's story. This is a mother whose own cries have not been heard. There were, we thought, two crying children in the living room. The mother's distant voice, her remoteness and remove we saw as defenses against grief and intolerable pain. Her terrible story had been first given factually, without visible suffering, without tears. All that was visible was the sad, empty, hopeless look upon her face. She had closed the door on the weeping child within herself as surely as she had closed the door upon her crying baby.

This led to our first clinical hypothesis: *When this mother's own cries are heard, she will hear her child's cries.*

Mrs. Adelson's work, then, centered upon the development of a treatment relationship in which trust could be given by a young woman who had not known trust, and in which trust could lead to the revelation of the old feelings which closed her off from her child. As Mrs. March's story moved back and forth between her baby, "I can't love Jane," and her own childhood, which can be summarized, "Nobody wanted me," the therapist opened up pathways of feeling. Mrs. Adelson listened and put into words the feelings of Mrs. March as a child. "How hard this must have been. . . . This must have hurt deeply. . . . Of course, you needed your mother. There was no one to turn to. . . . Yes. Sometimes grownups don't understand what all this means to a child. You must have needed to cry. . . . There was no one to hear you."

The therapist was giving Mrs. March permission to feel and to remember feelings. It may have been the first time in Mrs. March's life that someone had given her this permission. And gradually, as we should expect—but within only a few sessions—grief, tears, and unspeakable anguish for herself as a castoff child began to emerge. It was finally a relief to be able to cry, a comfort to feel the understanding of her therapist. And now, with each session, Mrs. Adelson witnessed something almost unbelievable happening between mother and baby.

You remember that the baby was nearly always in the room in the midst of this living room-kitchen therapy of ours. If Jane demanded attention, the mother would rise in the midst of the interview to diaper her or get her a bottle. More often, the baby was ignored if she did not demand attention. But now, as Mrs. March began to take the permission to remember her feelings, to cry, and to feel the comfort and sympathy of Mrs. Adelson, we saw her make approaches to her baby in the midst of her own outpourings. She would pick up Jane and hold her, at first distant and self-absorbed, but holding her. And then one day, still within the first month of treatment, Mrs. March, in the midst of an outpouring of grief, picked up Jane, held her very close, and crooned to her in a heartbroken voice. And then it happened again, and several times in the next sessions. An outpouring of old griefs and a gathering of the baby into her arms. The ghosts in the baby's nursery were beginning to leave.

These were more than transitory gestures toward rapprochement with the baby. From all evidence to Mrs. Adelson's observing eyes, mother and baby were beginning to find each other. And now that they were coming into touch with each other, Mrs. Adelson did everything within her capacity as therapist and developmental psychologist to promote the emerging attachment. When Jane rewarded her mother with a beautiful and special smile, Mrs. Adelson commented on it and observed that she, Mrs. Adelson, did not get such a smile, which was just the way it should be. That smile belonged to her mother. When a crying Jane began to seek her mother's comfort and found relief in her mother's arms, Mrs. Adelson spoke for Jane. "It feels so good when mother knows what you want." And Mrs. March herself smiled shyly, but with pride.

These sessions with mother and baby soon took on their own rhythm. Mr. March was often present for a short time before leaving for work. (Special sessions for father were also worked out on evenings and Saturdays.) The sessions typically began with Jane in the room and Jane as the topic of discussion. In a natural, informal, nondidactic way, Mrs. Adelson would comment with pleasure on Jane's development and weave into her comments useful information about the needs of babies at 6 months or 7 months and how Jane was learning about her world and how her mother and father were leading her into these discoveries. Together the parents and Mrs. Adelson would watch Jane experiment with a new toy or a new posture, and, with close watching, could see how she was finding solutions and moving steadily forward. The delights of baby-watching, which Mrs. Adelson knew, were shared with Mr. and Mrs. March, and, to our great pleasure, both parents began to share these delights and to bring in their own observations of Jane and of her new accomplishments.

During the same session, after Mr. March had left for work, the talk would move at one point or another back to Mrs. March herself, to her present griefs and her childhood griefs. More and more frequently now, Mrs. Adelson could help Mrs. March see the connections between the past and the present and show her how "without realizing it," she had brought her sufferings of the past into her relationship with her own baby.

Within four months Jane became a healthy, more responsive, often joyful baby. At our ten-month testing, objective assessment showed her to be age-appropriate in her focused attachment to her mother, in her preferential smiling and vocalization to mother and father, in her seeking of her mother for comfort and safety. The Bayley developmental testing showed uneven but impressive progress. Jane was two months advanced on social interaction items and at age level for fine motor performance for her corrected age. Lags of from one to two months on vocalization and gross motor items placed her below her corrected age, but still within the normal range.

Mrs. March had become a responsive mother and a proud mother. Yet our cautious rating of the mother's own psychological state remained: "depressed." It was true that Mrs. March was progressing, and we saw many signs that the depression was no longer pervasive and constricting, but depression was still there, and, we thought, still ominous. Much work remained.

What we had achieved, then, in our first four months' work was not yet a cure of the mother's illness, but a form of control of the disease, in which the pathology which had spread to embrace the baby was now largely withdrawn from the child; the conflictual elements of the mother's neurosis were now identified by the mother as well as ourselves as "belonging to the past" and "not belonging to Jane." The bonds between mother and baby had emerged. And the baby herself was insuring those bonds. For every gesture of love from her mother, she gave generous rewards of love. Mrs. March, we thought, may have felt cherished by someone for the first time in her life.

All this constitutes what we would call "the emergency phase of the treatment." Now, in retrospect, we can tell you that it took a full year beyond this point to bring some resolution to Mrs. March's very severe internal conflicts, and there were a number of problems in mother-child relationships which emerged during that year; but Jane was out of danger, and even the baby conflicts of the second year of life were not extraordinary or morbid. Once the bond had been formed, nearly everything else could find solutions.

OTHER CONFLICTUAL AREAS

We shall try to summarize the following months of treatment. Jane remained the focus of our work. And following the pattern already established, the therapeutic work moved freely between the baby and her developmental needs and problems and the mother's conflicted past.

One poignant example comes to mind. Mrs. March, in spite of new-found pleasure and pride in motherhood, could still make casual and unfeeling plans for babysitting. The meaning of separation and temporary loss to a 1-year-old child did not register with Mrs. March. When the mother took part-time work at one point (and the family poverty gave some justification for additional income), Mrs. March made hasty and ill-thought-out sitting arrangements for Jane and then was surprised, as was Mr. March, to find that Jane was sometimes "cranky" and "spoiled" and "mean."

Mrs. Adelson tried in a number of tactful ways to help the Marches think about the meaning to Jane of her love for mother and her temporary loss of mother during the day. She met a blank wall. Both parents had known shifting and casual relationships with parents and parent-substitutes from their earliest years. The meaning of separation and loss was buried in memory. Their family style of coping with separation, desertion, or death was "Forget about it. You get used to it." Mrs. March could not remember grief or pain at the loss of important persons.

Somehow once again we were going to have to find the affective links between loss and denial of loss, for the baby in the present, and loss in the mother's past.

The moment came one morning when Mrs. Adelson arrived to find the family in disorder: Jane crying at the approach of a now-familiar visitor, parents angry at a baby who was being "just plain stubborn." Thoughtful inquiries from Mrs. Adelson brought the new information that Jane had just lost one sitter and started with another. Mrs. Adelson wondered out loud what this might mean to Jane. Yesterday she had been left, unexpectedly, in a totally new place with a strange woman. She felt alone and frightened without her mother, and did not know what was going to happen. No one could explain things to her; she was only a baby, with no words to express her serious problem. Somehow, we would have to find a way to understand and to help her with her fears and worries.

Mr. March, on his way to work, stopped long enough to listen attentively. Mrs. March was listening too, and before her husband left, she asked him to try to get home earlier today so that Jane would not be too long at the sitter's.

There followed a moving session in which the mother cried, and the baby cried, and something very important was put into words. In a circular and tentative way, Mrs. March began to talk about Aunt Ruth, with whom she had lived during her first five years. There had not been a letter from Aunt Ruth for some months. She thought Aunt Ruth was angry at her. She switched to her mother-in-law, to thoughts of her coldness and rejection of Mrs. March. Then came complaints about the sitters, with the theme that one sitter was angry because Jane cried when her mother left. The theme was "rejection" and "loss," and Mrs. March was searching for it everywhere in the contemporary scene. She cried throughout, but somehow even with Mrs. Adelson's gentle hints, she could not put all this together.

Then at one point Mrs. March left the room, still in tears, and returned with a family photograph album. She identified the pictures for Mrs. Adelson. Mother, father, Aunt Ruth, Aunt Ruth's son who had been killed in the war. Sorrow for Aunt Ruth. Nobody in the family would let her grieve for her son. "Forget about it" is what they said. She spoke about her father's death and her grandfather's death in the recent past.

Many losses, many shocks, just before Jane's birth, she was saying. And the family always said, "Forget about it." And then Mrs. Adelson, listening sympathetically, reminded her that there had been many other losses, many other shocks for Mrs. March long ago in her infancy and childhood. The loss of her mother, which she could not remember, and the loss of Aunt Ruth when she was 5 years old. Mrs. Adelson asked how Mrs. March had felt then, when she was too young to understand what was happening. Looking at Jane, sitting on her mother's lap, Mrs. Adelson said, "I wonder if we could understand how Jane would feel right now if she suddenly found herself in a new house, not just for an hour or two with a sitter, but permanently, never to see her mother or father again. Jane wouldn't have any way to understand this; it would leave her very worried, very upset. I wonder what it was like for you when you were a little girl."

Mrs. March listened, deep in thought. A moment later she said, in an angry and assertive voice, "You can't just replace one person with another. . . . You can't stop loving them and thinking about them. You can't just replace somebody." She was speaking of herself now. Mrs.

Adelson agreed, and then gently brought the insight back on behalf of Jane.

This was the beginning of new insights for Mrs. March. As she was helped to reexperience loss, grief, and feelings of rejection in childhood, she could no longer inflict this pain upon her own child. "I would never want my baby to feel that," she said with profound feeling. She was beginning to understand loss and grief. With Mrs. Adelson's help, she now began to work out a stable sitter plan for Jane, with full understanding of the meaning to her child. Jane's anxieties began to diminish, and she settled into her new regime.

Finally, too, we learned the dread secret which had invaded the transference to Dr. Zinn and caused her to take flight from psychiatric treatment. The morbid fear of being alone in the same room with the doctor, the obsessive sense of sin which had attached itself to Jane's doubtful paternity, had given us the strong clinical impression that Jane was "an incestuous baby," conceived long ago in childhood fantasy, made real through the illicit relationship with an out-of-wedlock lover. By this we meant nothing more than "an incestuous fantasy," of course. We were not prepared for the story that finally emerged. With great shame and suffering, Mrs. March told Mrs. Adelson in the second year of treatment her childhood secrets. Her own father had exhibited himself to her when she was a child and had approached her and her grandmother in the bed they shared. Her grandmother had accused her of seducing her elderly grandfather. This Mrs. March denied. And her first intercourse at the age of 11 took place with her cousin, who stood in the relationship of brother to her, since they shared the same house in the early years of life. Incest was not fantasy for Mrs. March. And now we understood the obsessive sense of sin which had attached itself to Jane and her uncertain paternity.

JANE AT 2 YEARS OF AGE

During the second year of treatment, Mrs. Adelson continued as the therapist for Mrs. March. Dr. Zinn had completed his residency, and Mrs. March's transference to Mrs. Adelson favored continuity in the work with the mother. William Schafer, psychologist on our staff, became the guidance worker for Jane. (We no longer have separate therapists for parent and child, but in this first case we were still experimenting.)

It is of some considerable interest that in the initial meetings with Mr. Schafer, Mrs. March was again in mute terror as her morbid fear of "a man" was revived in transference. But this time Mrs. March had made large advances in her therapeutic work. The anxiety was handled in transference by Mr. Schafer, and brought back to Mrs. Adelson where it could be placed within the context of the incestuous material that had emerged in treatment. The anxiety diminished, and Mrs. March was able to make a strong alliance with Mr. Schafer. The developmental guidance of the second year brought further strength and stability to the mother-child relationship, and we saw Jane continuing her developmental progress through her second year, even as her mother was working through very painful material in her own therapeutic work.

Were there residues in Jane's personality from the early months of neglect? As a 2-year-old, Jane was an attractive, busy little girl who presented no extraordinary problems in development. The only residue we could detect was a momentary stoppage of play at times when Mrs. March became temporarily uncomfortable, as in an unfamiliar social setting or when recalling particularly painful memories.

For the rest, Jane was a bright, vocal, sociable child. Her affectionate ties to her mother and father appeared to us as appropriate for her age. She was remarkably free from signs of withdrawal, self-absorption, or separation anxiety. In spontaneous doll play, we saw a strong positive identification with her mother and with acts of mothering. She was a solicitous mother to her dolls, feeding, dressing them with evident pleasure, murmuring comforting things to them. Bayley developmental testing showed continued progress. She had retained her age adequacy on social interaction and fine motor items. Gross motor development was now also at age level. Language, which had previously been a major area of concern, now showed only a slight delay of one month.

It was in doll play at 1:10:0 that Mr. Schafer first heard Jane speak a full sentence. Her doll was accidentally trapped behind a door with a spring catch, and Jane could not recover it. "I want my baby. I want my baby!" she called out in an imperative voice. It was a very good sentence for a 2-year-old. It was also a moving statement to all of us who knew Jane's story.

For us the story must end here. The family has moved on. Mr. March begins a new career with very good prospects in a new community that provides comfortable housing and a warm welcome. The external circumstances look promising. More important, the family has grown closer; abandonment is not a central concern. One of the most hopeful signs was Mrs. March's steady ability to handle the stress of the uncertainty that preceded the job choice. And as termination approached, she could openly acknowledge her sadness. Looking ahead, she expressed her wish for Jane: "I hope that she'll grow up to be happier than me. I hope that she will have a better marriage and children who she'll love." For herself, she asked that we remember her as "someone who had changed."

Greg

Within the first weeks of our new program we were asked to make an urgent call and an assessment of Greg, then 3½ months old. His 16-year-old mother, Annie, refused to care for him. She avoided physical contact with the baby; she often forgot to buy milk for him, and she fed him Kool-Aid and Tang. She turned over the baby's care to her 19-year-old husband, Earl.

Annie's family had been known to social agencies in our community for three generations. Delinquency, promiscuity, child abuse, neglect, poverty, school failure, psychosis had brought every member of the family to our community clinics and courts. Annie Beyer at 16 now represented the third generation of mothers in her family who actually or psychologically abandoned their babies. Annie's mother had surrendered the care of her children to others. As did *her* mother. And it was, in fact, Greg's grandmother, Annie's mother, who called our agency for help. She said, "I don't want to see what happened to me and my babies happen to Annie and her baby."

Vivian Shapiro of our staff called for an appointment and made a home visit immediately. Mother, father, and Greg were present. Mrs. Shapiro was greeted by a cold and silently hostile adolescent mother, a sad, bewildered boy who was the father, and a solemn baby who never once in that hour looked at his mother. Greg was developmentally adequate for his age, Mrs. Shapiro estimated, and her impressions were later sustained by our developmental testing. This spoke for some minimum adequacy in care, and we had good reason to believe that it was Earl, the father, who was providing most of Greg's care. At nearly every point in the one-hour session when Greg required care, Annie summoned her husband or picked up the baby and gave him to his father. He settled comfortably with his father and, for father, there were smiles.

During most of this session, and for many others that followed, Annie sat slumped in a chair. She was obese, unkempt, and her face registered no emotion. It was a mask which Mrs. Shapiro was to see many times, but when Annie brought herself to speak, there was barely controlled rage in her voice.

She did not want our help. There was nothing wrong with her or her child. She accused her mother of a conspiracy against her and, in her mind, Mrs. Shapiro was part of the conspiracy. Winning Annie's trust was to become our most arduous therapeutic task of those first weeks. To maintain the trust, after it was given, was equally difficult. It was a great advantage to Mrs. Shapiro, as it has been for all of us, to have come to this work with broad clinical experience with children and adolescents. An adolescent girl who defies her would-be helpers, who challenges, provokes, tests mercilessly, breaks appointments, disappears to another address, will not cause an experienced social worker to turn a hair. Mrs. Shapiro could wait to earn Annie's trust. But there was a baby in peril, and within only a few visits, we understood how great the peril was.

We began with the question to ourselves, "Why does Annie avoid touching and holding her baby?" To find the answers, we would need to know more about Annie than she was willing to give in those early hostile hours. And always there was Greg, whose own needs were imperative, and who could not wait for his teenage mother to make the therapeutic alliance, which is slow-paced in adolescence. It was surely not ignorance of the needs of babies that distanced Annie from her child. Doctors and public health nurses had given wise counsel before we ever met the Beyer family. She could not use the good advice.

AN ILLUMINATING HOUR

In the sixth home visit, something of the therapist's caring for Annie as a lonely and frightened child came through. Annie began to speak of herself. It made her angry, she said warily, when her husband, when people, thought she wasn't doing enough for her baby. She knew she was. Anyway, she said, she had never liked holding a baby very much . . . ever since she was a little girl. When she was little, she had had to take care of her younger sister. She would be given the baby and told to hold her. She much preferred leaving the baby on the couch.

And then, led on by tactful questions, she began to speak of her childhood. We heard about Annie, as a 9-year-old girl, responsible for the cleaning, cooking, and care of other siblings—after school hours. For any negligence in duties, there were beatings from her stepfather, Mr. Bragg.

Annie spoke of her childhood in a flat, dull voice, with only an edge of bitterness in it. She remembered everything, in chilling detail. And what Annie told the therapist was not a fantasy and was not distorted, since the story of Annie's family had been factually recorded by protective agencies and clinics throughout her community. There was the mother who periodically deserted her family. There was the father who died when Annie was 5 years old. And there was Mr. Bragg, the stepfather, alcoholic, probably psychotic. For trivial misdemeanors he dragged Annie off to the woodshed and beat her with a lath.

When Mrs. Shapiro spoke to the feelings of Annie as a child, of anger, fear, helplessness, Annie warded off these sympathetic overtures. She laughed cynically. She was tough. Her sister Millie and she got so they would just laugh at the old man when it was over.

In this session, in the midst of Annie's factual account of childhood horrors, Greg began a fretful cry, needing attention. Annie went to the bedroom and brought him back with her. For the first time in six visits Mrs. Shapiro saw Annie hold Greg closely cuddled in her arms.

This was the moment Mrs. Shapiro had been waiting for. It was the sign, perhaps, that if Annie could speak of her childhood sufferings, she could move protectively toward her baby.

The baby clutched his mother's hair as she bent over him. Annie, still half in the past and half in the present, said musingly, "Once my stepfather cut my hair to here," and pointed to her ears. "It was a punishment because I was bad." When Mrs. Shapiro said, "That must have been terrible for you!" Annie, for the first time, acknowledged feelings. "It was terrible. I cried for three days about it."

At this point, Annie began to talk to the baby. She told him he was smelly and needed to be changed. While Annie was changing him, Greg seemed to be looking for something to play with. There was a toy beside him on the couch. It was, of all things, a toy plastic hammer. Annie picked up the toy hammer and tapped it, gently, against the baby's head. Then she said, "I'm gonna beat you. I'm gonna beat you!" Her voice was teasing, but Mrs. Shapiro sensed the ominous intention in these words. And while still registering, as therapist, the revealed moment, Mrs. Shapiro heard Annie say to her baby, "When you grow up, I might kill you."

It was the close of the session. Mrs. Shapiro said those things that would quiet the turbulence in Annie, supporting the positive strivings toward motherhood, allying herself with those parts of the ego of this girl-mother that sought protection against the dangerous impulses.

But this, we knew, as we talked together in an emergency session back at the office, would not be enough to protect the baby from his mother. If Annie had to rely upon her therapist as an auxiliary ego, she would need to have her therapist in constant attendance.

AN EMERGENCY CLINICAL CONFERENCE

The question was, how could we help Annie and her baby? We now knew why Annie was afraid to be close to her baby. She was afraid of her own destructive feelings toward him. But we had read these signs from the breakthrough of unconscious impulses in the tease games with the baby. We could not interpret sadistic impulses which were not yet conscious to Annie herself. If we cooperated with the ego to maintain these sadistic impulses in repression, Annie would have to distance herself from her baby. And the baby was our patient too. Our most vulnerable patient.

We were attentive to small positive signs in this session. *After* talking about her childhood terrors, even though the affect was flat in the telling, Annie did pick up her baby and hold him close and cuddle him. And this was the first time we had seen closeness between mother and baby in six sessions. If Annie could remember and speak of her childhood suffering, could we open pathways which would free her baby from her own past and enable her to mother Greg? If Annie could be helped to examine her feelings toward the baby, if we could elicit the unspeakable thoughts, would Annie be able to reach out to her baby?

From the standpoint of an exercise in pure theory and method, we were probably on the right track in our thinking. The case considerations were derived from psychoanalytic experience. But this was not a psychoanalysis. As psychoanalytic consultant, Selma Fraiberg recalls that she suddenly found herself bereft of all the conditions and the protections against error which are built into the psychoanalytic situation.

First of all, the conditions of this therapy on behalf of a baby and his adolescent mother made it imperative to move quickly to protect the baby. Under all normal circumstances in therapy, we believe in cautious exploration: an assessment of the ego's capacity to deal with painful affects, an assessment of the defensive structure of the patient. Also, as experienced therapists with adolescents, we knew that to win the trust of this hostile girl might easily take months of work. And the baby was in immediate danger.

We were attentive to the defenses against painful affect which we saw in Annie. She remembered, factually, the experiences of childhood abuse. What she did not remember was her suffering. Would the liberation of affect in therapy increase the likelihood of acting out toward the baby or would it decrease the risks? After thorough discussion of alternatives, we decided, with much trepidation, that the chances of acting out toward the baby would be greater if the anxiety and rage were not elicited in treatment. Selma Fraiberg recalls: "Speaking for myself, I clung to the belief that it is the parent who cannot remember his childhood feelings of pain and anxiety who will need to inflict his pain upon his child. And then I thought: 'But what if I am wrong?'"

Then we would also be confronted with another therapeutic problem in this once-a-week psychotherapy. If we worked within the realm of buried affects, we could predict that the therapist who conjures up the ghosts will be endowed in transference with the fearsome attributes of the ghost. We would have to be prepared for the transference ghosts and meet them squarely every step of the way.

As we reviewed these conference notes one year later, we were satisfied that our treatment formulations had stood up well in the practical test. We now know, through the progress of our treatment, that the main lines of the work were well considered.

But now we shall have to take you with us on a detour from the treatment that turned out to be as important for the outcome as the psychotherapeutic plan.

Before any part of this treatment plan could be put into effect, Annie took flight from the therapist.

ANNIE LOCKS THE DOOR: A FLIGHT FROM TREATMENT

You remember that our emergency conference had followed the critical sixth session interview in which Annie began to speak of her childhood beatings. The seventh session was a home visit in which a number of Annie's relatives came to visit, and there was no opportunity to speak with Annie alone. In the eighth session, Mrs. Shapiro arranged to speak with both Annie and Earl about continuing visits and to invite them to raise questions with her about how we might best be able to help the Beyers. Earl said emphatically that he wanted Mrs. Shapiro to continue visiting them. He said that he felt Mrs. Shapiro was helping them to see things about Greg's development that they would never have been able to see themselves. Annie remained silent. Then, when Mrs. Shapiro inquired about Annie's wishes, Annie said, with some hesitation, that she would like Mrs. Shapiro to continue to come. She would like to be able to talk about the baby and about herself.

In this hour Annie herself picked up the narrative which had begun in the sixth session. She began, however, by speaking of her fears that Earl drives too fast, that he might have an accident. A child needed a father. Greg needed a father. This led her to speak of her own father, her natural father, with some affection. After her father died when Annie was 5 years old, nobody ever really cared for her. There had been several men in the household who lived with Annie's mother. There were six children, born to four different fathers. Millie was her mother's favorite. Annie said bitterly, "They didn't want me. I didn't want them. I didn't need anybody." She spoke again of Mr. Bragg and the beatings. At first she used to cry, but he wouldn't stop. Then later, she would laugh, because it didn't hurt any more. He beat her with a lath. He would beat her until the lath broke.

After her father died, Annie's mother disappeared. She went to work in another city, leaving the children with an old woman. To punish the children, the old woman locked them out of the house. She remembered one night when she and Millie were locked out in the freezing cold and huddled together. Her mother never seemed to know what was going on. Even when she returned to her family, she went to work, and even when she wasn't working, she didn't seem to be around.

To all this Mrs. Shapiro listened with great sympathy. She spoke of a child's need for protection. How frightening to a child to have no one to protect her. How much Annie missed her mother and a mother's protection. Perhaps she would be a different kind of mother to Greg. Would she feel she had to protect him? "Of course," Annie replied.

And very gently, Mrs. Shapiro spoke of the deep unhappiness and loneliness in Annie's childhood, and how difficult it was to be a young mother who had missed so much in her own childhood. Together, Mrs. Shapiro and Annie would talk about these things in their future visits.

It was, Mrs. Shapiro felt, a good visit: clarification of the role of the therapist, an acknowledgment that Annie and Earl wanted help for themselves and for their baby. For Annie, the beginning of the permission to feel along with remembering. A permission that she was not yet ready to take. But this would come.

And then, following this visit, Annie refused to see Mrs. Shapiro. There were numerous broken appointments. Appointments would be made, but Annie would not be at home. Or Mrs. Shapiro would arrive, with all signs of activity in the house, and Annie would refuse to answer the door. Annie literally locked the door against Mrs. Shapiro.

It was no consolation during a period like this to understand the nature of transference resistance while the patient barricades the door against the therapist. It is far worse to know that there are two patients behind the door and that one of them is a baby.

As the memories of childhood terrors emerged in that last session, the original affects must have emerged—not in the treatment hour, but afterward—and the therapist became the representative of fears that could not be named. Annie did not remember or experience her anxiety during the brutal bearings by Mr. Bragg, but anxiety attached itself to the person of the therapist, and Annie took flight. Annie did not remember the terror of being locked out of the house by the woman who cared for her when her mother deserted the family, and to make sure that she would not remember, the ghosts and the ego conspired to lock Mrs. Shapiro out of the house. Annie did not remember the terror of abandonment by her mother, but she reenacted the experience in transference, creating the conditions under which the therapist might have to abandon her.

We were, ourselves, nearly helpless. But this is not to say that the psychoanalytic insight was without value. To understand all this gave us a measure of control in the countertransference. We were not going to abandon Annie and her baby. We understood the suffering behind the provocative, tough, and insolent adolescent posture, and could respond to the anxiety and not the defense.

The only thing we lacked was a patient who could benefit from the insight. And there was the baby who was more imperiled than his mother.

During the two-month period in which Mrs. Shapiro was locked out of the house, reports from grandparents, visiting nurse, and others increased our alarm. Annie showed phobic symptoms. She was afraid to be alone in the house. And she was pregnant again. Greg looked neglected. He was suffering from recurrent upper respiratory illness and was not receiving medical care. The paternal grandparents were alarmed for Greg and reported to Mrs. Shapiro that Annie was playing rough games with Greg, swinging him from his ankles.

Our own alarm for Greg brought us to a painful decision. In our hospital and in our community we are ethically and legally bound to report cases of neglect and suspected or actual abuse to Protective Services. In a case where treatment alternatives are rejected by the family (as in Annie's case) the report is mandatory. The law is wise, but in the exercise of our legal responsibility we would bring still another tragedy to the Beyer family.

This was a critical moment, not only for the family but for Mrs. Shapiro and for our entire staff. There is no greater irony for the clinician than that in which he possesses the knowledge and the methods to prevent a tragedy and cannot bring this help to those who need it. Clinically speaking, the solution to the problem resided in the transference resistance. Exploration of the negative transference with Annie would prevent further acting out. We all know how to deal with transference ghosts in an office with a patient who gives even grudging cooperation with our method. How do we deal with the negative transference when the patient has locked herself in a house with her baby and their ghosts and will not answer the door?

The considerations for Greg were paramount now. Mrs. Shapiro wanted to prepare Annie and Earl for the painful alternative which lay before us, a referral to Protective Services. But Annie refused to answer the door when Mrs. Shapiro called.

As a sad alternative, Mrs. Shapiro prepared a letter which was sent to Annie and Earl and to both sets of grandparents. It was a letter which spoke for our concern and deep caring for both of the young parents and for their baby. It cited the many attempts we had made to reach the family with our help and our wish, still, to help this young family. If they felt we could not help them, we would need to seek help for them elsewhere, and we would request the help of Protective Services. A reply was requested within the week.

We learned within a few days of the impact of this letter on Annie and Earl and the grandparents. Annie cried for the entire weekend. She was angry at Mrs. Shapiro. She was frightened. But on Monday she called Mrs. Shapiro. Her voice was exhausted, but she managed to say that everything in Mrs. Shapiro's letter was true. She would see Mrs. Shapiro.

EXTENDED TREATMENT

This was the beginning of a new relationship between Annie and Earl and Mrs. Shapiro. Step by step, Mrs. Shapiro dealt with Annie's distrust, her anger toward Mrs. Shapiro and all "helping people," and clarified her own role as a helping person. Mrs. Shapiro was on the side of Annie and Earl and Greg and wanted to do everything possible to help them—to find the good things they wanted and deserved in life, and to give Greg all the things he needed to become a healthy and happy child.

For Annie, the relationship with Mrs. Shapiro became a new experience, unlike anything she had known. Mrs. Shapiro began, of course, by dealing openly with the anger which Annie had felt toward her, and she made it safe for Annie to put anger into words. In a family pattern where anger and murderous rage were fused, Annie had only been able to deal with anger through flight or identification with the aggressor. In the family theater, anger toward the mother and desertion by the mother were interlocking themes. But Annie learned that she could feel anger and acknowledge anger toward her therapist, and her therapist would not retaliate and would not abandon her.

It was safe to experience anger in transference to the therapist, and within this protected relationship the pathways of anger led back to childhood griefs and terrors. It was not an easy path for Annie. Yes, she acknowledged in a session soon after Mrs. Shapiro began visiting again, yes, she had felt bad about the therapist coming to see her. Yes, she resented her. "But what's the use of talking? I always kept things to myself. I want to forget. I don't want to think."

Mrs. Shapiro, with full sympathy for Annie's suffering and the need to forget, discussed with Annie how trying to forget did not get rid of the feelings or the memories. Annie would only be able to make peace with her feelings by talking about them to Mrs. Shapiro. Together, through talking, the therapist would be able to help Annie feel better.

Annie did not reply in words. At this point in the session she picked up Greg and held him very close, rocking him in her arms. But the tension within her was transmitted to Greg; she was holding him too tightly and the baby began to protest. Yet we had seen Annie reach *spontaneously* for her baby, and this was a favorable sign. (Her awkwardness was to diminish over time, and we were later to witness a growing pleasure in physical intimacy with her baby.)

In successive sessions, Annie took the permission to speak of her feelings. And the story of childhood privations, of brutality and neglect, began to emerge once again, as if the narrative begun two months ago could now be resumed. But this time Mrs. Shapiro knew what had caused Annie to take flight from treatment two months ago, and her own insight could be employed in a method which would prevent flight or acting out and would ultimately lead to resolution. It was not the telling of the tales which had caused Annie to take flight, but the unspoken affect which had been maintained in isolation from the memories. Annie, you remember, had described her stepfather's beatings in exact and chilling detail, but the affect was isolated. She laughed cynically throughout that early session. Somewhere between the factual reporting of beatings and neglect and the flight from Mrs. Shapiro, affect which had been maintained in partial repression had emerged, and anger, fear, simple terror sought an object, a name for itself, and the name was Mrs. Shapiro.

This time, with the start of treatment, properly speaking, Mrs. Shapiro elicited affect along with the telling and made it safe to remember. When the story of childhood horrors emerged now, Mrs. Shapiro offered her own commentary. "How frightening to a child. You were only a child then. There was no one to protect you. Every child has a right to be taken care of and protected." And Annie said, with bitterness, "The mother is supposed to protect the children. My mother didn't do that." There was a refrain in these early hours which appears in the record again and again. "I was hurt. I was hurt. Everyone in my family is violent." And then another refrain. "I don't want to hurt anybody. I don't want to hurt anybody." Mrs. Shapiro, listening attentively, said, "I know you don't want to hurt anybody. I know how much you have suffered and how much it hurt. As we talk about your feelings, even though it is painful to remember, it will be possible to find ways to come to terms with some of these things and to be the kind of mother you want to be."

Annie, we saw, got both sides of the message. Mrs. Shapiro was on the side of the ego which defended against the unconscious wish to hurt and to repeat the hurts with her own child. At the same time, Mrs. Shapiro was saying, in effect, "It will be safe with me to speak of the frightening memories and thoughts, and when you speak of them you will no longer need to be afraid of them; you will have another kind of control over them."

Mrs. Shapiro also anticipated with Annie the possibility of negative transference feelings that might arise during sessions where painful memories would be revived. Mrs. Shapiro said to Annie, "It may be

187

that in talking about the past, you will feel angry toward me, without knowing why. Perhaps you could tell me when this happens, and we can try to understand how your feelings in the present are connected to memories in the past."

For Annie, however, it was not easy to tell anyone she was angry. And she resisted putting into words her affect, so clearly evident in her face and body language. When Mrs. Shapiro asked Annie what she thought Mrs. Shapiro might do if Annie became angry with her, Annie said, "Sometimes I get close to people—then I get mad. When I get mad they leave." Mrs. Shapiro reassured Annie that she could accept Annie's angry feelings and that she would not leave. With permission now to express anger, Annie's rage emerged in succeeding sessions, often in transference, and very slowly anger toward the objects of the past was reexperienced and put into proper perspective so that Annie could relate to her present family in a less conflicted way.

During all of these sessions, Mrs. Shapiro's watchful eye was upon Greg, always in the room. Would the rage spill over and engulf Greg? But once again, as in the case of Jane, we became witness to extraordinary changes in the young mother's relationship to Greg. In the midst of anger and tears, as Annie spoke of her own oppressive past, she would approach Greg, pick him up, enclose him in her arms, and murmur comforting things to him. We knew then that Annie was no longer afraid of her destructive feelings toward the baby. The rage belonged to the past, to other figures. And the protective love toward Greg, which now began to emerge, spoke for a momentous shift in her identification with the baby. Where before she was identified with the aggressors of her childhood, she now was the protector of her baby, giving him what had not been given, or rarely given, in her own childhood. "Nobody," said Annie one day, "is ever going to hurt my child the way I have been hurt."

Mrs. Shapiro, in her work, moved back and forth between the story of Annie's past and the present. She helped Annie see how fear of the parental figures of her childhood had led her to identify with their fearsome qualities. And as Annie moved toward a protective relationship with her own baby, Mrs. Shapiro fortified each of these changes with her own observations. Sometimes, speaking for Greg, Mrs. Shapiro would say, "Isn't it good to have a mommy who knows just what you need?" As Greg himself, now mobile, began to approach his mother more and more for affection, for comfort, for company, Mrs. Shapiro drew Annie's attention to each move. Greg, she pointed out, was learning to love and trust his mother, and all of this was due to Annie and her understanding of Greg. Annie was holding Greg now, cradling him protectively in her arms. We saw no more "playful" threats of beating and killing, such as we had witnessed months ago. Annie was feeding the baby and using Mrs. Shapiro's tactful suggestions in providing the elements of good nutrition in the baby's diet.

In this family without traditions in child rearing, Mrs. Shapiro often had to be the tactful educator. In Annie's and Earl's families, even a 7-month-old baby was regarded as being capable of malice, revenge, and cunning. If a baby cried, he was "being spiteful." If he was persistent, he was "stubborn." If he refused to comply, he was "spoiled rotten." If he couldn't be comforted, he was "just trying to get someone's goat." Mrs. Shapiro always asked the question "Why?" Why is he crying, why is he being stubborn, what could it be? Both parents, perhaps initially surprised by this alien approach to a baby, began to assimilate Mrs. Shapiro's education. More and more, as the weeks and months progressed, we saw the parents themselves seeking causes, alleviating distress by finding the antecedent conditions. And Greg began to flourish.

This is not to say that within a few months we had undone the cruel effects of Annie's own childhood. But we now had access to this past. When Annie's voice sometimes became shrill and she gave brusque treatment to Greg, Annie knew as well as Mrs. Shapiro that a ghost from Annie's childhood had invaded the nursery again. And together they could find meaning in the mood that had suddenly overpowered her.

As the baby progressed and Annie's conflicted past became sorted out, we began to see one figure emerge in Annie's .childhood who stood for protection, tolerance, understanding. This was Annie's natural father, who had died when Annie was 5. In Annie's memory he was kind and fair. He never beat her. He would never have allowed other people to be cruel to her, if only he had remained with the family. And as she spoke of her own father, love and a remembrance of his loss overwhelmed her. Whether Annie's memory of her father was accurate or not does not matter, of course. What does matter is that in the chaos and terror of her childhood there had been one person who gave her a sense of love and protection. In searching her past for something good, for some source of strength, this is what she found, and Mrs. Shapiro kept this good memory alive for Annie. We now understood another part of the puzzle. When we had first known the Beyer family, you remember, Annie had not only refused to care for her baby but regularly turned him over to her husband, the baby's father, for care. All of this had changed in the intervening months as Annie learned, through her therapist, how a mother too can be a protector to her child.

Greg himself began to show a strengthening of his bond to his mother within the early months of work. At 10 months of age, just before Mrs. Shapiro left for vacation, his behavior toward his mother showed selective response and seeking of her, much smiling and seeking contact with her, approaches to mother for comfort and for company. But there was still some fear of mother, we saw, when her strident voice stopped him in the middle of some trivial misdemeanor.

During these months, we should now recall, Annie was pregnant. She rarely spoke of the coming baby to Mrs. Shapiro. It was as if the pregnancy was not real to her. There were no fantasies about the baby. She was fully preoccupied with her own self and with Greg, who was becoming the center for her.

In July, when Mrs. Shapiro was on vacation, Annie delivered a stillborn child. When Mrs. Shapiro returned, Annie was sad and burdened with guilt. The death of the baby she thought was a punishment to her. She had not wanted the baby, and she thought God did not want a baby to come into the world who would not be loved. Many hours were spent in putting together the experience of loss and self-reproach.

It was during this period too that Annie began to understand with help why she had not been ready for another baby. She was, indeed, drawing upon all of her impoverished emotional resources to give care and love to Greg, and in giving she felt depleted. Many times we had the impression that she was sustaining herself through the warmth and caring of her therapist, borrowing strength, augmenting the poverty of her own experience in love through the relationship to her therapist. This was always a professional relationship, of course, but for a girl who had been emotionally starved and brutalized, this professional caring and understanding seemed to be experienced as the giving of love.

The unsatisfied hungers of childhood were persistent ghosts in this household. Often when the therapist arrived, Annie and Earl were watching television. Their favorite TV shows were children's programs and animated cartoons. This was not for Greg's sake, we must assure you, since Greg himself had no interest in these shows. During the summer of the Watergate hearings, which were carried on nearly every channel, of course, Mrs. Shapiro saw Annie and Earl switch from channel to channel until they found a program they liked. It was "The Jolly Green Giant."

When Mrs. Shapiro brought carefully selected toys for Greg (as we always do for our children when we know that the parents cannot provide them), Annie wore a conflicted look on her face. It was envy, Mrs. Shapiro realized, and longing. On one occasion, when Mrs. Shapiro brought some simple plastic toys for the baby, Annie said, in a voice full of feeling, "It's my birthday next week. I'll be seventeen." Mrs. Shapiro understood, of course. Annie wished the present were for her. The therapist, quickly responding, spoke of Annie's coming birthday and her wish that it be a very special day. Annie said, "I never had a birthday. I never had a party. I'm planning to have one for Greg in August. My mother will probably forget my birthday." (Her mother did forget.) And for Annie's birthday, Mrs. Shapiro brought a small, carefully chosen present for her.

On Greg's birthday, Mrs. Shapiro brought a toy bus for the baby. Annie opened the package. She was enraptured. She examined each of the little figures, opened the bus door, placed all the little people on the seats, and only when she had finished playing with it did she give it to Greg and share her excitement with him.

THE LAST GHOST: THE MOST OBSTINATE ONE

The last ghost to leave the nursery was also the first ghost to enter it. And its name, of course, was "identification with the aggressor." Even in its most formidable aspect after the first months of therapeutic work this ghost no longer threatened the baby. That is to say, there was no longer serious danger of abuse of Greg by his mother. We saw how the strengthening of the love bonds between Annie and her baby protected the child from physical abuse. We also saw how Annie's remembrances of her own suffering became a form of protection to her baby. She would no longer inflict her pain upon her child.

At the end of the first year of treatment, then, Greg showed favorable signs of developmental progress and attachment to his mother. But the ghost still lingered, and we saw it in many forms that still endangered Greg's development.

As Greg became active, independent, curious, and mischievous in his second year, Annie's repertoire of disciplinary tactics appeared ready-made from the ruins of her childhood. Maternal and protective and affectionate as she could be when Greg was quiet, obedient, and "good," there was a voice for disobedience or ordinary toddler mishaps which was strident, shrill, and of a magnitude to shatter the eardrums. Greg at these moments was frightened, and Mrs. Shapiro drew Annie's attention to the baby's reactions on many occasions. And then very quickly, it seemed to us, Greg acquired a defense against the anxiety produced in him by mother's anger. He would laugh, giddily, a little hysterically, we thought. And this, of course, was exactly the defense which his mother had acquired in her childhood. Greg was 16 months old when we witnessed the appearance of this defense.

Very clearly an important component of Annie's defense—"identification with the aggressor"—had not yet been dealt with in the therapy. Annie had not yet fully experienced in therapy her childhood anxiety and terror before the dangerous, unpredictable, violent, and powerful figures of the past. From analytic experience we knew that the pathogenesis of the defense known as identification with the aggressor is anxiety and helplessness before the attackers. To reach this stratum of the defense structure through psychoanalysis is often a formidable task. How shall we reach it through our once-a-week psychotherapy-in-the-kitchen?

We examined the pathways available to us. Annie's voice, Mrs. Shapiro had observed, would shift in a single moment from a natural conversational voice, which was her own, to the strident, ear-shattering voice which seemed to be somebody else's. But Annie seemed not aware of this. The alien voice was also incorporated in her personality. Could we employ the on-the-spot manifestations of this pathological identification in a two-phase interpretive process? First, to make the voice ego-alien, identify it; then, to interpret it as a defense against intolerable anxiety and lead Annie to reexperience her own childhood sense of terror and helplessness?

There was no difficulty finding the occasion in a home visit. The occasion, as it happened, appeared with startling clarity in a visit shortly after we examined the technical problems in our conference.

Greg, 17 months old, was in his high chair, eating his breakfast. Mother kept up a stream of admonitions while he ate: "Don't do that. Don't drop the food off." Then suddenly, responding to some trivial mishap in the high chair, Annie screamed, "Stop it!" Both Greg and Mrs. Shapiro jumped. Annie said to the therapist, "I scared you, didn't I?" Mrs. Shapiro, recovering from shock, decided this was the moment she was waiting for. She said, "Sometimes, Annie, the words and sounds that come out of your mouth don't even sound like you. I wonder whom they do sound like." Annie said immediately, "I know. They sound just like my mother. My mother used to scare me." "How did you feel?" Annie said, "How would you feel if you were in with a bull in a china shop? . . . Besides, I don't want to talk about that. I've suffered enough. That's behind me."

But Mrs. Shapiro persisted, gently, and made the crucial interpretation. She said, "I could imagine that as a little girl you might be so scared that in order to make yourself less scared, you might start talking and sounding like your mother." Annie said again, "I don't want to talk about it right now." But she was deeply affected by Mrs. Shapiro's words.

The rest of the hour took a curious turn. Annie began to collapse before Mrs. Shapiro's eyes. Instead of a tough, defiant, aggressive girl, she became a helpless, anxious little girl for the entire hour. Since she could find no words to speak of the profound anxiety which had emerged in her, she began to speak of everything she could find in her contemporary life that made her feel afraid, helpless, alone.

In this way, and for many hours to come, Mrs. Shapiro led Annie back into the experiences of helplessness and terror in her childhood and moved back and forth, from the present to the past, in identifying for Annie the ways in which she brought her own experiences to her mothering of Greg, how identification with the feared people of her childhood was "remembered" when she became the frightening mother to Greg. It was a moment for therapeutic rejoicing when Annie was able to say, "I don't want my child to be afraid of me."

The work in this area brought about profound changes in Annie and in her relationship to Greg. Annie herself began to leave behind her tough, street-child manner, and the strident voice was muted. As the pathological identification with her own mother began to dissolve, we saw Annie seeking new models for mothering and for femininity, some of which were easily identified as attributes of Mrs. Shapiro.

And Greg himself began to respond to the changed climate of his home. As we should expect, the fear of mother and the nervous laugh as a defense against anxiety began to disappear. Since there were, in fact, strong bonds between mother and baby, there was much that Annie could now employ in an education of her son without fear. .

Mrs. Shapiro enlisted the mother as observer of Greg's attempts to communicate with her. Concrete suggestions and demonstrations were offered in a supportive, noncritical way. This time Annie was able to use the developmental guidance in a less defensive and more constructive way, working in alliance with the therapist on behalf of Greg. Within a month of the time Greg's need for help in language was first identified, he began to use language expressively and was soon well within the normal range of the Bayley Scale.

Treatment continued for two years, which is some time beyond the point where Greg had achieved adequacy in all areas of functioning and Annie and Earl themselves had become competent and devoted parents. In large measure, the work of those two years was supportive of the two young parents who were coping with the stresses of "growing up" themselves, of completing their own adolescence, at the same time as they were learning to become parents of a kind they had never known in their own experience. Annie and Earl continued to seek guidance from Mrs. Shapiro in many areas of child rearing and yet were making good and wise decisions on their own as Greg moved into each new developmental stage. Treatment was terminated when Greg was 3 years old, when Annie herself told Mrs. Shapiro that she now felt good about her ability to manage without help. It was understood that at any time in the future that she needed to call Mrs. Shapiro or visit she would always be most welcome.

FOLLOW-UP

Since Annie and Earl kept in touch with Mrs. Shapiro from time to time, we have a follow-up report augmenting the story of this family.

The outcome of treatment for Annie, for Earl, and for Greg has been hopeful. In 1977, Greg—now close to 5 years of age—is seen in follow-up as a healthy, buoyant little boy, affectionate and endearing. A new baby brother, now 2 years old, testifies to the good mothering he is receiving and the good climate of his home. The marriage of Annie and Earl has become stable—and it is the only stable marriage in both their extended families. Annie herself is a proud and competent young woman. Last year Annie, the high-school dropout, enrolled in a class in child development. She was surprised, she told Mrs. Shapiro, to discover how much she knew.

She is consulted by all members of her family, including her mother, as family crises continue to occur. She dispenses wise counsel and keeps her own head. She thinks her mother and sisters all need therapy and has done her earnest best to persuade them, but not yet with success.

The Questions—and a Hypothesis

We began this chapter with a question: "What is it, then, that determines whether the conflicted past of the parent will be repeated with his child?" Morbidity in the parental history will not in itself predict the repetition of the past in the present. The presence of pathological figures in the parental past will not, in itself, predict identification with those figures and the passing on of morbid experience to one's own children.

From the clinical studies of Mrs. March and Annie Beyer and from many other cases known to us in which the ghosts of the parental past take possession of the nursery, we have seen a pattern which is strikingly uniform: These are the parents who, earlier, in the extremity of childhood terror, formed a pathological identification with the dangerous and assaultive enemies of the ego. Yet if we name this condition in the familiar term, "identification with the aggressor," we have not added to the sum of our knowledge of this defense. Our literature in this area of defense is sparse. Beyond the early writings of Anna Freud which named and illuminated this defense in the formative period of childhood, we do not yet know from large-scale clinical study the conditions which govern the choice of this defense against other alternatives, or the dynamics which perpetuate an identification with the enemy, so to speak.

We are on sound grounds clinically and theoretically if we posit that a form of repression is present in this defense which provides motive and energy for repetition. But what is it that is repressed? From a number of cases known to us in which "identification with the aggressor" was explored clinically as a central mechanism in pathological parenting, we can report that memory for the events of childhood abuse, tyranny, and desertion was available in explicit and chilling detail. *What was not remembered was the associated affective experience.*

Annie for instance, remembered her childhood beatings by her stepfather, and she remembered her mother's desertion. What she did not remember was terror and helplessness in the experience of being abused and deserted. The original affects had undergone repression. When the therapeutic work revived these affects, and when Annie could reexperience them in the safety of her relationship to the therapist, she could no longer inflict this pain upon her child. Mrs. March could remember rejection, desertion, and incestuous experience in childhood. What she could not remember was the overwhelming anxiety, shame, and worthlessness which had accompanied each of these violations of a child. When anxiety, grief, shame, self-abasement were recovered and reexperienced in therapy, Mrs. March no longer needed to inflict her own pain and her childhood sins upon her child. With the reexperiencing of childhood suffering along with the memories, each of these young mothers was able to say, "I would never want that to happen to my child."

These words strike a familiar note. There are many parents who have themselves lived tormented childhoods who do not inflict their pain upon their children. These are the parents who say explicitly, or in effect, "I remember what it was like. . . . I remember how afraid I was when my father exploded. . . . I remember how I cried when they took me and my sister away to live in that home. . . . I would never let my child go through what I went through."

For these parents the pain and suffering have not undergone total repression. In remembering, they are saved from the blind repetition of that morbid past. Through remembering they identify with an injured child (the childhood self), while the parent who does not remember may find himself in an unconscious alliance and identification with the fearsome figures of the past. In this way, the parental past is inflicted upon the child.

The key to our ghost story appears to lie in the fate of affects in childhood. Our hypothesis is that access to childhood pain becomes a powerful deterrent against repetition in parenting, while repression and isolation of painful affect provide the psychological requirements for identification with the betrayers and the aggressors. The unsolved mystery is why, under conditions of extremity, in early childhood, some children who later become parents keep pain alive; they do not make the fateful alliance with the aggressor which defends the child ego against intolerable danger and obliterates the conscious experience of anxiety. We hope to explore these problems in farther study.

The theory posited here, however incomplete, has practical implications for psychotherapy with parents and children in those families where the ghosts of the parental past have taken up residence in the nursery. In each case, when our therapy has brought the parent to remember and reexperience his childhood anxiety and suffering, the ghosts depart and the afflicted parents become the protectors of their children against the repetition of their own conflicted past.

VIII

Billy: Infant-Parent Psychotherapy on Behalf of a Child in a Critical Nutritional State

VIVIAN SHAPIRO

SELMA FRAIBERG

EDNA ADELSON

IN THIS CHAPTER, we describe the treatment of Billy, who was referred to our infant mental health program at 5 months of age in a grave nutritional state. The baby was starving. His growth curve showed an ominous downward plunge which our pediatricians read as the profile of an infant moving toward the critical (and sometimes irreversible) state which is broadly covered by the term "failure to thrive." *

Extensive diagnostic study of Billy revealed no organic cause for growth failure. His psychological status was equally alarming to the medical staff. And Billy's parents, a 17-year-old mother and a 21-year-old father seemed, themselves, to be depleted and without hope. There appeared to be no connection between the young parents and their baby.

At the time of referral, the progressive decline in Billy's growth and

* A description of the "nonorganic failure to thrive" syndrome and a concise summary of the literature appears in the introduction to the case of Nina (Chapter V).

psychological development would require hospitalization for the baby if the pathological tendencies could not be reversed in a few weeks. Billy's weight had not yet declined to the critical point "below the third percentile." A referral was made to our program by the well-baby clinic with the hope that a collaborative pediatric and psychiatric treatment of the baby and his parents could avert hospitalization and bring about a favorable resolution. These hopes were realized in the work that followed.*

Billy at 5 Months

Billy Douglas was referred to our program when he was 5 months old. Billy vomited after each feeding. He had not gained weight in three months. At birth he had been a full-term, healthy baby, whose weight of 8 pounds put him at the 70th percentile. At 5 months he weighed only 14 pounds 5 ounces, which placed him at the 25th percentile. He had become a tense, morose, somber baby who looked, in the doctor's words, "like a little old man." A pediatric resident at the Child Health Center had worked intensively with Billy and his young mother for two months. There were extensive diagnostic studies which revealed no organic causes for growth failure. The doctor realized that the mother was becoming increasingly depressed.

Kathie Douglas was an anxious 17-year-old girl who had married Billy's 21-year-old father, John, only two months before Billy's birth. She was often unable to carry through with suggestions regarding food and medication. The pediatrician called in a public health nurse to see Billy and his mother at home weekly. Despite their best efforts, however, the doctor and the nurse observed that Kathie and Billy were not responding to their advice. At 5 months Billy's situation was critical. He was regressing, and hospitalization was being considered. Further, Kathie seemed even more depressed, distant, and sometimes confused.

At this point the medical team asked our help in making a psychological assessment of Billy and his family and in providing treatment, if possible.

---

* Vivian Shapiro was the primary therapist. Edna Adelson and Selma Fraiberg were consultants. "I" in this chapter refers to Vivian Shapiro.

Assessment

Our first task, then, during this medical emergency, was to make a psychological assessment of Billy and his family. As therapist, I began twice-weekly visits to the home for direct observation of the baby, his parents, and their modes of interaction.

Under ordinary circumstances we devote approximately five weekly one-hour sessions to the clinical evaluation period. In Billy's case, the nutritional and psychological perils were so great that we knew after the first three visits (one-and-a-half-weeks) that intervention in the form of some concrete guidance to the mother must begin before the psychological complexities were fully understood. These earliest visits, however, gave us vital clues which we could pursue in the emergency period.

INITIAL OBSERVATIONS OF BILLY AND HIS PARENTS

When I first arrived at the Douglases' small apartment, I met a timid, sad-faced, 17-year-old girl, who was Billy's mother, and a gaunt young man, Billy's father, barely out of his teens, who was so uneasy that he did not acknowledge my presence until almost the end of this visit.

My first impression of Billy brought the doctor's words to mind. Billy looked like a little old man. He was in his crib, up on his hands and knees, staring at the door, when I entered the room with his mother. His eyes met mine with an intense stare and a fixed smile. His stare never wavered.

Billy was motorically very precocious and was able at 5 months to turn over quickly, to creep, to grasp and manipulate objects. All of his movements and efforts at communication had an urgency that was unusual in a baby of this age. When I held him for a moment, I could feel the strain and tension in his body.

Billy seemed unusually aware of sounds. In particular, his mother commented that Billy responded quickly to any sounds related to feeding. She illustrated this by opening the refrigerator door while Mr. Douglas held the baby. Billy almost jumped out of his father's arms, his mouth opened, anticipating food, and his whole body strained toward the refrigerator. As his mother approached him with an eyedropper with vitamins, Billy, still in his father's arms, leaned back, opened his mouth, his hands became inert, and he looked like a starving baby bird awaiting food from his mother. Mother and father seemed uncomfortable with Billy. They treated him like a newly arrived stranger whom they had to approach cautiously and from a distance.

In early home visits, I saw that Billy spent his day amusing himself either on the floor or in bed. He was capable of spending a lot of time in solitary play with toys. There were few signs of human attachment. Even though he could creep, Billy rarely approached his mother. He rarely made eye contact with her. He rarely smiled unless mother used gross tactile play. When he fussed, his mother put him to bed with a pacifier and honey.

Billy's mother said sadly that Billy did not enjoy cuddling. She said that when she held him in her arms, he seemed to turn away from her. In fact, neither mother nor father held Billy in a close ventral position. They held him so that he was constantly facing away from them.

Already it was obvious to us that this baby and his parents were out of synchrony with each other. There was none of the normal spontaneity or joy in mutual gazing which one would expect between parents and baby at this age. Billy was a somber, tense baby who seemed to be starving. His mother was also morose and somber and, as we shall see, both parents were hungry and starving in their own way.

We soon learned that this new family was in a state of great stress and deprivation. They were living in poverty, supported only by Mr. Douglas's small earnings and food stamps. In addition to the financial stress, Mr. and Mrs. Douglas had lost the support system of their extended families by their move to a strange city. They felt abandoned and overburdened. There simply were not enough financial or emotional resources in this new family unit to satisfy the needs of mother, baby, and father.

Billy's mother at 17 seemed pathetically young and childlike. Her schoolgirl face, her T-shirt bearing a high school insignia, gave her the appearance of a girl surprised by the events that had brought her to motherhood.

In response to my comment that this year must seem different from last year when she was still at school, Kathie spoke of her feelings of loss. She missed her home town, her high school friends. She missed going to school. So much was unfinished and now everything had come to an end. In her mind, Kathie was not Mrs. Douglas, she was a misplaced teenager keeping house. All this emerged in a sad and distant voice. I was struck by the depth of Kathie's depression, which was evident in her posture as well as in her words. Her range of affect was constricted. Her movements were slow. Her speech was halting, and she seemed distant and sometimes confused. She rarely made eye contact with me.

The full weight of Kathie's depression soon became evident. She said that most of the time she was holding back feelings of rage that were so strong that "if I let go, I would kick the walls out of the house." She was having many somatic complaints, headaches, backaches, and gynecological problems, and she was also overweight. She sadly spoke of herself as feeling and looking like a fat old lady. She felt guilty about imposing on her husband for his time and attention.

John Douglas was also very young. At 21, he was haggard, thin, frightened, and harrassed by difficulties he could no longer cope with by himself. He was much more hesitant than Kathie to engage in any interaction with me. He literally turned away from me during my first few meetings with him. When he did talk to me, it was through a teasing question to Billy. "Billy, do you want to go home with her?" We believe he was simultaneously expressing his ambivalence about Billy and questioning my attitude toward his own worth as a parent. The first time he directly looked at me and smiled was about a month after I started visiting when he told me that Billy seemed happier, that he liked to play more.

Billy's state and his feeding problem made intervention imperative, yet after two sessions in the home, we had not yet observed a feeding, which would provide us tangible clues. Although I had arranged to come at mealtimes, Kathie avoided feeding Billy in my presence. She was, perhaps, not yet sure of me, not yet ready to reveal herself in the situation in which she was most inadequate. It was in the third session that Kathie volunteered to let me see how Billy was fed.

HOW IS BILLY FED?

As part of our assessment, a video play session was arranged at our office playroom. We customarily videotape a play session and Bayley testing at this point in an assessment. This is done only with the consent of parents, of course, and we do everything possible to make the taping nonintrusive. We never invite intimate discussions at these times. We do not use video for treatment sessions, but we find that the taping of play sessions and testing is almost always of great interest to parents, and the playback of the tapes for the parents is valued both by them and by us as an opportunity to observe the baby and themselves. In Billy's case, because of the urgency of the feeding problem, a formal Bayley testing was postponed until nutritional adequacy was achieved at 7½ months.

This session was primarily planned so as to permit the baby's own play as well as spontaneous mother-baby interaction. What occurred gave us a sobering picture of the isolation and the estrangement of baby and mother. As if he were alone in the room, the baby engaged in solitary exploration of toys and furniture. He never once sought his mother with his eyes. He was mobile, but never crept toward his mother. His mother looked distant and self-absorbed.

Then Billy uttered sounds of complaint. His mother said that it was time for his bottle and volunteered to feed Billy. She said, "Watch what he does when I show him the bottle." She placed the bottle on the floor, several feet away from Billy, who was on hands and knees. Billy's face registered alertness and urgency—no smile, but urgency. And the 5-month-old baby began to creep the long distance toward the bottle. He reached for it unsteadily, but could not quite grasp it at first. Finally he did grasp it, mouth open hungrily, but it was bottom up. He could not quite orient it. At last he got the nipple into his mouth. He sucked solemnly, greedily.

While I watched this scene, masking my own inner pain and horror, the schoolgirl mother explained that this was the way Billy took his bottle. "He likes it that way. He likes to have his bottle alone, on the floor."

After a while I suggested that Mrs. Douglas sit with Billy in our rocking chair and feed him. The second observation gave us another piece of the puzzle. Kathie now held Billy loosely in her arms. Billy was still supporting his own bottle. The mother, looking tired and apathetic, said that Billy usually finished his bottle in four minutes. "Sometimes, however, if the bottle is slow, it takes an hour." She talked as though it were solely his feeding, not something that she had anything to do with. She herself looked distant and empty. Our impression was that although Billy was in his mother's arms, he was still feeding himself. There was no mutual gaze, and little tactile contact. The mother was right: The baby turned away from her. She looked uneasy and sad and sometimes irritated.

Later in this visit Kathie started to rock herself in the rocking chair while holding Billy loosely in her arms. She looked like a little girl rocking herself, almost a parallel play situation: The hungry adolescent mother rocking and nurturing herself, allowing her baby to drink his bottle in her arms. Yet, as cold as the scene appeared to us, Kathie seemed to get some pleasure from this unusual closeness between herself and Billy. While watching this videotape later, she commented that this was in fact a good feeding, a better feeding than usual.

WHY CAN'T KATHIE FEED HER BABY?

As a treatment team we reexamined the videotape and the detailed notes of the home visits. We asked ourselves, "Where shall we begin? This is a schoolgirl mother who cannot feed her baby and who avoids physical contact with him." To encourage intimacy in feeding leads at best to mechanical compliance, as we saw on tape, but there were few rewards for mother or baby.

Yet we knew that we must promote this intimacy and proper feeding and must, at the same time, seek the answers to the crucial diagnostic questions that would lead to help. What lies behind the avoidance of physical contact? Is it the destructive rage which Kathie had expressed in her first session: "I could kick the walls out of this house?" Is it the mother's own unsatisfied hungers, which have led her unconsciously to withhold love and nourishment from her child? Was there something else on the mother's face and in her voice and manner as we watched the video story? Perhaps an aversion to feeding? Disgust?

We would have to find out much more. But a teenage girl, even under more favorable circumstances, does not give her trust so readily to a helping person. We would need time to explore the dimensions of this conflict. But this teenage girl was a mother; her baby was our patient too—and the baby was in great peril.

No case report can ever do justice to the feelings of the therapist who works with infants and their parents. There is an urge to rescue the baby who is in danger, to mother him oneself. There are deep reproaches, even anger, toward the schoolgirl who is starving her baby, which must not be expressed and which must be dealt with by the therapist lest they intrude in the work. In this situation we were helped by the fact that all of us are child therapists. We saw the mother herself as a child, an unfinished adolescent who still needed a mother herself. She was frightened, helpless, hungry, depleted. This did not imply that I, the therapist, must become a mother or a mother-substitute, but if we understood the child who was the mother and responded to her feelings of anguish and deprivation, we might earn her trust. Only on this basis was there hope for treatment.

In the home visits that followed the illuminating feeding session, Kathie began to respond to my deep concern for her as well as the baby. She began to speak of deep revulsion at the feeding of Billy. She was repelled by Billy's vomiting, she confessed, and had been since his birth. She was sickened by the sight, the messiness. I saw for myself the horror and panic which came over Kathie when she anticipated—or only imagined—that the baby was going to spit up or vomit.

At the end of a bottle feeding (Billy was taking his bottle on the floor), Kathie hurriedly picked up Billy to burp him. We would expect, of course, that she would hold Billy upright against her shoulder. Instead, she rushed to the bathroom with the baby, faced him over her arm so that he was hanging over the bathroom sink—and Billy vomited his meal into the sink. In this way Kathie avoided her worst fears that the baby would throw up in her arms. And the strategy that she employed virtually guaranteed that the upside-down baby would throw up his dinner!

Until I discussed my observations with Kathie, it had not occurred to the mother that she was precipitating the baby's vomiting. In her mind the only alternative was dreadful: to have the baby vomit in her arms.

Thereafter Kathie could tell us more. She had noticed that when Billy was 3 months old and had begun taking solids in his diet, the color and texture of the vomit had changed. She was so repelled that she reduced Billy's solids to a minimum as a way of avoiding the revolting mess. We now had another vital clue: The decline in Billy's weight curve had started at 3 months.

What, in fact, constituted Billy's daily food intake? Kathie was not sure. During the first visits I often heard Billy's piteous cries of hunger. When I said to both parents that Billy seemed very, very hungry, they were astonished. The father said, "Do you think he is still hungry? I think he is just like me. I could never be satisfied. I could eat everything that was given to me right now." The mother said resentfully that Billy never seemed satisfied, he was always begging for food. "If we gave him everything he wanted, he'd eat us out of house and home."

It soon became clear that neither of these young parents had any real sense of how much food Billy needed. Actual hunger was part of their daily experience and they had to severely limit their own appetites in many ways. At some level both Kathie and John seemed to feel that Billy would simply have to share in their hunger. Apparently, they did not fully understand that his life was at risk.

Treatment Plan for the Emergency Period

The period that we speak of as "emergency treatment" lasted for two months. It is really synchronous in time with the assessment period. During this period Billy began to eat normally, the vomiting virtually ceased, and he began to gain weight in a stable and satisfactory manner.

Our initial assessment gave us many of the vital clues to Billy's feeding problem. Billy was starving; but he was not "refusing" food, he was being deprived of food. The vomiting, according to our observations, was induced by his mother's unique procedures for burping, which were in turn related to her dread of being defiled by vomit.

The psychological picture was beginning to emerge: A teenage mother who avoided contact with her baby; a baby who crept toward his bottle on the floor and fed himself; a mother who had a deep inner revulsion against messiness and possibly toward her own destructive rage; a mother who was an adolescent with unsatisfied bodily and psychological hungers.

The baby was in nutritional peril and in great psychological peril, for in none of our observations did he show signs of attachment to either of his parents. At an age when preferential smiling and vocalization should emerge toward the baby's partners, we saw none. At an age when the baby normally seeks eye contact with his partners, we saw gaze avoidance. At an age when a mobile baby seeks partners through his own mobility, Billy sought no one. He did not enjoy closeness in his mother's arms, and was stiff and resistant in the arms of any human partner. His mental abilities seemed well within the Bayley ranges, which testified to some minimal adequacy in experience. But what could not be measured through any existing scale was the effect of emotional impoverishment and unsatisfied body hungers in this baby, now almost 6 months old.

At this point we faced a therapeutic dilemma. As clinicians we knew that the psychopathology of these young parents, and particularly the mother, would not be accessible to us within a few weeks, but the baby could not wait for the resolution of his mother's neurosis.

In this medical and psychological emergency we formulated our plans for the first phase of treatment. We would concentrate on the feeding problem, giving direct advice and guidance. We would do everything possible to promote the attachment of baby and mother. We would use our clinical insights to guide us during this emergency period, but we would not expect to gain full understanding of the parental psychopathology at this time.

The transference to me as therapist would be fully utilized in this emergency period. This was an adolescent girl with her own developmental needs. My own professional caring could be a form of nurturance for this young mother. The adolescent need for identification models could be employed in a sensitive offering of this professional help.

THE THERAPEUTIC RELATIONSHIP

I will briefly summarize the clinical work of this period which helped mother resolve some aspects of the feeding problem.

The therapeutic sessions with Billy and his mother took on a pattern that was set by Kathie. She had chosen a meeting time at home shortly before Billy napped. At the beginning of each visit, the focus was on Billy. Either Kathie or I would observe, or Kathie would feed him or have some questions—more often complaints—about Billy. Usually, midway through the visit, Kathie would put him to bed, and the remainder of the time would be hers.

I found out very quickly that if I responded to Kathie's own needs and feelings, either covertly or overtly expressed by her, Kathie would soon—and often in the same session did—attend to some of Billy's needs. For example, when I acknowledged that I understood how hard it was for Kathie to try to hold a baby who turned away, she was able to hold Billy—though with tears in her eyes—instead of putting him down.

Many aspects of the positive transference became available in helping Kathie on behalf of Billy. Kathie was initially very dependent and related to me as a child to a mother. (For example, when I visited, I had to let myself in, hang up my coat, and find a place to sit down, while Kathie often continued to sit slumped in a chair in the living room.) I responded to Kathie's need for a mother, while taking care, of course, to offer her another kind of "caring for Kathie" which was part of a therapeutic relationship.

I sympathized with Kathie's sense of loss in leaving her own family and in leaving childhood as an unfinished adolescent. I responded to Kathie's feelings that no one cared for her and that she was physically deteriorating. I helped to arrange free medical service for Kathie at a health clinic which had been available but which she had not been able to seek out. I encouraged her in her efforts to finish high school, and praised her for any accomplishments regarding her own efforts to continue her artwork.

We knew that Kathie felt inadequate. She had been told she was by her mother, and in a sense by Billy himself as he repeatedly seemed to reject her food. I was very careful not to compete with Kathie in any way for Billy's attention, nor did I actually intervene and do things for Billy, even though at times I could hardly restrain myself. It was important for Kathie to feel that I, as a child consultant, identified with her as a mother facing problems in caring for her baby and that I had confidence that Kathie, with my help, could give Billy what he needed in order for him to be a healthy baby. Together we observed Billy, his preferences and his dislikes, and took joy in any of his accomplishments. Billy's accomplishments were always related back to Kathie's efforts. I especially shared my observations with Kathie of any special feeling that Billy expressed toward her, as his mother, such as a preferential smile or a reaching out to her. Kathie's feeling of failure was so strong that she was amazed when Billy preferred to go to her rather than to me. She clung to any bit of evidence that Billy liked her. When she saw the videotaped scene of herself in the rocking chair with Billy, she said, "That looks so peaceful, Billy looks so contented."

GUIDANCE: INFANT NURTURE AND MOTHER NURTURE

Within this framework, and relying very largely upon the positive transference, I introduced suggestions for feeding and burping Billy that were effective in a very short time. While these issues are treated topically in the pages that follow, they were actually concurrent and interwoven in every session.

The first concrete changes came in Kathie's willingness to try to hold Billy for a feeding. Kathie had said that Billy did not like to be held, she knew this because he turned away. I commented that even though Billy turned away, his body seemed to be more relaxed and I thought this indicated that he did like his mother to hold him. It was obvious that Kathie's bland, sad face could not hold Billy's attention when she was trying to feed him in her arms. One time, as I watched Kathie trying to do so, Billy repeatedly turned away. Seeking a tactful way to guide Kathie to a livelier exchange with her baby, I asked her if she ever told Billy stories. She said, "No." I asked if I could tell Billy a story while Kathie held him, and she agreed. I began my story, "Once upon a time there were three bears," using what Stern (1973) describes as "normal baby talk expression," elongation of smile, rise and fall of voice, exaggerated nuances. All of these are typical exchange behaviors between baby and mother. All were missing from Kathie's conversation with Billy.

Billy and his mother *both* loved the story. Billy began to smile and make eye contact with me and his mother, as together we watched him. Kathie so enjoyed this herself, as both child and mother, that she herself began to tell Billy stories and, of course, Billy quickly began to respond. However, this took so much effort on Kathie's part that she was often fatigued and once again lapsed into her silent behavior.

A major concern was the burping process. I had made many suggestions to Kathie about burping Billy and had tried to help Kathie understand how her method would precipitate vomiting. It was only when I actually stood beside her, however, and shared with her the tension she was feeling, as she put Billy gently over her shoulder with the diaper underneath him, that she was gradually able to begin burping Billy in a normal fashion.

Kathie began to feed Billy the bottle in her arms on a regular basis. She was still not feeding him solids. During a number of interviews it became clear that this was part of more complicated feelings about feeding Billy. At this point we identified two fears: Kathie's fear that "Billy would eat the family out of house and home" and that he would throw up endlessly.

While we recognized that these fears were deeply rooted in Kathie's personality, we knew that we could not uncover the origins of these fears in the emergency period. And Billy's needs were paramount. We would have to help Kathie in a concrete, educational way to provide caloric adequacy for Billy.

I was able to use the positive transference in supporting Kathie step by step in a feeding program for Billy. It was futile, of course, to challenge Kathie's irrational belief that Billy would "eat the family out of house and home" or that he would "throw up endlessly." I only sympathized with Kathie's fears and led her gently into a collaboration on Billy's behalf.

With pencil and paper and measuring cups, Kathie and I worked out quantities and sample feedings. We soon saw that Kathie could follow this regime. Long afterward we are still wondering how this was possible in view of the fact that food quantities were still bound up with profound conflicts in Kathie. Our best guess is that the objective, "on paper" feeding plan relieved Kathie of the responsibility for dealing with her own unconscious and dangerous impulses toward her baby. "Siding with the ego," I as therapist was lending my own quiet authority to support Kathie's positive strivings to mother and her defenses against the destructive wishes.

In many discussions with me, Kathie expressed her fear and revulsion at Billy's throwing up. I acknowledged that I could understand how especially difficult it was for Kathie to hold and feed Billy. I told Kathie that together we would pay special attention to insure that Billy would not throw up through overeating and that I wanted Kathie to observe carefully how much he ate and whether or not he threw up. With much relief at my understanding of her difficulty, Kathie agreed to place Billy on a solid feeding schedule, which she and I monitored carefully.

Figure 2. Growth Curves Relationed to Intervention

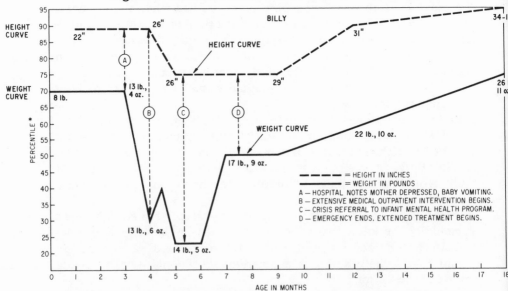

NOTE: * These percentiles for infant boys are based on the Anthropometric Chart of the Children's Medical Center, Boston.

Billy began to gain weight steadily. Vomiting virtually disappeared. By 7 months, Billy had gained 2 pounds 8 ounces and reached the 50th percentile in weight; the pediatrician was satisfied that Billy was no longer in nutritional peril.

THE FAMILY'S PROGRESS

During the time this work was progressing, we were, of course, concerned with the well-being of the whole family, Mr. and Mrs. Douglas and Billy. An important part of the work was the help given to Mr. Douglas. He came from a large, impoverished family and had suffered physical and emotional privations in his own childhood. As a young husband and father he was again struggling with poverty and hunger, and his depressed young wife drained his emotional resources. Each member of the family was hungry for physical and emotional sustenance. When John was home, he too shared his worries with me, and I responded with sympathetic understanding and with attention to his problems. I helped John and Kathie find ways to work out their present financial difficulties. I let them know that their hunger was my concern as well.

In summary, the work during the emergency period brought Billy to nutritional adequacy, and his parents had formed a strong alliance with me as therapist on behalf of their baby. Kathie, however, was still depressed, and we remained concerned about her and Billy.

The Extended Treatment Phase

REASSESSMENT

The period that we speak of as the extended treatment phase carried the work with Billy and his parents for a full year beyond the emergency period. While Billy had made progress, we still regarded him as a baby "at risk" in the psychological sense.

In the area of human attachments we saw much that we considered ominous. Billy did not respond to his parents in ways that were appropriate for a child of his age. He still avoided eye contact with his mother by turning away. He preferred play with toys rather than human partners. When he was hungry or in need, he still cried helplessly and piteously.

It seemed to us that Kathie was now able to follow much of my advice, but her responses were always mechanical. She was still unable to mother Billy in a harmonious and spontaneous manner; she still seemed estranged from her baby. She appeared to hold back food and only slowly responded to Billy's hunger cries. She was not empathic with Billy's attempts to communicate distress or hunger. The interaction between mother and baby was still erratic, and Billy could never really count on a pleasurable response from his mother. Very often Kathie teased Billy with food and seemed to be competing with him.

As part of our continuing assessment, when Billy was 7½ months old, we videotaped another playroom visit which included a Bayley Developmental Assessment and a spontaneous feeding. The Bayley showed that Billy was slightly above the median, in both mental and motor scores overall, but differentially lagged in beginning language items.

This tape spoke eloquently for the mother's ambivalence toward her baby and for a profound conflict in the mother which was now centered on the baby.

In one scene Kathie was holding Billy in her arms in a close and tender way while she was feeding him his bottle. Suddenly, she pulled the bottle away, tossed back her head, dropped some milk in her own mouth, and then engaged Billy in a teasing game in which she was competing with him for his bottle. She repeated this "game" several times in a five-minute interval. It was painful to watch, but more painful was our witness to the baby's reactions: He was laughing. He had become a partner in this sadomasochistic game.

We have learned to give such "baby games" serious clinical attention. Some of our most important clinical insights have been derived from observing parents at play with their babies. The parent in conflict frequently reveals the essence of the conflict in play, in the "harmless games" (Fraiberg 1974).

What we saw on tape, then, was a young mother competing with her own baby for his bottle. The moments of tender mothering were interrupted by an intruding thought, and feeding the baby became "teasing the baby," "taking food out of his mouth," "jealousy," "competition." As the staff watched this tape, we were struck by the thought that the mother behaved as if her baby were a sibling—and at that point the story began to come together for us.

THE GHOST IN BILLY'S NURSERY

By this time we had come to know a fair amount about Kathie and her own childhood. In the emergency phase of treatment, this was information we could register and store but could not put into use for Kathie's treatment. Kathie had regarded herself as the unwanted middle child of her family, the no-good child who could "never do anything right." While Kathie had spoken with some acidity about her mother and her older sister, she could barely control her rage when she spoke about Essie, her younger sister. "Essie got everything," she said bitterly. Her memories of Essie, which may have been distorted, linked Essie to food in many ways. One of the bitterest memories, possibly a screen memory, was of a time when Kathie's parents took Essie out for an ice-cream cone and left Kathie home to do the dishes. Essie was the good child, the child that Kathie's mother favored.

We knew that Billy had been the "intruder" in Kathie's current life, the unwanted baby, the baby who "spoiled everything" for her, the baby who was taking food out of her mouth. There was a ghost in Billy's nursery, we thought, and the name of the ghost was Essie. Essie was the first intruder, the first baby in Kathie's life, who deprived her of the good things in life, of mother, and, in symbolic terms, of food.

If we were right, the therapeutic problem for us was to get the ghost out of the baby's nursery. We would need to help Kathie deal with the repetition of the conflicted past in the present, to disengage Billy from the figures of the past.

THE CHILDHOOD CONFLICTS AND REPETITIONS IN THE PRESENT

Our treatment during this period united guidance on behalf of Billy and a therapy which explicitly focused on Kathie's conflicts in mothering and their origins in her own childhood conflicts.

The setting remained the same: home visits, scheduled twice weekly. Kathie was a willing and eager collaborator in her own treatment, to find out "why" she felt herself the victim of her own past.

Typically, the sessions would begin with Billy in the living room or the kitchen, and Kathie and I would speak about Billy's progress or discuss any of Kathie's questions. I continued, of course, to offer my observations, to help Kathie herself to observe Billy, to interpret his needs and his signals, and to praise his accomplishments and her own growth as a mother. Kathie's own need for my time sometimes brought her into competition with Billy. Billy always had "his" time, during part of each session, and sometimes when Kathie felt most urgently in need of time, she would say, "Shh, Billy, it's *my* turn now." Usually the visits were timed so that Billy's nap would divide the session and give Kathie some time for privacy.

In nearly every succeeding session her childhood grievances appeared with more and more intensity. But vitriolic anger toward Essie, the first intruder, dominated many of these hours.

The transference was employed both to open up the past and to offer Kathie, the "unfinished" adolescent, a new figure for identification and for undoing the powerful effects of her own mother, remembered as rejecting, critical, suspicious, and harsh, the "witch-mother" of early girlhood and adolescence.

The flow of memories converged again and again on the time following the birth of Essie, a period which marked a profound shift in Kathie's relationship to her own mother. Allowing for much distortion in adolescent memory, the figure of Essie, the baby who robbed Kathie of her mother and the figure of the mother who "rejected" Kathie for the new baby were persistent ghosts. Along with these memories came overwhelming feelings of grief, depression, mourning for herself as a neglected, unwanted child. These were the feelings which had been revived with the birth of Billy. In Kathie's living room, with her own baby, I often had the eerie feeling that I was witnessing another time, that Kathie was again the bereaved 5-year-old robbed for the second time by a baby. Kathie was locked once again in the infantile conflict.

The therapeutic relationship opened up many pathways for "undoing."

"My mother never listened to me" was Kathie's reproach, a recurrent theme in these hours, but I listened and responded to Kathie's feelings of grief and rage. "My mother said I was bad. It was bad to hate my sister." I acknowledged and accepted the feelings of jealousy and anger toward the sister "who got everything." "My mother never understood me." I explicitly told Kathie that I wanted to understand her. "My mother said I couldn't do anything right." I sided with Kathie who wanted to "do things right," and could give honest support to the many aspects of Kathie's growth as wife and mother in which she showed her good capacities. Since Kathie believed that her own mother did not find satisfaction in motherhood and did not provide a model for mothering that Kathie felt she could use, I shared many moments with Kathie when she achieved great satisfaction with Billy. Moreover, I offered an alternative model for mothering, which Kathie could use if she wished.

When muted or sullen anger appeared in the transference, I helped Kathie put her anger into words and to discover that the anger would not destroy me or the positive relationship we had developed and could, indeed, open pathways to the conflicted past and ways to find meaning in that anger.

We now select themes from the work of this period. In the process of treatment these themes were, of course, interwoven.

KATHIE, ESSIE, AND BILLY

The story of Essie, the first intruder, emerged as a central theme in Kathie's sessions when Billy was 8 months old. Kathie was still a reluctant mother to her baby, mechanically following the advice on feeding, now holding Billy for feedings and providing adequacy in caloric intake, but with little spontaneity or joy in her exchanges with the baby.

As memories of Essie emerged, accompanied by rage toward that first baby "who spoiled everything," and as grief for herself as a small girl was revived, we began to see for the first time a spontaneous reaching out to Billy. This is described in an excerpt from a visit with Kathie when Billy was 8 months old:

> I had asked Kathie if she could tell me what it was like for her when her own baby sister was born. She said, "I've told you I hated my sister, how she always came between me and my mother. I don't remember much. When my sister was little, I remember being outside of the house much of the time. I do remember a couple of things. I didn't want to play with her. I hated to be told to play with her, and I told my father that I hated her."
>
> At this time, Kathie had her hand raised and was shaking it in the air. (I think she was nonverbally imitating her father talking to her and was speaking for her father.) She said, in a deep voice, "No child of mine can hate another sister. You play with her."
>
> After a while Kathie continued: "The first time I really got angry with my sister was when my parents took my sister out for ice cream and left me to do the dishes. I was so mad, I decided to run away. My mother found me and dragged me back to the house. She was angry at me for leaving." I asked if she had told her mother how she felt. Kathie said she had told her mother that she had run away because she didn't want to be left at home when they went out. I asked if her mother had understood. Kathie said sadly, "She said she did, but"—and shook her head helplessly—"nothing changed."
>
> At this moment a dramatic shift occurred. Kathie got up, went to Billy who was playing on the floor, swept him up in her arms, brought him back to her lap, hugged him, and started to play pat-a-cake with him, in a warm, thoughtful manner. She looked over at me (I was facing Billy's back) and she invited me to come and see Billy's face. Billy was ecstatic. On previous visits I had suggested traditional baby games which Kathie could play with Billy. Kathie had never before picked up on this.

In this excerpt, then, we see that as Kathie reexperiences the rage toward Essie, she can turn toward her own baby and spontaneously show her affection for him. She plays a game with him with full enjoyment, and we recall the words she had used in the early part of this session when she spoke of Essie: "I didn't want to play with her. I hated to be told to play with her." As the affective pathways lead back to Essie, Kathie is able to disengage Billy from the first intruder and, as if some preconscious association had taken place around "play," she gives the "no" to Essie and the "yes" to Billy. Where Kathie's mother "didn't understand" and both parents sternly prohibited the expression of anger toward Essie, I understood and accepted the words "I hated her." The play with Billy was also, then, a gift to me, her therapist.

This was the first time that we saw this pattern. We were to see it many times in the sessions that followed. When Kathie expressed strong feelings of anger toward her sister or sadness in remembering the rejection by her own mother, she was able to reach out to Billy and hold him close to her. I could now become more active in interpreting to Kathie the displacement of feelings from Essie to Billy.

The ghost of Essie appeared in many disguises. For weeks I was puzzled by a complaint from Kathie: Billy, Kathie said, drove her to distraction when he followed her around the house. From my point of view, Billy's following of mother and touching base with her were a most welcome sign of the growing attachment between Billy and his mother. Kathie found it nearly intolerable and took a dim view of my ideas on the subject.

Then, in an interview when Billy was 8½ months old, Kathie quite unconsciously provided the vital clue. Kathie was delivering a tirade against Essie:

> "The worst thing that I hated—I was about 9 or 10—was when my sister followed me all around the house. She used to stare at me and whisper like me and repeat what I said. I used to tell my mother, but my mother said I was crazy and she could not understand what I was talking about. I couldn't stand it. I spent more and more time away from home. I wanted my mother to stop her, but my mother wouldn't." I asked her what it was that had bothered her so much. Kathie said that she didn't know, didn't care, she only hated it. She just didn't want to have anything to do with her sister at that time.
>
> After a few moments I asked her what it was like for her when Billy followed her around the house. Kathie said, "It's entirely different." Then she laughed. She understood. Kathie went to Billy and picked him up. She cuddled him, and put him on her lap so that he was lying on her knee, and tickled his back until Billy was laughing and giggling. He seemed delighted.

With this new insight, Kathie could now use more of the developmental and guidance information that was offered. For example, regarding Billy's following her, I explained that he wanted to keep her in sight at home because he was attached to her. At 8 months mother's presence was reassuring. As Billy grew, he would be able to remember her presence even if she was in another room. He would not have to follow her all the time.

Kathie's relationship to Billy was beginning to have moments of tenderness, spontaneity, and joy. She was making obvious progress in becoming a mother to Billy. She was manifestly enjoying Billy, proud of his achievements, gratified by his steady weight gain, and eager for his response to her.

However, although the teasing games with Billy receded during this period, I still caught glimpses of "teasing" that concerned us. On an educational level I had dealt directly with the teasing games during feeding. I pointed out that these were games that might lead to problems Kathie would not really want to see in Billy. I spoke of the meaning that food and love had for babies as well as for adults. What did these games mean to Billy? Kathie consciously made an effort to give up the teasing games and was partially successful. Yet the urge to tease Billy still broke through in a game she played with him, and more explicitly, in her withholding food from him when he was manifestly hungry, responding only to his most urgent cries.

Billy, meanwhile, was responding to his mother's efforts by sometimes showing preferential responses to her in significant ways. But one aberrant tendency remained. At 9 months of age he still avoided eye contact with his mother. Even in baby games with Kathie when she smiled and encouraged him, he turned his head away from her. In one sequence on tape, we saw Kathie playing pat-a-cake with Billy on her lap, facing her, and the baby—though participating in the game— averted his head to avoid eye contact with his mother. Kathie, encouraged by me, repeated the game until finally Billy rewarded her by smiling and cooing, but still turned away from her. I interpreted the smiling and vocalizing as his way of telling mother he enjoyed the game. Perhaps soon he would also give her the reciprocal gaze she so wanted as affirmation of his affection toward her. Kathie, we saw with sadness for her plight, had to work very hard to woo her baby after the many months of avoidance and neglect.

Then, when Billy was 11 months old, the meaning of the teasing games and a facet of Kathie's uncontrollable urge to inflict pain broke through in a session:

Kathie had recently returned from a visit to her own family and was angrily recounting what had happened. Once again Kathie did the dishes while Essie disappeared from the kitchen, and once again Essie got all of mother's attention.

Kathie said, "I hate my sister. She doesn't do anything. Just like now when my mother needs her. I have hated her ever since the time I was asked to take care of her and my little cousin together. I could have been with my friends, I really didn't want to do it, but I did. After a few days, my sister said to me, 'Bug off, we all hate you, we don't want you here.' "

In response to my question, "What did you do?" Kathie said, "I told my mother. She just shrugged it off." I asked, "How did you feel?" "I hated her." I said, "It really hurt, didn't it?" She replied, "Yes." Her face was red and she was very tense. I said, "It seems as though you are still angry." She said, "Yes."

Kathie continued, "I told you how I would try to get her into trouble, how I would make up stories, how I would tease her. I would tell my mother things that she would do. When she got me really mad I would shake her."

Kathie was so caught up in feelings of rage toward her sister in the past that without thinking she reached and grabbed Billy's arm and began shak-

ing him angrily saying, "I would shake her like *this* and like *this*." Billy started to cry, obviously scared. I was scared for him. His tears and my concern
brought her back to the present. She stopped abruptly. She was shocked and
said, "Sorry, Billy, I didn't meant to hurt you."

I said, "I can see how angry you feel at your sister, and now I understand
how you felt before." Kathie nodded. I asked her whether she sometimes got
mad at Billy in the way she got mad at her sister, as though he were like her
sister.

Kathie had an immediate response. She said, "No" in an emphatic voice
and moved away from me. "I never get mad at Billy that way." Soon Kathie
went over to Billy, started to play with him, got down on the floor, and for a
long time held him and cuddled him.

Thus the teasing and sadistic rage toward Essie emerged from memory and could also be observed in a direct displacement toward Billy.
After many interpretations, in this visit and others, of the repetition of
feelings from the past in the present, Kathie's quick denial finally gave
way to affirmation and insight.

The insight was very meaningful to Kathie and further freed Billy
from being the target of her feelings of anger toward her sister. During
the next visits we began to see a new depth in the relationship between
Kathie and Billy. Teasing of Billy was significantly reduced and began
to disappear. Kathie began spontaneously to reach out to Billy and, on
her own, began to interact with him in such a way that both of them
received great pleasure. Our observations also began to show some incidents of mutual gaze and approaches between Billy and Kathie.

KATHIE AND HER MOTHER

The competitiveness with Billy was only one of the many themes
that appeared throughout the work with Kathie. There was another important theme. We had often observed her seeming indifference to Billy's cries. Many times it seemed as if she and Billy were crying together. There was no mother present in the room. With great sadness and
anger Kathie would say that her mother had not understood her. Once
again I acknowledged that Kathie too had much need to be heard, to be
loved, and to be understood and nurtured.

I asked many times what it was that Kathie most wanted her mother
and perhaps me to understand. Gradually her true feelings emerged.
She did not want to be a mother, she had never wanted to be a mother,
and she was not ready to give up her role as a child. She had in fact not
really separated from her own family.

With great sadness Kathie told me of the very painful relationship
she had had with her own mother. She felt that her mother was never
satisfied with her, especially as a daughter. Kathie said that she had always been the family "boy," loved by her father and ridiculed by her

mother. As a little girl she had never played with dolls, but had always preferred to play with the neighborhood boys. As she approached puberty, she was accused by her mother of being too seductive. Nothing she did was right. With great hurt she described how her mother had said that she could never be as pretty as her older sister or as good as the younger sister. She began to go out with John, whom her mother had liked. During this time Kathie's mother had begun to enter menopause and was wishing explicitly for a grandchild. Kathie's older sister did not have any children. Kathie got pregnant and had Billy. Kathie, with hurt and anger, said that now her mother had a grandchild, but for her Billy's birth was not all that it was supposed to have been. The fantasy of renewed babyhood for Kathie never materialized. Now that Billy was born, he was the grandparents' pride, not Kathie. She was only 17 and faced with an entirely new role, that of motherhood, which she did not want.

In the work with Kathie, her ambivalence toward Billy now became overt. Even as she expressed her ambivalence, we began to see progress in her relationship with Billy. As she spoke of these feelings, she began to be able to respond to him.

Nearly every session was related to Billy's needs in one way or another. Billy was approaching 12 months of age, a time when he did not yet have words for needs. As Kathie would weep for herself and berate the mother who never heard her cries and needs, Billy oftentimes needed her.

At first Kathie was unable to interpret Billy's cries, and I would talk for him. For example, many times Billy was in his playpen and wanted to get out, but Kathie was unable to respond. I would talk for Billy, and say, "Mom, I'm trying to tell you that I want out of the playpen, but I don't have any words yet." Kathie would then respond. We had many discussions about the ways in which Billy tried to communicate with her without words. When Kathie did respond, I always rewarded her efforts. I might say, "Isn't it good to have a mommy who hears you and understands you? Even mommy has to be understood."

The first sign that Kathie was beginning to hear Billy and to be empathic with him was her ability to comfort him when he cried. She would pick him up in her arms, hold him closely, and pat his head. Eventually she anticipated his needs for both food and play. She took pride in his attempt to communicate and in her attempts to understand him, which I encouraged and reinforced. She began to identify more strongly as Billy's mother. In fact, she started to let me know that she knew Billy better than I, and I, of course, stepped back from the role of active interpreter.

As we traced the content of these sessions "on being a mother" and the therapeutic work in this area, we could see the effects of reexperiencing, "undoing," and insight in Kathie's own ability to be a mother.

When Kathie's own cries were heard by me she began to respond to her baby's cries. When Kathie's needs were "understood" by me, she began to interpret the signs of needs in her baby. When hostile feelings toward Billy could be put into words, they no longer exerted their influence in distancing Kathie from Billy; she was free to enjoy him. When the powerful ambivalence toward her own mother came into the therapeutic work, Kathie "completed" her own adolescence and became free of the "witch-mother" who impeded her own development as wife and mother.

Termination of Treatment and Follow-up

The major part of our therapeutic work was achieved by the time Billy reached his first birthday. Our work continued until he was 18 months old, when the family moved to another community. John found new work, which brought financial security to the family.

Billy, at 1 year of age, already reflected both the changes in Kathie which were brought about in her treatment and the developmental guidance which Kathie could now use on his behalf with spontaneity and self-assuredness.

There were no residual feeding problems; Billy at 12 months and at the follow-up (25 months) was a child who enjoyed food. He had no food idiosyncrasies or conflicts with his mother around feeding. There were no symptoms or disorders in the areas of orality or beginning autonomy. We watched carefully for signs of affective disturbances and saw none. We worried about possible residues from the sadomasochistic feeding games, which had so concerned us when Billy was 8 months old, but we could identify no sequelae in the second-year behavior picture.

In his second year, Billy was a cheerful, exuberant, busy little boy, curious, eager to learn, pleased with himself. Language development was excellent.

Most important of all, Billy's attachment to his mother was secure, mutually satisfying, and demonstrably joyous. In direct observations and in a number of vignettes on videotape we saw special smiles for mother, good eye contact, seeking of mother for comfort and protection, enjoyment of games and play with mother and father, and, equally important, a steady growth in self-confidence and independence.

Billy had become an endearing child to both his parents, and their pride and pleasure in him came through in nearly every visit. (He was also, objectively, an endearing child as others saw him.)

The therapeutic work with Kathie succeeded in freeing her and Billy from those aspects of a conflicted childhood that were being reenacted between her and her baby. In some measure, we believe, the work also resulted in the completion of Kathie's own adolescence. The resolution of infantile conflicts between Kathie and her mother freed her to become a mother and a wife in her own right. For not only did Kathie become a mother who enjoyed her child; we also saw many positive changes in her relationship to her husband, and the marriage gained in stability. While the work with Father had been less intensive, he, too, had worked through many conflicts regarding his now much treasured son.

FOLLOW-UP

When Billy and his parents were seen in follow-up at 25 months, we were satisfied that he and his parents had sustained the gains of treatment. With only minimal therapeutic support and guidance during the period that followed their move from our community, both parents showed growth as young adults and had brought wisdom and good judgment to their rearing of Billy. They were justifiably proud of Billy· and his achievements and spoke tenderly of his affectionate nature and his endearing ways of greeting his parents when he woke each morning.

Toilet training was proceeding smoothly. There was no sense of pressure in either Kathie or John. In Billy's play we discerned no anxieties in connection with the toilet or cleanliness.

Recalling Kathie's earlier revulsion toward vomiting and messiness, we were interested to see that none of this had carried over to the toilet training of Billy. Since our work had not dealt with the deeper layers of this revulsion in Kathie, we wondered why the area of toilet training had not been contaminated. Then I remembered that throughout the early critical period of the treatment, I had observed many diaperings of Billy and at no time had Kathie shown revulsion toward the baby's feces or cleaning the anal region. It was, then, specifically an oral revulsion on Kathie's part, in which food and vomit may have had anal determinants but were curiously not manifest in connection with anal functions.

One vignette from our last records of Billy and his family is cherished by all of us. I had made a visit to the new home of the Douglases when Billy was 20 months old. Billy remembered me well and was very much a delighted child seeing an old friend. At one point he left the room and returned with a handful of Chinese noodles which he pressed in my hand. Kathie said, "He likes you. He always does this. He likes to share his favorite foods with people he likes."

Three years later, when Billy was 5, the family came to see me at the Child Development Project. Billy had entered kindergarten, and the proud parents wanted to share their pleasure with me. At school Billy was apparently an outstanding student. The teacher had wanted to know what preschool program he had attended that accounted for his special social and intellectual abilities. His mother proudly told me, "I was the preschool program." Billy was tall, handsome, warm, verbal, and with a twinkling eye and good sense of humor. There was warmth, openness, and trust between Billy and his parents that was delightful to see. In the visit it was apparent that Kathie and John had worked hard to continue successfully their own growth as young adults. The parents spoke gratefully of the help they had received almost five years ago, which they realized had enabled them all to come through a most difficult time. Most of all, they enjoyed Billy tremendously, and he obviously felt good about them and about himself.

BIBLIOGRAPHY

Fraiberg, S. 1974. "The Clinical Dimensions of Baby Games." *Journal of the American Academy of Child Psychiatry* 13: 202–220.
Stern, D. N. 1973. "Mothers and Infants at Play," in *The effect of the Infant on the Caregiver*. New York: John Wiley, Lewis, M., and Rosenblum, L., eds., pp. 187–213.

IX

An Abandoned Mother, an Abandoned Baby

EDNA ADELSON

SELMA FRAIBERG

THIS CASE REPORT differs in focus from other clinical studies in this volume.* It was originally prepared in response to questions from our colleagues. The questions were: "How are psychotherapeutic principles adapted in your treatment when an infant and mother are both patients and when the therapy itself is conducted largely through home visits?" "What transpires in typical therapeutic sessions in this form of treatment?"

The format chosen for the presentation of the case of Beth and Trudy emerged in response to these questions. Two early sessions of the treatment were selected for presentation and the events of those sessions are described in clinical detail. When the report was presented, the work on this extraordinarily difficult case was only six months in progress and the outcome could not be known. Yet we felt it served to illustrate how an infant's needs and behaviors resonate with his parent's repressed memories and how this interaction, in turn, can provide the impetus and the material for psychotherapy. For the readers of this volume we have added a brief epilogue in which we report Trudy's progress at her third birthday, when treatment ended.

---

* Edna Adelson was the therapist; Selma Fraiberg was the supervisor. The first-person singular refers to Edna Adelson.

221

Introduction to Beth and Trudy

Beth was an unmarried teenage mother. Her history was reported to us by the hospital social worker who made the referral when Trudy was 4½ months old. Trudy had been diagnosed as a "failure to thrive" baby, a baby who was being starved. Beth herself had once been a starving infant. She had been found in the streets of a war-torn country, abandoned and unfed. After an unknown period in an orphanage she was adopted at age 2½ by an American family who had several children of their own. Beth was an unhappy and difficult child. She ate poorly and vomited. She was fearful and cried a good deal, but she could not be held or comforted. There were sleeping problems, then behavior problems, and eventually learning problems. She was a marginal student, rebellious and unpredictable at home. Before she was 17 she was pregnant.

Beth's pregnancy and delivery were normal, and the baby was a healthy 7 pounds at birth. The baby was to be placed for adoption in order that Beth could return home and complete high school. Instead, Beth came home with the baby, only to find that her mother refused to let her stay if she kept Trudy. Beth would not give her baby up. She applied for Aid to Dependent Children (ADC) and moved into a low-cost housing apartment. Beth was depressed, unable to take care of herself or Trudy. At 1 month of age, Trudy was eating and sleeping poorly,

Figure 3. Weight Changes Related to Intervention

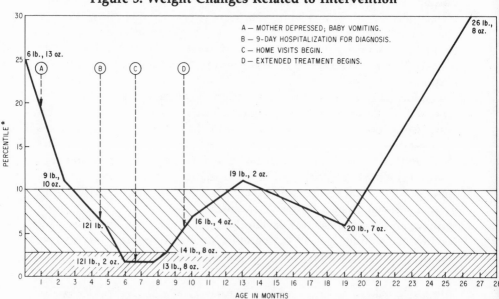

NOTE: * Birth percentile based on Colorado Intrauterine Growth Charts; other percentiles based on the Anthropometric Chart of Children's Medical Center, Boston.

vomiting, and crying; she had become a vivid re-creation of Beth's own past deprivation and terror. At 2 months of age, Trudy entered a day-care nursery. Group care by day was thus added to the neglect at home. Beth was scolded and given advice by her family, the daycare staff, and the pediatrician. Beth appeared sullen and defiant, and the baby's condition worsened. Trudy became increasingly apathetic. Fear for Trudy's survival grew when her weight fell toward the 3rd percentile of the normal growth curve. (See Figure 3.)

At 4½ months of age, Trudy was hospitalized for medical examination and more adequate feeding. Beth seldom visited. After ten days of good nursing care Trudy still vomited and had not gained any weight. The primary diagnosis was "failure to thrive due to low caloric intake and severe maternal deprivation." The question of a malfunction of the esophagus was raised, but no organic cause was found. When Trudy was discharged, the hospital staff referred her to the Child Development Project, and the case was assigned to me. But Beth would not meet me. Trudy returned to the daycare nursery and Beth to school. Some friends, Tom and Don, moved in with Beth and joined the chorus of voices urging her to tend to the baby. Nothing changed. The sad story of Beth's own abandonment and deprivation was being replayed. Again Beth had lost her mother. Again a small baby hungered and cried and no one heard, no one helped.

The help offered through the Child Development Project was not wanted. Indeed, we were not sure we could help since so many of those who already knew Beth described her as hard to reach. She was said to be the most difficult child in her family, the most difficult adolescent mother at the daycare center, the most difficult mother of a "failure to thrive" baby seen at the hospital. Whenever I called the high school or pediatric clinic, no one knew where Beth was or when she would come to leave or retrieve the baby. She had no telephone, so there was no way to get in touch with her. I located Beth at last when the pediatrician let me know the baby had a clinic appointment. By then Trudy was 6 months old. Since I knew her condition was so morbid that the next steps would be hospitalization and notification of Protective Services, I hurried to reach the clinic before Beth and Trudy were gone. Trudy was a desolate sight. Her tattered clothes were damp from vomit. Scraggly dark hair framed a gaunt, wary face. Beth was cornered, glowering at the hospital staff who were giving her up for lost, who could even take her baby away.

Beth's fear and doubt of me were heightened by the circumstances of our meeting. Her past was filled with broken or disappointing relationships, meaning that a formidable negative transference had to be dealt with immediately. My acknowledgment of Beth's fury, disappointment, and distrust enabled her to visit me twice that week. She made constant demands on me. She changed the meeting times. I agreed. She asked for Trudy's hospital records. I got them. She wanted to scold the hospital social worker. I summoned her. Beth came, bringing the baby and also the daycare counselor.

It was dreadful to see how things were for mother and for baby. Trudy was no longer normal, and there was no way for Beth to deal with this. On each visit Trudy sat or lay on the couch vomiting copiously. She drifted to sleep with glassy, unclosed eyes. When Beth cried out loudly that no one listened to her or understood her, Trudy stiffened and cried out too. But Beth could not understand or help her baby. Her rough handling made Trudy cry more, so Beth left the baby alone. The daycare counselor cuddled Trudy, who calmed and smiled with the awful smile of a baby with marasmus. As Beth's desperation and anxiety mounted during the visits, she too deteriorated; her thinking became confused, at times bizarre.

I did not offer any advice on diet or feeding at this time because I felt it would go unheard. It seemed wiser to wait until direct observations could provide me with a better sense of Beth's conflicts about offering food to her baby. However, I did express my wish to understand how this situation had come to be. I said Beth could talk to me and I would listen.

The Past and the Present

Beth accepted my permission to recall and to speak of her feelings, and on her next visit she came alone. She wanted me to know in what ways Trudy was just like her. She reviewed the parallels: Beth had vomited as a child, now Trudy vomited; Beth had been in the hospital with pneumonia, now Trudy was getting very sick. Beth knew something was wrong. She insisted it was "medical" and that there must be an answer. It was evident that Beth could name the similarities between her and her baby, but she could not recover the affective links by herself. I encouraged her to tell me more about herself. Beth said she was adopted. She was told that she had been left to wander alone because her own true mother could not feed her. As she spoke, it was plain that she did not see the parallel with her own inability to feed Trudy. Beth spoke on: After she left the orphanage and reached this country, she was malnourished and fell ill. In response I began to summon up the crying child of long ago. With much feeling I spoke of how it must have been for a frightened little child to take such a long trip, to find herself among strangers, to face a world completely different from all she had ever known. I said she must have cried a good deal. Beth fell silent. Then she said that she wished she could see her own old hospital records in addition to Trudy's.

I said that Beth thought something in the past could explain things now; such questions and memories about the past often come back when a mother has a new baby. Beth's thoughts then moved to her becoming a mother, deciding to remain a mother, and being cast out by her adoptive mother. She pondered her decision to keep her baby. She had not meant to, but once Trudy had been born she found she could not do to her baby what had been done to her. She could not give her away. She paused, reaching to touch my knee, to ask if she was boring me. Assured that I would listen, she continued with an outpouring about her pregnancy and delivery. There was much sadness in her voice. She was near tears as she told of the terrible fight with her mother, who shouted, "No one will let you keep the baby! What have you got to give a baby anyway?" Beth, deeply hurt, had hidden her tears from her mother and left. She had been thrown out again to fend for herself.

After asking my permission to talk once more, she reviewed the delivery of the baby. As she spoke, she seemed to glow; her voice was touched with awe. She said that when the baby was born and she heard the baby cry, it was a feeling too hard to describe, a feeling she would never forget. The cry of her newborn had made a powerful claim on Beth. Beth had then returned home to make the same claim on her mother, who could neither accept the baby nor deal with her frightened daughter's pain and tears. Beth told of Trudy's current crying. These screams made her so tense she did not know what to do. She asked if I would come to the house to see if I could help when the baby cried, maybe at bath time. I agreed. I felt I was being asked to hear two crying voices, Beth's and Trudy's. There were two lost babies who were given up and thrown out. The positive transference was growing. Our hope was that when I could help Beth experience similarities in affective experience with her baby, make them real for her, Beth would be able to give to Trudy that which had not been given to her.

Beth must have regretted her invitation, for no one was home when I arrived. I left a note and waited for word. On the day of Trudy's next checkup the hospital called with bad news. Beth was too tired to come in, so she sent the baby with her friends, Tom and Don. And Trudy was losing weight. I went to the house at once, and this time Beth was at home. That visit, the fifth, when Trudy was 0:6:22, will be reported in some detail. It will demonstrate some of the ways in which treatment proceeds when the baby remains the focus and is physically present.

The Fifth Visit

Beth and I stepped over bags of trash to settle on the crumbling mattresses in the dark living room. Beth knew the baby was thinner and feared the worst. The boys soon arrived and Tom laid the sleeping baby beside her mother in the rumpled bedding. Beth appeared cold and indifferent. She ignored the baby and lit a cigarette. Tom reported on the checkup, emphasizing that the doctor wanted the baby to have whole milk because she needed the calories. In the course of the next hour, with many interruptions, a tragic story emerged. As I listened, I realized that Beth was actively starving the baby. She was giving her very dilute skim milk in a desperate effort to halt the vomiting. But worse, Beth became completely out of touch when I asked when Trudy had eaten last. With alarming vagueness Beth thought the baby had eaten half a jar of some kind of food, maybe yesterday or the day before.

I fell silent as Tom argued with Beth about another kind of neglect; she never went to the baby when Trudy cried and did not want anyone else to hold her. Tom was sure you should pick a baby up. He said, "You have to let a baby know you care." Then, turning to Beth, he said, "You know, your brother once told me that you screamed and screamed when you were a baby." Beth's coolness gave way to furious outrage. "What do you know about it! When I was two I went from that orphanage all the way to a new home. It was a long, terrible trip and I didn't know anybody when I got here. Nobody could understand me and I was frightened!" She continued, as if old pictures were flashing before her. "Everyone looked different and I was scared." I spoke then to establish a link between that screaming child who was now a mother and her screaming, neglected baby who was one of my two patients. I said that it would be very hard for a small child to be alone among strangers. Crying and crying would be the only outlet for her when they did not understand her needs and she did not understand them. I felt that Beth heard me and registered the double reference.

She half listened as the boys continued a fine discussion of child care. Beth seemed absorbed in thought and when she next spoke, it was to ask, "Could memories from long, long ago, memories that are forgotten, still be in the back of someone's head?" And she placed her hands on her head as if to find just where they could be. She wanted to know *how* a mother's nervousness and old worries could get passed on to a baby. And again she rummaged through the bits of her history, and once again I underscored the feelings of abandonment. I said it must have been a dreadful experience for a tiny baby. I said she must have cried and cried.

By this time Tom, too, wanted to know how something from long ago could affect a mother's ability to care for her baby now. I took this chance to describe the project and explain therapy. I told them we thought it was not *what* happened that mattered so much, even though that might have been very sad. We thought it was how a small child *felt* and whether anybody was there to understand that frightened child, whether she had been able to share her feelings and be comforted long ago. There was quiet. Beth lay exhausted on a heap of pillows. I said, "Beth thinks the answer lies somewhere in the past. She is trying to figure it out, and this is a courageous and difficult thing to do. Looking back at frightening times means facing great pain inside and scary feelings." I said it took time to believe it was safe to talk to me. But people really could. They could get angry at me and know it would not hurt me. They could tell me their worries and know I would not be damaged or turn away. I said I could listen because I knew I could help. Other mothers and their babies had been able to change and have things be better. Tom was sober, then angry at all those who had not listened or explained things to them in the months before. And Beth joined him to list all the times no one believed her or understood what was wrong.

Something had been touched in Beth. But though she was beginning to reexperience something of her own past, she could not transform it into empathy for her child so early in the therapy. This was made clear by what happened next. Trudy stirred and wakened. Beth said the baby would sleep more. She could not consider that Trudy might be hungry. While I was attentive to opening up every possibility for change in Beth, that change could only take place over time. I also had an obligation to the baby. I could not let her starve while we took weeks or months to gain insights.

Since Beth could not read Trudy's signals, I would. I said firmly that the baby must be very hungry right now; she had not eaten for a long time. Beth sat Trudy up abruptly and vanished into the kitchen. Trudy cried out. The boys tried to distract her with play. They did not connect Trudy's distress with her mother's sudden disappearance. As Trudy wept, they told me how unhappy she was all the time. She no longer enjoyed anything, and it was getting worse. I was sympathetic and, when it was tactful, suggested they leave so that mother and baby and I could give full attention to the feeding. They made their polite farewells.

I could see the tension mount for Beth as she began an awkward spoon feeding. I could also see Trudy's readiness to give up, to fall back to sleep unfed. I crouched beside them and worked to prevent a disruption, to help the essential exchange continue. I spoke aloud for mother and for baby, playing both parts. I provided the signals, established the rhythm, named the delicious pleasure. It was a silly mundane monologue: "Mom, I liked that and I'm ready for some more." "Isn't that a good baby, to open her mouth so wide?" "Won't she grow to be beautiful, eating all the good food that Mommy gives her?" "Such a good girl!" I sensed that Beth took all these comments as being addressed to her. Toward the end of the feeding, I became quiet because Beth was starting to imitate me. She called the baby "good girl" and made small "num num" sounds to her. Beth opened her own mouth with each spoonful she gave to Trudy. She was joined in the act of feeding and was enjoying her baby's satisfaction, if only for these few brief moments. Beth kept going through the pitiful remains in three encrusted jars, about half a cup altogether. Trudy ate it all, with no spitting up. As I supplied psychological nurturance for the ghost of a baby who once starved for food and much more than food, the positive transference helped Beth begin to provide adequate nutrition for her baby who was starving now.

The visit was not yet over. Beth had asked me to come because the baby's cries made her so tense. When the feeding ended Beth found a way to lead us back to that question. Trudy was playing quietly near her mother when Beth disappeared again, going to the kitchen. Trudy screamed but Beth remained out of sight. I called out, "Beth, being left with a stranger will make Trudy cry more and more. What should I do?" No reply. I called again, "We have to keep Trudy from crying so the food will stay in her tummy, so she won't spit up." Beth returned. She said the one thing that always worked was to hold the baby, but she had other things to do. I coaxed and soothed until Beth held Trudy long enough to let her become quiet and resume play. Then I tried to find out what kept Beth from holding her crying baby. When Trudy made a few fretful sounds, I asked if this was the crying that was so difficult for Beth. "Oh no!" Beth said. "The cry I mean is something much worse, much harder to listen to." Beth reached out to touch me before voicing her intense feelings. "I get so angry! That crying makes me so furious!" Beth tensed her arms in a pantomime of barely controlled violence. "I get so that I feel . . . it's awful. . . . I just want to throw her away!" Here was another link. The mother who had once been thrown away was confessing the urge to throw her baby away—to do after all what had been done to her.

Having heard Beth's confession, I could then make her a promise. I would do all I could to find a way to help her with these frightening feelings, to find relief, to keep things safe for her and her baby. And then I gave my attention to Beth's hunger. I said I thought *she* was not eating well and this worried me just as much as Trudy's not eating. I suggested a plan for the rest of the week. I would come at lunchtime each day to help Beth and Trudy have a quiet feeding, to keep the food in Trudy's stomach. The next medical checkup would show us if it worked. If it did not work, we would think of something else. Beth said I was welcome any time.

A Critical Period for Mother and Baby

Day by day I listened to whatever Beth wanted to tell me, including her fears that if the baby died, Beth would go crazy. I said I would keep trying to help so that these terrible things would not happen. And I helped her continue to feed her baby gently. Trudy ate and did not spit up all week.

When we all went to the next checkup Trudy had gained nine ounces. We had shown that Trudy could stop vomiting, could gain when her mother fed her. At first Beth could not believe it. Then as the good news was repeated, she was beside herself with excitement. She came to me to have her long hair brushed from her face. Then, with Trudy sitting high on her shoulders, Beth dashed to the mirror to see herself and her baby together. She said, "Look, Trudy. Say, 'I'm so happy! I feel so good!'"

I persuaded Beth that Trudy needed her at home for a while, and a leave from school was arranged. Full-time care of a sickly baby was difficult for Beth. Trudy was still fussy and was not always ready to eat when Beth offered food. There were more stormy exchanges between Beth and her mother. Beth grew angry with me about it all, and I let her know that the anger at me was all right and that I would come even if Trudy did not eat. I would come so she could tell me what worried her. In truth, I was very concerned for Beth herself. She seemed anorexic and often out of touch. I asked her to keep notes for me; her own written diary became one way for her to hold onto what happened while I was not there, to show me how much she tried, how hard it was. The next day Beth called to ask my help in planning to have her class assignments sent from school. She also wanted to tell me of a bad dream she had had that afternoon. I said it sounded as though her mind was working on something, trying to figure something out, and we could talk about it the next day.

With Beth's call to me at night about a bad dream (to be described later), material emerged about her loneliness and night fears which led to a solution of Trudy's sleep problems. From the start I saw Beth treat

Trudy's sleep with the same lack of empathy she showed for Trudy's hunger. The baby was left wherever she happened to fall asleep—on the floor or on the mattress. Frail as she was, she was never covered, and this was the coldest part of winter. Thus far no advice from anyone had helped Beth establish a familiar comforting sleep routine for her baby. Change did not come until Beth had had many opportunities to deal with her own feelings about nighttime.

The Eleventh Visit

The eleventh session, when this material first emerged, will be a second illustration of the baby's place in the therapy, a therapy aimed at separating the baby from her mother's conflicts. Trudy was now 7 months old. As a prelude, I should report how I had used food as a diagnostic tool the week before. At every visit I brought a variety of baby foods to help us discover Trudy's preferences. I also brought a simple lunch for Beth and myself. Trudy was fed and I ate. But Beth was unable to feel her own hunger; she ate one piece of celery, one slice of green pepper. Each day I left the untouched food with her. I watched for an awakening of Beth's appetite as a sign of her awakening affect. On the eleventh visit it came. Beth welcomed me with a picnic feast. She was humorous, delighted with herself, pleased by my deliberately open pleasure in the food she was giving her therapist. She made a fine sandwich and ate it all. While we ate, I read Beth's notes to me. They confirmed my impression that Trudy's progress was slowing. Though Beth was home all day, she had difficulty timing the feedings and soothing the fussy baby. I suspected too that she was again being rough in handling Trudy. When Beth was deeply troubled, the baby was neglected or bound up in her mother's inner conflict. Trudy had no lunch this day, only a graham cracker to eat by herself. Hints about her need for something other than salami or Coke were ignored. I took this behavior as a hint to me to pay attention to what was on Beth's mind. I spoke of what she wrote in her good notes, how hard she found it to manage everything by herself, how tiring that job was, how her sleep was spoiled by the bad dream she mentioned in her phone call.

Beth described the dream. It was about a family gathering and an uncle who was ungrateful for much help received from Beth's mother. He was outspokenly prejudiced against foreigners. There were men who were violent with their arms—her uncle, her father—and she made efforts to protect a small baby. And there was an angry fierce little dog who nipped. Beth said it was all weird and frightening. I said it must have been terrible in the dream to be trying to protect the baby and to feel so frightened and helpless. Then Beth told me she has always been afraid of what might happen in the dark and will do almost anything to avoid being alone in the apartment at night.

As a child she was scared at night by the pranks of friends. She was terrified at bedtime when her mother made her turn out the lights. She was upset by her father's stories of bears in the woods who would "eat you up if you were not good." She believed him. She was afraid of the woods outside her apartment. There might be someone out there, someone who would come banging on the door and insist on taking Trudy away; she had read about such things. We can conjecture that the dream and the memories and fantasy were representations of unre-membered childhood experience, with the kidnapper standing for one fantasy of how a mother lost her baby, how a little child lost her moth-er. I did not interpret this dream, but responded to the helpless terror which was so real for Beth that she could remember how her heart had pounded.

She continued with a confession and a question. First she had to tell me she lied last week when I asked if she and the baby slept well. She had said they had because she was not able to tell me how scared she really was at night. Sometimes she kept the baby up so as not to be alone. Poor Beth, I thought. No wonder she could not use advice about sleeping schedules. Having confessed, she next had something to ask me. "How do you raise a child not to be afraid of the dark? I don't want Trudy to be afraid like me." She said her mother turned out the lights at a certain time to force the children to get used to the dark. I said I thought Beth would find a way to help Trudy not fear the dark by let-ting Trudy know her mother was near, by helping Trudy fall asleep in a comfortable way. Beth named her dilemma. She wanted Trudy to sleep, did not like holding a fussy baby, but she also needed to have her near for company. And as Beth spoke she picked up the baby and held her very close, as if she was hanging onto Trudy for her own com-fort. Trudy, no longer so fearful of her mother, enjoyed the rare close-ness and settled down to explore her mother's face and shirt.

I interpreted Beth's ambivalence, her feeling two ways about the baby. It was not long then before Beth used the baby in another way to make her own fears real and to ask me once more what to do with a crying baby. Beth stood Trudy up at her knee and then, with no warn-ing, she forced the baby to the floor. Trudy braced herself stiffly on hands and feet and cried out in terror. And Beth turned to ask me, "How do they learn to balance anyway? Why is she crying?" I tried to answer both her questions by combining developmental information with the affective parallels between the baby's present fright caused by

Beth and Beth's story of being frightened by her own mother, a mother whom Beth described as never doing anything for a crying child.

I explained that Trudy was already learning to balance nicely when she sat by herself. We could both see this progress. And Trudy would learn to balance in other ways when she was ready. Trudy could not creep yet, but she would soon be moving about on her own very well. Just now she was crying because, not having gotten onto her hands and knees by herself, she did not know what would happen next. I said it was like having the light turned out when you are not ready, the way Beth's mother used to do. That was scary.

Beth's several fears had been heard, and she must have experienced an inner relief because she offered comfort to Trudy right away. She gathered her terrified baby to her and lay beside her on the bed to comfort her with a bottle. And as Beth herself relaxed she reflected about connections between her moods and Trudy's. Maybe Trudy had been fussy this morning because Beth was "uptight," hurrying to dress and get to school for her assignments. I asked if it was the hurrying, or was it having to face her teachers? That was it. They did not believe her, did not understand that now she had a good reason for missing classes. She said it was so hard for her to explain herself, to talk to other people. I sympathized, but pointed out that she had found words today to say some very difficult things and was able to help me understand just what she meant. If she could continue in this way, I thought things would change. As I drove away, I felt that a working alliance was forming which would enable us to answer Beth's question about how a mother's worries were passed on to her baby. As Beth's worries were voiced and heard, there could be moments of safer closeness between her and her baby.

Trudy Begins to Thrive

During the next weeks Beth's caregiving remained haphazard, but was no longer so neglectful. Trudy's progress was erratic but unmistakable. The most concrete measure, Trudy's weight gain, continued and held even through a feverish illness. As her physiological state stabilized, there were rapid gains in development. She was still very tense at times. But she became lively, happier, and prettier. Her vocalizations became more normal. In her walker she scooted about after her mother, exploring things along the way. Trudy invited more social responses, and Beth could not always resist. This development was matched by

Beth's greater openness to her own thoughts and feelings. As her sense of self became more coherent, the days were less confusing and unpredictable to her. She could do her own observing and thinking between sessions. Twice-weekly visits were enough.

Beth could talk about the loneliness she felt for her family. She knew when the feeling was there and recognized her efforts to block it by drink or marijuana. Not only could she say she sometimes wished she had not kept the baby, but she could say it without endangering her ability to care for the baby. She was no longer using Trudy as a shield against the darkness. She asked why, after so many discouraging months, a few weeks had made such a difference? She answered it herself in a touching note to me. She wrote, "I think I know why things are getting better. It is not just because I am staying home with the baby. It is because I am talking to you and you listen. Trudy and I want to thank you."

With the intensified transference came ambivalent feelings toward her family. Beth missed them, but many of her memories of life at home had a nightmarish quality. The furniture had been destroyed when the kids were left to run wild. The yard was strewn with garbage, prompting neighbors' complaints and causing public humiliation. Nevertheless her feelings about home were warm. She struggled to make that clear to me. She said it was like a combination of a love story and a horror movie. When I said that whatever happened, I knew Beth and her mother loved each other very much, she felt I understood.

The way had been opened for positive affect. As Beth felt herself become a valued person to her therapist, she could make her baby a valued part of herself. And this too had a concrete representation.

On the fifteenth visit, two weeks after Beth first told me of her night fears, she had something special to show me. At the end of the hour she led me on tiptoe to the bedroom—as if to see a newly arrived baby. Trudy was asleep in her crib. Beth could let her sleep by herself. But I noted a much more significant transformation. Until now this room had been a place for discards, the crib hidden in a tangle of torn and matted blankets with no proper space for a baby at all. It had been a home away from home for a thrown-away mother and her thrown-away baby, surrounded by trash. Today the room and crib were tidy, with a vaporizer to help Trudy sleep more comfortably. As we stood there, Beth picked Trudy up to have her wave good-bye to me. With her baby in her arms she told me she was making something for Trudy, a pretty pink blanket. For Trudy the night would become a time of comfort, warmth, and healthy, contented sleep.

The clinical hypothesis from the first was that Beth was attempting to rediscover her past through her baby. Her own conflicts about motherhood and abandonment prevented her from meeting Trudy's vital needs or reading Trudy's emotional signals. Beth was blocked from normal exchanges of affect with her baby just as she was blocked from awareness of the repressed affects belonging to her deprived orphan past. The clinical method derived from the diagnosis. We posited that Beth would be able to empathize with sensitivity, to respond promptly and appropriately to Trudy, without conflict that endangered Trudy if we could work to revive Beth's most painful affects: her longings and bodily hungers, her fear of loss and abandonment, her inner over-whelming rage which inhibited closeness to her baby. In our experience, if a mother can be helped to separate the baby from her own internal conflicts, we can provide a climate in which the mother's capacity to nurture becomes available to her long before her inner conflicts can be resolved.

In the examples given we have tried to demonstrate how the clinical work is carried out by including the baby directly in the sessions and combining developmental guidance with interpretations timed so that they refer to the infant-mother couples of both the immediate present and the distant past. Promising changes for the baby can often be made rather rapidly. Therapy addressed to the parent's conflicts will require much work over much time. Nevertheless, mother and baby can come together with increasing affection and spontaneity, as occurred in the months leading to Trudy's first birthday.

Trudy's First Birthday

The physical emergency lessened as Trudy's weight rose well above the 3rd percentile by 12 months. The psychological emergency lessened as a more secure attachment to her mother developed. She continued to score at age level on the Bayley, and continued to be somewhat delayed in her vocalizations. The grossly aberrant behaviors disappeared. The screaming, vomiting, fearful infant was gone. At 1 year, Trudy was truly attractive, offering her mother a beautiful smile and warm hug, or toddling around to discover and explore her small world. She was a lovable and beloved baby. We understand her good developmental and emotional progress to be related to Beth's freer capacity to mother her baby. It is this picture of a beloved, protected, adequate baby one must keep in mind as we summarize Beth's own dangerous turmoil when her graduation and Trudy's birthday drew near.

Frustrating attempts to find a good sitter for the baby so Beth could complete high school brought up material about frightening, mean adults and helpless children, about what could happen to a little child when mother is not there: fear, injury, possibly death. So many bad memories of the early school years troubled Beth that she wanted to get rid of them, forget about them. Her ambivalent longings for her adoptive mother increased. Transference resistance led to broken appointments. When this behavior was interpreted and when I promised I would not turn from her, she said, "But I ran away from you lots of times in the beginning. I'm glad I met you. I knew I needed your help."

Her graduation was in real doubt. But her poor record, her low self-esteem, the disappointment to her mother—all were denied. Instead, there were changes in her living arrangements, changes in sitters, constant planning and replanning for herself and her baby. The tension mounted, and Beth began to plan the first of many impossible trips. Going away and throwing away became themes in the sessions. Belongings were damaged, thrown away, or had to be returned to the store. At the same time there were questions about the baby's health; maybe she too was damaged. I heard mutterings about leaving the baby.

My spring vacation, at a time when Beth's mother would be away, intensified the wish to go someplace, be with someone. Beth spoke of her confusion about her past. She had travel dreams that were so real she used to believe them and tell others and be laughed at or called a liar. She did not want her own baby to be so confused. She would take her baby on real trips. I said that Trudy would not become confused because Trudy would always know who her mother was, where her mother was, and where home was. And this comment prompted another of Beth's questions. How come the baby was gaining weight even though her appetite was down, and mother herself was upset and feeling poorly? I said what mattered was how the baby was fed and who fed her, and that I knew Beth was giving her baby much more than food, giving her many things that only a mother can give to her baby.

The therapy saved Trudy from being abandoned by her mother. Beth's plans for flight now included the baby. Beth acted out her early abandonment in many ways. She left her apartment a shambles and moved to a stinking hovel with a gang of young burglars. Simultaneously she planned to live with several different families far away. From week to week she did not know where she would be, whether she would be on her own, or if someone would want to take her in and care for her and the baby. The plans always fell through; there was no home waiting for her. One night she called to tell me she was going to sign adoption papers for Trudy to give her a good home. There was another call in the night, after a broken appointment. Beth had been to the state prison to visit a kidnapper, someone who took children from their families.

With interpretation of Beth's attempts to picture her own past, to make real her nightmare fantasies of how babies and mothers become separated, this acting out decreased. There were exchanges of real pictures between Beth and me. For graduation I gave Beth a book of sketches of street scenes of our small city. This gift was especially chosen for a girl whose birth certificate read "abandoned on the street," streets she could not remember. For Trudy's birthday, Beth wanted a complete record of the baby's Bayley tests at 4, 8, and 12 months so that years from now she could show her "how smart she was." These were given to her. I also took instant photographs of Trudy's birthday party to confirm and document the event. Trudy's advances into toddlerhood, her evident ability to listen to and understand her mother, combined with the documentation of Trudy's present to evoke orphanage memories in Beth, memories of the time when she was a toddler, when things happened that she could not understand. A few sessions later these memories brought to light mementos from that other time, that other place: well-worn toys, very special photographs. A gentler, more beloved part of Beth's past was brought to light.

Epilogue

This case report was meant to serve as one example of the intervention model developed in the infant mental health program at the Child Development Project. Beth is a young mother whose history of early abandonment and starvation, followed by later developmental and psychological difficulty, foreshadowed a very disturbed adolescence. Her pregnancy at 17 years, and her extreme neglect of her baby, were part of her acting out of long-standing inner conflicts, a repetition of the past abandonment with dangerous consequences for both mother and baby. When some of the affect associated with the past trauma was elicited from Beth, and as she saw herself valued by her therapist, pathways were opened to positive affect. It was possible in only one month to help Beth begin to nurture her baby instead of starving her. Trudy's chance for adequate ego development had been restored; her aberrant behaviors had become more normal by her first birthday.

We had reached a point in treatment when many clinics might consider their goals achieved with Trudy's reassuring weight gain and her adequate developmental test scores. But we felt justified in continuing treatment since our objectives were different. It was true that Trudy was showing a growing warm attachment for her mother and a sturdiness and verve that gave promise of a chance for healthy ego development. And it was true that the positive changes in Trudy were rewarding for Beth, giving her what every parent seeks: hope for a rebirth of the self. Nevertheless, even though Beth's continued conflicts were no longer inflicted so directly upon her child, we felt they both remained at risk. We continued treatment until we felt Trudy's development had stabilized sufficiently so that the stress of events and changes in the future would present less of a threat to her. At one year the initial emergency was over and the way had been prepared for an extended treatment which lasted two more years.

Beth and Trudy were to live in seven homes before the work ended. With the wisdom of hindsight we can see patterns that were not so clear while the work was in progress. Looking back, it seems that each home provided a setting in which Beth could try to recapture different aspects of the conflicts rooted in her past. As she moved from place to place, she was also attempting to move out of a troubled adolescence into adulthood and motherhood. Beth moved when a house became objectively dangerous for herself and Trudy, or when a steady relationship led to the kind of personal closeness she or her friends could not handle. With each move, which was always in some sense a running away, I had to search to find two lost children, to locate Beth and Trudy, rebuild the positive transference, and restore the working alliance with Beth. I often found myself in the role of a mother who would not let her patient-children be lost or abandoned, and my commitment to Beth and Trudy was repeatedly put to the test.

The summer Beth spent with the gang of young delinquents was a period of extremely low self-esteem when she placed herself with a group of abandoned and motherless outcasts. It was as if she had found a representation of the dimly remembered orphanage, and it was in that parentless household she first showed me her orphanage souvenirs. She wanted me to hold each toy and picture, to see what I would see in them. She was giving me a very private and precious part of herself. What I saw, and what I told her, was that someone unremembered by Beth had wanted to give her a chance at a better life. Someone had helped her get ready for the long trip to a new home and sent her on her way with tender attention and hope. Beth had originally defined herself to me as abandoned and unloved. But now we had evidence that she had been lovable, she was not such a completely bad little girl. After this glimpse of a better self Beth made several futile efforts to rescue her fellow tenants from great dangers. Then she rescued herself and Trudy, escaping from scenes of fire and gunplay to move to a more peaceful home with a real family. Trudy was then 14 months old and making good progress.

In the new house Trudy was delighted to be in the midst of a family with three young children. She was treated as a pet, and all looked promising at first. The new home was similar to her grandparents', where, despite all the disagreements, Trudy had her place. But the parallels to the family home that were so attractive for Trudy were disastrous for Beth. Surrounded by a warm and friendly family who knew and welcomed her, she found herself overcome by a painful yearning for her real mother. Beth could not cope with the longing to be mothered or with her fear of that longing. She created constant turmoil with her motherly landlady. There were battles, threats, accusations of neglect on both sides.

It was as if she were recalling in a most primitive preverbal fashion the early history of her adoption at 2½. She was disappointed, insatiably demanding, and could not live up to her own expectations. She behaved in all ways like the impossible, angry, ungrateful child she thought she had been, the child no one could understand or take care of long ago. At the same time she was also being an utterly impossible adolescent, antagonistic, unreachable, building herself up to a crisis and a rejection similar to what had occurred when she was first shut out of her parents' home with her new baby. Beth began to be afraid of the dark again, to have bad dreams, and to take flight. She sank into a deep depression. She would not let anyone take care of her, nor could she take care of Trudy while she was buffeted by such deep ambivalence. Once more Trudy became a neglected fellow orphan, a shield against night terrors. Beth kept Trudy up at night to ward off her own fears. She left Trudy unclothed and shivering. Soon Trudy caught a cold that dragged on for weeks. Her appetite decreased and she stopped gaining weight. She weighed 19 pounds 2 ounces at 14 months and only 1 pound 5 ounces more at 19 months.

Beth remained the psychological center of Trudy's world. But for playfulness and for happy sociability Trudy waited for the other children to come home from school, or turned to other adults and to me. Her developmental and intellectual progress continued, but she looked sickly and wan. Beth was more worried than she dared say. She feared all would be lost and began to miss appointments with me. The growth curve (see Figure 3) illustrates this repeat of the initial problem, a repeat that occurred between Trudy's 14th and 19th months. Trudy's physical status was a reflection of a complex set of conflicts from which her mother could not protect her. This period of decline, when Trudy's place on the growth curve dropped from the 11th to the 6th percentile was less severe than the failure to thrive of a year ago. But it confirmed our sense that the continuing risks called for further work.

Once again the essence of the work lay in using events as they occurred on the visits to help Beth deal with both positive and negative transference feelings. She felt flooded by unmanageable longings and overwhelming disappointments in herself and in all those who came close but turned out not to be the one person she really sought, her true mother. We were able to examine the conflict she created with most mothering figures; it was so repetitiously reenacted that she could see how much her past intruded into the present. With the insights that came from this period of work it seemed as if she had gained enough understanding to make alternate plans for herself and Trudy. This time instead of impulsively fleeing, she made a well-planned move that let her, and Trudy, anticipate the change. She chose to live in a comfortable apartment near old school friends. An important step had been taken in the uneven process of separation from her adoptive mother. There would be many more ups and downs, but from then on Trudy's health would be good, and her weight gain would hold steady despite other crises.

By the time Trudy was 2 years old she was a healthy, active toddler. There was no physical evidence of her earlier failure to thrive. Her weight was at the 25th percentile and her height nearing the 75th. She was somewhat reserved and often serious, but when things were relaxed, she could be playful and express a full range of usually well-modulated feelings. Her language, which had been so delayed at 1 year, was now advanced and well used, as was a full range of inventive symbolic play. Her mother's presence reassured her unless Beth herself was very upset about something. We saw no evidence of pathological symptomatology. But what was still lacking was harmonious reciprocity and pleasure shared between Trudy and Beth. Trudy was ready, but Beth was not; she held herself back from full affection, and Trudy did not turn to her for comfort in extreme distress. Tantrums over unexpected leave-takings could be easily calmed by me, but Beth could not yet empathize with Trudy's troubled feelings over sudden separation. Those feelings were still too shaky for Beth herself to manage.

Over the course of the next year many of Beth's feelings about separation, deprivation, failure, and abuse were brought into the sessions and dealt with. Whenever significant interpretations could be based upon ongoing observations of Trudy, and connected to Beth's attempts to remember the vivid overwhelming feelings from her own childhood, Beth was able to empathize with her child, to protect and nurture her, to free Trudy from Beth's past fears and worries.

Trudy's obvious readiness to respond and to understand her mother, to offer her affection as only a child can, was a constant reminder to Beth that all had not been lost in those dreadful early months. Though she might feel discouraged, she did not need to feel her own difficulties would be visited upon Trudy and repeated for her.

Much had happened by the time Trudy was 3. Beth was working and had met a young man, Rick, who wanted to marry her and keep Trudy. Trudy was doing well in a good nursery school. In play sessions she had no trouble showing what she wondered about, worried about, or was confused by—and she readily made use of explanations offered by me and by her mother with my help. Beth was a full partner in the play sessions, because she had many of her own unanswered questions left over from childhood—and these too were attended to—questions about sex differences and the beginnings of motherhood. There was a greater freedom between Trudy and her mother, and Trudy counted more and more on Beth to understand a little girl's problems.

The last months of treatment were devoted to helping Beth and Trudy prepare for a trip to a new life. Rick had a chance to work for his firm overseas and wanted Beth and Trudy to go with him. For Trudy it was yet another move, but one that she had time to get ready for, with her mother's full support and explanation. For Beth it was a dream come true, since the move would bring her near the country of her birth. Extra visits were planned to give her time to sort out what all this meant to her. I told her some of the history I'd learned of events in her native land when so many families were separated in the upheaval of mass flight. Beth gave a great deal of thought to this, poring over maps and illustrated books that showed where she had once been and where she was now going. Her fantasies of her unknown and unknowable mother were transformed. Perhaps she had not been purposely abandoned. Perhaps it had been an unavoidable tragedy, as sad for her mother as for herself. She connected that early history to current news of the Asian boat people, facing desperate dangers, trying for a new life. Beth's sense of self-worth took a turn for the better, and she could even fantasize a happy outcome for her unknown mother—who might have landed somewhere safe and made a good life for herself. Having done this much Beth could then look ahead to good possibilities for herself and her child who would not be separated. Their trip to a new land need not be dangerous. They were not being cast out. They were going to someone who waited and wanted them to be there with him.

This trip, of course, was a fortuitous opportunity for additional acting out for Beth, but one that moved her a bit further along in separating fact from fiction. This would be a real trip—not one of the dreams that filled her childhood. She was relieved to know that her mind could hold onto the facts that went into her learning about the new place, as well as onto the travel arrangements. People were not making fun of her for wishful thinking; they believed her, and the family pitched in to help her prepare.

During the next year there were letters from far away to the family back home, and to me. In her letters to me Beth, who had barely been able to write a complete sentence all through school, wrote at length about her coping in a new land, with new language and customs. She wrote of her feelings and of Trudy's as well. She wrote with motherly pride and concern. She was thinking about things psychologically, facing depression and doubts. There was an ebullient letter announcing her marriage to Rick, with an outpouring of gratitude for all that therapy had meant. Then the letters stopped.

This is as far as we can carry the story of Beth and Trudy. They have been on their own for a year. There is no way to know what the letters did not say. It seems reasonable to think that Beth was working hard to keep in touch with the mode of self-examination that characterized the therapy—and to use it for herself and Trudy. She had internalized a nonblaming introspective style of looking at problems when she recognized them. Trudy seemed to be turning to her mother for pleasure and for understanding. Trudy had a fair chance at continuing her good development if she did not have to face too many crises in the near future.

X

Make Way for Abby

ALICIA F. LIEBERMAN
PETER BLOS, JR.*

MRS. HARRIS consulted us during the eighth month of her first and planned pregnancy because she found herself overwhelmed by intense anxiety and unexpected negative feelings about it. She was afraid that these feelings would affect her ability to mother her baby. Her husband, she said, did not understand her persistent worries. He was confident that he and his wife would be good parents, but nothing that he said could calm her anxiety.

In the course of our assessment period it became clear to us that the pregnancy had evoked for Mrs. Harris many disturbing memories of the past and that there was danger, as she feared, that the baby might become engulfed in old conflicts.

The Assessment Period

Mr. and Mrs. Harris were a couple in their early thirties. Both were physically attractive, he with a boyish charm, she with a serene dignified bearing which did not reveal her intense anxiety. The Harrises had been married for six years. Both had graduate degrees and were currently employed in their professions.

*Alicia F. Lieberman was the therapist in this case; Peter Blos, Jr., was the supervisor.

Mrs. Harris described herself and her husband as "driven people" who found it difficult to relax. They were immersed in multiple activities and did not want to diminish their commitment to any of them. This conflict was most noticeable in Mrs. Harris's attitudes toward motherhood and work outside the home. She said that both were important to her, but she feared that motherhood was incompatible with pursuing a career and felt torn by feelings that she would deprive her baby of full-time mothering if she worked and deprive herself of the satisfactions of her career if she did not.

Feelings of fatigue, dependency, shame, and embarrassment replaced her familiar feelings of self-confidence, independence, and pride. She now felt tired and clumsy, and longed for her former energy and the full, productive schedule from which she had derived a strong sense of competence and well-being. Mrs. Harris said that she felt at a loss because she could no longer take her body and activity level for granted. Sometimes she was too exhausted to get up for a drink of water but could not ask her husband for help because she thought that he was proud of her self-sufficiency and would be disappointed by this display of helplessness. She would remain thirsty sometimes for as long as an hour, waiting for her husband to perceive her need for a glass of water. When he failed to do so she felt angry and neglected. Bitter arguments then ensued. Mr. and Mrs. Harris could not understand what triggered these arguments, and they felt overwhelmed by the increasing and inexplicable tension in their relationship. For Mrs. Harris, these arguments provided a powerful confirmation of her fear that she and her husband would be unable to cope with the presence of a baby.

Mr. Harris had a different view of the situation. He believed that he and his wife would adjust well to the new demands posed by parenthood. He wished his wife could follow the example of other women who were relaxed and at peace during their pregnancies. He spoke wistfully of his own mother, describing her as a "supermom" who derived satisfaction and pleasure from raising children and caring for her husband and home. Mr. Harris knew his wife could not be happy with such domestic pursuits, but he wished that she could cheerfully accept being dependent on him for a few months. He wanted to take care of her.

Yet Mr. Harris acknowledged sharing some of his wife's misgivings. In particular, he worried about changes in their life-style and the inevitable readjustment of priorities that the baby's birth would entail. However, he saw no point in dwelling on these concerns. He believed that it was unfair for such worries and uneasy feelings to exist and wished one could simply take a pill to make them disappear. He concluded that since there was no pill, they should simply stop worrying because "endless" anticipatory talk would not help.

Following this logic, Mr. Harris repeatedly told his wife that they would solve problems as they occurred, and he tried to reassure her that everything would be "all right." Mrs. Harris saw these reassurances as a rejection of the reality of her feelings. In desperate attempts to make him understand, she described her concerns again and again until Mr. Harris felt overwhelmed. He then felt unable to maintain his reassurances and withdrew in an attempt to recover his calm. Mrs. Harris interpreted his withdrawal as a confirmation of her fear that he would desert her emotionally. She would then have to cope alone both with the baby and with her own anxiety. Mr. Harris, on his part, thought that his wife's anxiety indicated that she was not committed either to him or to their baby.

A condensed excerpt from the narrative record illustrates this recurrent pattern:

> Mrs. Harris said she knew through her experience that many children bear the consequences of their parents' negative feelings and are constantly scolded and even spanked. She feels angry about the pregnancy and is afraid that her anger will affect the baby. She wants to take the anger away from the baby and channel it in a different direction so that the baby will not be harmed. She does not know whether she can do that.
>
> Mrs. Harris spoke intensely, looking at her husband. He nodded his head repeatedly, saying, "That's right, that's right," but he seemed distracted. At one point he closed his eyes and immediately afterward shook his head and opened his eyes again. It looked for a moment as if he had fallen asleep. Mrs. Harris saw this and stopped talking abruptly, then looked away toward the window. There was a long and tense silence. He then said, very softly, "Did I put you off?" She nodded her head yes. He said, "What did I do?" She did not reply but started crying silently. He repeated his question several times. She did not answer, only nodding her head as if she could not speak. He leaned toward her with a very concerned expression and touched her hand. She finally said that when he shakes his head like that she always has the feeling that he is rejecting her. He said that he was actually agreeing with her, that he had felt overwhelmed for a second by the weight of all their feelings. Perhaps he had expressed those painful feelings the wrong way, perhaps he should try to talk about them rather than close his eyes and shake his head. He went on to explain that he now felt bewildered by her reaction because the punishment did not "fit the crime." He had felt momentarily weak and had shown his weakness, and she reacted as if he was going to walk out of the room and refuse to face the problem. He added that when this happens he feels his only alternative is to try to be stronger, never to show any weakness because his weakness scares her so. . . . Mr. Harris turned to me and said that episodes like this were occurring with increasing frequency.

As the therapist began to understand the pattern of the self-perpetuating miscommunication and the resulting emotional estrangement between husband and wife, she took an active stance. She could point out how much each wanted to help the other and how bewildered Mr.

Harris became when his efforts to be supportive were misunderstood. Mr. and Mrs. Harris could then start to understand how their own fears and suspicions distorted their perception of each other. In the fourth session, the mutual distrust having diminished, new and significant information emerged about Mrs. Harris's early history and the circumstances of the baby's conception.

Mrs. Harris was the eldest of four children and the only girl. She described her mother as a dependent, ineffectual, yet harsh and demanding woman who had always been dissatisfied with her role of housewife and mother. Mrs. Harris had been closer to her father, whom she described as a quiet, melancholy man, a "friend of kittens and puppies and children," who paid little attention to himself but liked to make other people happy. He had died about one year ago following a chronic illness for which he had long neglected medical evaluation. Eight months before his death, a medical examination revealed that the disease was already too advanced for successful treatment. He had been able to recognize the seriousness of his condition, but his wife refused to acknowledge it and continued to act as if his recovery was only a matter of time. Mrs. Harris attempted to explain the situation to her mother but desisted after her mother repeatedly refused to listen. Mrs. Harris then became the only person with whom her father could share his feelings about his impending death. Father and daughter became very close, and Mrs. Harris perceived herself as her father's confidante in the last months of his life. She became pregnant shortly after he died.

As she spoke of these events, Mrs. Harris went on to recall the circumstances surrounding her brother's birth when she herself was 10 years old. In the last weeks of her mother's pregnancy, Mrs. Harris had contracted a childhood illness which was then transmitted to the mother, who had to be hospitalized. The mother delivered shortly afterward but remained hospitalized in a serious condition. Her children were told that she might die.

While her mother was hospitalized, the 10-year-old daughter was expected to keep house and take care of the baby and of her younger brothers. Mrs. Harris recalled that the baby cried often and that there were frequent consultations with the doctor about his irritability. Mr. Harris, who had never heard this story, expressed sympathy for what his wife had endured. But Mrs. Harris, speaking a little dryly, said she had had no choice and then closed the matter by remarking that it was time to leave since the time was up.

There had been another baby, then, in Mrs. Harris's past, and there had been another time when Mrs. Harris was a mother to a baby. She had been only 10 years old at that time, but she had performed successfully the difficult task of caring for the baby and her other younger siblings. Mrs. Harris told the story factually. She did not mention the feelings that we could surmise she experienced in such a situation—feelings of being alone, inadequate, awed by responsibility. She seemed unable now to remember herself as a child with a child's feelings.

In the course of these first five sessions it was clear to the therapist that Mrs. Harris's troubled feelings about the coming baby and the evocation of painful memories from her past could indeed be impediments to mothering and to the course of the baby's development. The therapist suggested a plan of treatment in which she and the parents would work together to understand these feelings and to find ways of protecting both the child's development and the parents' own pleasure in their baby. The work would continue after the infant's birth for as long as necessary. Mrs. Harris gave immediate consent to the plan. Mr. Harris expressed some doubts about their need for treatment but quickly accepted his wife's plea that they should do everything in their power to ensure the best possible beginning for themselves and their child.

Abigail Is Born

A few days after treatment had been agreed upon, Mrs. Harris called to tell the therapist that she had delivered a girl the previous evening. Calm and businesslike, she described the baby, Abigail, and the delivery. It had been a natural childbirth, and Mr. Harris had stayed with his wife throughout the labor and delivery. Everything had gone smoothly, and the baby was healthy and lovely. Mrs. Harris declined the therapist's offer of a hospital visit because her room did not provide enough privacy. An appointment was made for a home visit a week later.

VISITS TO THE HOME

The first home visit took place in the late afternoon. The parents were sitting close together on a sofa with Abigail in a bassinet at their feet. They showed Abby to the therapist with obvious pleasure. She was indeed a beautiful baby. Mrs. Harris pointed out the reddish streaks in Abby's otherwise dark hair and compared them to her husband's red hair. Both Mr. and Mrs. Harris spoke softly, in muted tones. In the late afternoon light, the quiet and subdued mood contrasted strikingly with the anxiety and stress of the previous weeks.

Abigail was a placid and responsive baby who ate and slept well, cried seldom, and was easily soothed. One of Mrs. Harris's first comments to the therapist was that she worried sometimes that the baby was too quiet. She felt that her experience with the quiet Abby was in sharp contrast with her memories of her irritable newborn brother when she was a 10-year-old mother to him. Other things had also gone better than expected. Her milk supply had been established without difficulty, and Abby was already nursing well. The baby's schedule was spontaneously quite regular. Mrs. Harris felt relaxed and rested.

With everything going so smoothly, Mr. and Mrs. Harris felt they no longer needed treatment. The therapist suggested they meet again before making a final decision.

In the second home visit a week later areas of concern started to emerge. Mrs. Harris began to fear that things were going well only temporarily and that serious problems would soon appear. She felt uncertain about her ability to respond appropriately to her baby's cues, and was often unable to decide whose needs—Abby's or her own— should receive priority. This uncertainty was most noticeable with regard to feeding schedules. Mrs. Harris had been advised by the nurses to guide Abby gradually toward a regular feeding schedule, but she interpreted this advice as an imposition on Abby and therefore selfish on her part. Mrs. Harris also noticed that Abby was often alert and responsive after the 2:00 A.M. feeding, and she felt guilty about her wish to return to bed when Abby was clearly "ready to play."

THE THERAPIST'S OBSERVATIONS

The therapist could confirm these concerns in her own observations. She saw that Mrs. Harris was efficient in her ministrations to Abby but seemed self-conscious and lacking in spontaneity and pleasure, as if she held back from the baby. This seemed to include more than a new mother's awe or uncertainty. Mrs. Harris did not initiate playful games with the baby. Although usually responsive to Abby's signals, she became oblivious to them when she herself was in distress—for example, when she talked about her own mother's lack of interest and pleasure in Abby's birth. Mr. Harris, in contrast, showed spontaneous joy as well as emerging competence in his care of Abby.

In many ways, then, Mrs. Harris was a competent mother, and her baby was thriving. But something was holding back spontaneity and joy. There were hints in the mother's communications to the therapist that she was having troubled memories of the baby brother she had mothered as a child, but the affective links were missing. These memories were still reported in a matter-of-fact manner.

For the father, there seemed to be no intrusive memories, and the only complaints he registered came in the form of surprise and regret that the arrival of a baby should consume so much of the parents' time. He was finding that there was literally no time left for the ordinary things of life, let alone for quiet and private moments with his wife.

Yet the relationship between Mr. and Mrs. Harris was much less strained now than during the assessment period. In many respects, they did not differ from most couples with their first baby in discovering great changes in their lives and new demands upon their resources. Mr. Harris, who characteristically threw himself into work and home responsibilities with great zest, now worried that he would be falling short if he did not devote eight full hours to his family as well as eight full hours to his work.

As they spoke of these concerns, the Harrises decided that they wanted treatment to continue but requested that sessions be scheduled every two weeks rather than weekly. Later, as other issues entered the treatment, they were seen weekly until the treatment ended when Abby was 9 months old.

The Treatment Period

The first problem that Mrs. Harris brought to treatment had involved questions of "self-demand" versus "schedule" in feeding Abby. Mrs. Harris made her own decision to breast feed exclusively on demand, and she used as guidelines Abby's own fairly regular cycles of wakefulness, hunger, and sleep. (Feeding issues did not surface again for many weeks.)

The second issue was how to respond to the baby's crying. The two parents differed in their views. Mrs. Harris firmly believed that a baby's cries should be invariably and immediately responded to. She was shocked and dismayed by her husband's attitude as he played the devil's advocate: What if he and his wife were doing something else? Weren't parents entitled to their fun too? Wouldn't a baby be spoiled if parents responded to her cries too much or too quickly?

The therapist helped both parents by leading them into inquiries about the meaning of crying in an infant. What was the baby "telling" us through her cries? Once both parents began to consider that a baby communicated something through crying, the discussion with the therapist led naturally into other questions. The therapist explained that when parents respond to crying, the baby acquires a sense that she is heard and that her needs are being met, and in this way an inner security gradually develops. Mr. and Mrs. Harris reacted differently to this information. Mr. Harris found it illuminating and accepted the therapist's suggestions without reservation. Mrs. Harris asked in a worried voice whether responding to Abby's cries would at least also serve to promote inner security and self-reliance as the baby grew. The therapist responded to the undercurrent of anxiety and asked Mrs. Harris if she worried that her efforts to be a responsive mother would not have the results she hoped for. Then, for the first time, Mrs. Harris revealed a recurrent feeling that she was to blame for Abby's periods of fussiness. The crying made her feel inadequate and incompetent as a mother, as if Abby were telling her that she could do nothing right. On the other hand, she thought that the baby's periods of contentment were due purely to chance.

This was a poignant communication. The mother felt that her baby's cries were an accusation against her as a good mother. As Mrs. Harris came back to this theme again and again, it was clear that she felt she had to be constantly on guard against negative or hostile feelings. She felt guilty whenever Abby's wishes were even slightly overlooked or postponed.

On days when Mrs. Harris felt that she was not fully attuned to her baby, she even wondered whether Abby would still smile at her when she awoke. Mrs. Harris was afraid that unless she was fully devoted to and constantly involved in caring for her daughter, Abby would feel neglected, their relationship would fail, and Abby would not love her. Her terror was that some small fault in maternal devotion would lead to an irreversible process of alienation between her and her child.

EXPECTATIONS THAT CAN'T BE MET

When Abby was 16 weeks old she became ill with a severe cold. Mrs. Harris panicked. She knew how quickly infants' illnesses become serious, and she became frantic thinking that the cold might develop into croup. She read and reread her baby books but was unable to gain any relief. As she described her anguish, she said, "The worst part was when Abby looked at me with a pale and sad smile, as if asking for relief, and I could not give her any." The therapist asked what she felt when Abby looked at her with that "pale and sad smile." The mother replied that she felt incompetent, unable to meet Abby's expectations.

The therapist asked if she had experienced those feelings before. With sadness, Mrs. Harris recalled that her parents had always pressured her to achieve. She did not mind her father's pressure so much because his demands were understandable and predictable. Her mother, she felt, was irrational and unpredictable. She seldom showed interest in Mrs. Harris's activities but would often yell at her for "hours" for trifling misbehaviors. At these times, Mrs. Harris felt that she could never do anything right. In fact, she explained with a choked voice, she and her brothers thought it was their own fault that they could never satisfy their mother. As these early memories and feelings were recalled, the therapist suggested a connection between Mrs. Harris's current feeling that she could not please Abby and her earlier feeling that she was to blame for her mother's dissatisfaction.

In the course of several sessions the theme of "I can't please her" recurred again and again. Sometimes Mrs. Harris reacted to her daughter as if the baby were actually her mother, a stern and critical judge who could not be satisfied. At other times she was afraid that she herself resembled her mother and behaved toward Abby in an arbitrary and controlling manner. Abby then reminded Mrs. Harris of herself as a small child. Through the work of this period Mrs. Harris began to remember herself and her mother with profound feeling.

As treatment continued, it became clear that Mrs. Harris feared that Abby would one day disappoint her. As she watched Abby develop and acquire new skills, she wondered to herself whether her daughter was precocious in comparison with other babies. Mrs. Harris interpreted these comparisons as a worrisome indication that she was expressing her own competitiveness by pushing Abby to achieve. She started to entertain the idea of returning to work, reasoning that she would defuse this conflict and protect Abby by using work rather than her daughter as a channel for her competitiveness.

With the therapist's help, Mrs. Harris began to explore her fear of pressuring Abby to achieve. She readily acknowledged that she did not want to be harsh and demanding as her mother had been. But she was afraid that Abby's achievements might not suffice to please her. If she were dissatisfied with her daughter's performance, she might be led to continuous nagging, and then Abby would no longer love her. This realization triggered memories of her feelings of guilt for not loving her mother. She then recalled the feelings her mother had elicited: helplessness, alienation, lack of love. However, she could not remember having felt angry. Looking at Abby comfortably cuddled in her mother's arms, the therapist said gently, "Such a little baby, and all these fears about losing her love." The mother's eyes filled with tears. After a long silence, she said in a choking voice that her fear of being dissatisfied with Abby and losing her love were really an expression of her dissatisfaction with herself. Nothing gave her pleasure; she could not enjoy what she had or feel that her achievements were real. She was more like her mother than she wanted to be. With this realization, Mrs. Harris started to consider the possibility of individual psychotherapy for herself.

We can now partially retrace both the struggle Mrs. Harris had been engaged in and her efforts to spare her baby. Her own pregnancy had reawakened the feelings of helplessness, inadequacy, and futility that she had experienced as a child in trying to please her mother. The "unsatisfied" crying baby, Abby, evoked these old feelings which were now expressed in the thought "I cannot be a good mother." Before she had feared the loss of her own mother's love; now she anxiously anticipated the loss of her baby's love. At this juncture in the treatment, her identification with the aggressor (mother) could become conscious and be expressed in the thought, "I am just like my mother." But this defense still shielded Mrs. Harris from becoming aware of the original anger toward her mother. Anger was still experienced as "pushing" or "forcing" Abby, in identification with her mother. Thus the only way to protect the baby would be to get a "better" caregiver and return to work. The remorse at not being a good mother would be, unconsciously, just payment for the guilt of her hostility.

Although Mr. Harris did not experience the same conflicts in his relationship with Abby, he resembled Mrs. Harris in many ways. He too had longed for a close, accepting relationship with his parents. He too felt that his anxieties and self-dissatisfaction prevented him from fully enjoying his own achievements. In the sessions described above, Mr. Harris listened attentively to his wife and spoke about his own similar feelings. The couple's discovery that they experienced many comparable feelings brought them closer together and provided support for mutual change.

ABBY AT 5 MONTHS

As the infant-parent treatment proceeded, the therapist carefully followed Abby's development through direct observation and reports from the parents. "Baby-watching," the pleasures of infant observation, were a regular part of most sessions. The therapist conveyed to the parents her developmental observations, and the parents were encouraged to report Abby's newest achievements. The reality of the baby, her unfolding abilities, and the pleasure in her latest behavior were an integral part of this therapeutic method.

At 5 months Abby was an alert, sociable baby who responded differentially to her parents, readily explored available toys, and was busy practicing the individual components of crawling. Mr. and Mrs. Harris were thoroughly absorbed in their baby. Although still more restrained than her husband, Mrs. Harris showed spontaneous delight and engaged in long and mutually rewarding exchanges with her daughter. The earlier conflicts about responsiveness to crying and about eating and sleeping schedules were no longer a source of concern. Mr. and Mrs. Harris seemed to deal flexibly with temporary episodes of distress in Abigail's behavior. Mrs. Harris appeared to have succeeded in keeping her troubled feelings from contaminating her behavior toward her child.

A FEEDING PROBLEM APPEARS

This encouraging picture was disrupted when Abby was 22 weeks of age and solids were introduced into her diet. For a few weeks there had already been some concern, but things were now worsening. Abby ate puréed fruits with pleasure but turned her head away when Mrs. Harris offered her cereal. Mrs. Harris then attempted to force the cereal into Abby's mouth. After a few days Abby started refusing even the puréed fruits, and she spit up when Mrs. Harris persisted. Several times both parents stood in front of Abby trying to persuade her to eat. Feeding had become a battleground.

Mrs. Harris felt ridiculous. The pediatrician had reassured her that there was no urgent need for solids and that a gradual introduction adapted to Abby's acceptance of new foods would be adequate. Mr. Harris was willing to accept this advice. Mrs. Harris agreed that the advice made sense, but she could not stop worrying about dietary deficiencies leading to very unpleasant and painful tests. Her fears, she knew, were unfounded, and she was bewildered by their intensity and pressure.

The therapist pointed out that she might feel ridiculous and bewildered because she was unable to cope logically with a routine issue in child rearing. Mrs. Harris nodded and recalled her anxiety and feelings of incompetence when Abby had been sick. As the therapist led her to focus on how she felt when Abby turned away and refused to eat, Mrs. Harris said, "Helpless." It was as if Abby controlled her by refusing to yield to her wishes. When she could not persuade Abby to comply, she herself became angry and felt compelled to *force* Abby to eat.

Naturally, neither the therapist nor the Harrises believed in "forcing" Abby to eat cereal. But clearly something Mrs. Harris could not put into words was urging her to force food upon her baby.

In the sequence that follows we can see how the themes of "forcing" and "being forced" (active and passive) make their way into the mother's story. The therapist, attentive to the repetition of the theme of "forcing," moves away from Abby's feeding for a brief interval to explore the meaning of that theme:

> Mrs. Harris said that when Abby refuses to accept solids, she cannot help worrying about the possibility of iron deficiency and anemia. She then tries to coax Abby, and when the baby cries, she feels that Abby is dissatisfied, that there is something missing. I said, "As if you are not giving her what she wants." Mrs. Harris said that this is also the way she felt at work, with

her boss and others. I said, "And when you feel that Abby is dissatisfied, it must be harder, because your relationship with her is so much more important to you." Mrs. Harris nodded and said that she wanted Abby to develop her own rhythm and feels bad when she imposes something on her baby. She said it was so hard to be a parent. If at least she knew of anybody who liked their parents, it might make the task easier.

Mr. Harris then started to talk about how angry he had been at his parents for trying to instill good table manners in him. Now he was grateful that they had forced him to eat well and perhaps even wished that they had done a better job of it. I said that perhaps Mr. and Mrs. Harris worried sometimes that Abby might not like them if they imposed something on her, just as they did not like their parents for trying to impose manners or other things on them (at a much later age, of course).

Mrs. Harris then spoke in an intense voice about her mother's arbitrary rules. She said that her mother used to make scenes about Mrs. Harris's attempts to do anything. And it wasn't even "big" things: It wasn't as if Mrs. Harris wanted to smoke or drink or drive around with boys. It was things like whether she should read in bed after nine thirty when she was 16 years old. I asked Mrs. Harris how those rules made her feel. She said, "Furious." She then went on to talk very rapidly about how she had been so obedient throughout her childhood, until she was 13 years old or so. She did not remember ever doing something that her parents did not want her to do. Whatever her parents said was the law, and she never, never rebelled against them. It was only in adolescence that she started getting very angry at her mother and began to have confrontations with her. The worst part was that her mother would not allow her to raise her voice. Her mother would tell her to do something, Mrs. Harris would rebel against it, and then the mother would forbid her to rebel. Mrs. Harris said heatedly that the whole situation really made her quite furious.

I said it was puzzling that she had been such an obedient child during her childhood and then had become such a rebellious and angry adolescent. I wondered where all the anger had come from in a rather sudden way. Mrs. Harris acknowledged that this was indeed puzzling and was silent for a while. Then, shaken by her discovery, she remembered an episode that she placed at 3 years of age. She was being held in a harness and was screaming furiously because she wanted to get out of the harness and roam around in the park. Her mother did not let her out. I said that it seemed as if there were things that had made her angry even as a little girl, that she had been forced to do what the mother wanted regardless of what she felt. Mrs. Harris said that the most infuriating part of her childhood was that she had no choice, that her mother would even forbid her to express her feelings. Not only was she forced to do things that she did not want to do, she was also forced to pretend that she had no feelings about it. I said, "And then that triggered precisely those feelings of anger that your mother wanted to avoid." Mrs. Harris nodded with tears in her eyes. There was a silence. Then slowly and painfully, she said, "And what is sad is that she tried hard. She had the best intentions, and yet she failed at so many things. That is what worries me. We also have very good intentions." I said, "And you are afraid of failing?" Mrs. Harris nodded and there was another silence. Then I said, "Could it be that failing is so frightening because then it would mean that Abby would be angry at you, just as you feel angry with your mother?" Again Mrs. Harris nodded with tears in her eyes.

The predicament was clear. Mrs. Harris did not want to be controlled by Abby as she had been controlled and rendered helpless by her mother. Yet, in fighting her feelings of helplessness, she became as harshly controlling as her mother had been. The fear of Abby's anger and of losing her love was rooted in Mrs. Harris's own childhood anger and rejection of her mother.

"Forcing" Abby was for Mrs. Harris a return of the repressed impulse to retaliate in kind when the old anger toward her mother was aroused by Abby's demands. As Mrs. Harris relived these feelings, the therapist helped her to see the connections between the past and the present. Finally, Mrs. Harris was able to see that Abby was neither controlling nor rejecting her when she turned away. Abby was simply telling her mother that she did not want to eat cereal at that particular time. This realization led Mrs. Harris to a more relaxed attitude toward the introduction of solid foods, and the feeding problems quickly subsided.

ANXIETY AND THE LINKS TO THE BABY BROTHER

In the last period of treatment Mrs. Harris's fear of being overwhelmed by nameless dangers came into the center of the work. The fear that she would be found helpless before dangers that she could not control appeared in many forms in her sessions with the therapist. The exploration of these fears led Mrs. Harris to memories of the birth of her younger brother whom she had mothered when she was a child herself, and the nameless fears could now be named. It was the first baby, her brother, who had evoked the feelings of helplessness and the sense of a great burden which she was unable to bear.

This period of treatment began with the exploration of diffuse feelings of danger and the need to anticipate all possible dangers in order to forestall them. Mrs. Harris feared that her accomplishments as a mother would be short-lived, and that as Abby's signals became more complex, she would be at a loss to interpret them correctly. She imagined problems that might arise when Abby was of preschool age and asked her husband to rehearse with her how to deal with them. This pattern appeared also in areas unrelated to Abby. The prevailing theme seemed to be a fear that she might be faced with events that she would be unable to master. Her fear of losing control prompted Mrs. Harris to be always on the alert lest seemingly routine occurrences signal the onset of dangerous and irreversible events. The following condensed excerpt illustrates the mother's predicament.

> Mrs. Harris started to talk about how, when she was pregnant, she was afraid that she was too old to have maternal instincts. She was afraid that she

was "too old to be a mother." When Abby was born, she found that she did have maternal instincts after all and felt relieved and confident. But this confidence did not last long. She now had different questions. She wanted to know whether Abby would give her clear cues about what she wanted, and whether she, Mrs. Harris, would be able to interpret those cues correctly. I said that somehow the hurdles she had already overcome seemed trivial when she looked back at them, but that the future tasks seemed overwhelming and she feared that she could not master them. She nodded sadly and said that she always needed to plan things well in advance and to the last detail because she feared that at the last minute something might go wrong and she would fail. She was often overprepared for her work, but she could never learn from this experience, and the relief that she felt when she saw she was in control of the situation did not last. I commented that she had done a good job of reading Abby's cues and responding to them, but here too she felt that her success might be temporary and that she might fail in the future. In a slightly sarcastic tone, Mr. Harris said that was why he and his wife always wanted concrete answers, even though they knew that there were few concrete answers about how to respond to a baby. Mrs. Harris said sadly that she never felt safe, that something might always happen that would disrupt her ability to cope.

As Mrs. Harris became aware of the pervasiveness of this pattern, she tried to discover how it was linked to her past. She recalled that her father expected her to be outstanding in everything she did. He pressured her to take four advanced courses in high school and study music and diving in the afternoons. She began to experience severe headaches, and her parents were advised by the family doctor to reduce the academic and achievement pressures.

As one memory led to another, Mrs. Harris recalled vividly the burdens that had been placed on her when her youngest brother was born. She remembered the intense guilt she felt about "giving" her illness to her mother and the mother's subsequent hospitalization. She recalled spending hours alone with her brothers at night, while her father visited her mother at the hospital. Often she was afraid that something would happen in her father's absence and she would not know what to do. Mrs. Harris was puzzled when she remembered how outwardly serene she had been during that painful period. She did not cry or complain but performed all the duties expected of her, including buying everything the newborn would need when he was brought home from the hospital.

Now we could link these childhood fears that she would not be able to do what was expected of her with her need as a grown woman to anticipate all possible contingencies so that she would not be overwhelmed. She remembered that she constantly asked her father for reassurance that she would be able to do what she had been asked to do. Her father reassured her, but his words did not help. On the contrary, his reassurances only made her more anxious. Mrs. Harris could now acknowledge that she feared her father did not know how truly incompetent she was in caring for her baby brother, just as during her pregnancy she had feared her husband did not know how unable she would be to mother her baby. When the therapist asked what Mrs. Harris had thought would happen if she did not live up to her father's demands, she answered, crying: "I was afraid he would not love me." She then recalled her father's punishments. If she repeatedly displeased him, he would order her to bring him a switch with which to hit her. Being incompetent or refusing to please thus represented for Mrs. Harris another terrible danger: rebellion, the loss of her father's love, and painful physical punishment.

The themes of self-dissatisfaction, sense of incompetence, and conflicts over control came up again and again in different contexts and with a variety of affects, ranging from pain to anger. These feelings appeared first in connection with the daily relationship with Abby and were linked in the course of treatment to Mrs. Harris's feelings about her parents and to her own experiences as a child. As Abby was freed from her mother's childhood conflicts, Mrs. Harris began to find unexpected joys in her relationship with her child.

MOTHER'S WORK

Mrs. Harris's increasing commitment to and pleasure in her motherhood were seen most concretely in her plans about returning to work. At the beginning of treatment, Mrs. Harris was eager to return to work as soon as possible, certainly no later than six months after delivery. When Abigail was 3 months old, Mrs. Harris announced she wanted to use the treatment sessions partly to work out a good childcare arrangement which would allow her to resume working. She explained that she and her husband were having financial difficulties because of outstanding debts, but in addition she also wanted to protect Abby from the pressure of her competitiveness. (The therapeutic work that resulted in her understanding the displacement of the impulse to pressure Abby has been reported earlier.)

The date originally set for Mrs. Harris's return to work approached and then passed without her mentioning it. The next time the topic came up, when Abby was 7 months old, Mrs. Harris expressed her *reluctance* to go back to work. While still interested in her career, she felt that there were many years ahead to devote to it, whereas the time she spent now with Abby was precious and irreplaceable. When the therapist reminded her of her previous attitude, Mrs. Harris could hardly believe that she had ever been eager to return to work. In fact, neither she nor her husband could readily remember how trapped Mrs. Harris had felt at the prospect of becoming a mother.

However, financial considerations finally prevailed. The changes in Mrs. Harris's attitude toward her role as a mother were clearly expressed in her preparations to return to work. She refused, without any conflict, her employer's offer of a full-time position. Moreover, she firmly explained to her employer and colleagues that her priorities were now different and that she could no longer be counted on to work after hours. Privately, she decided that she would leave this otherwise ideal job if work conditions proved to interfere with the time she spent with Abby. Mrs. Harris and her husband worked out a schedule that would minimize the pain of separation for Abby. Mr. Harris agreed temporarily to change his work schedule in order to stay with Abby two mornings a week while Mrs. Harris was at work; thus Abby would have to be left at a sitter's home only three mornings a week. As Abby became used to the new routine, she could stay with the baby sitter five mornings a week. The baby sitter, selected with care, was a neighbor who stayed home with her own 1½ year old. Mr. and Mrs. Harris familiarized Abby with the sitter and her home for a few weeks before starting the actual baby-sitting arrangement. All the details that would minimize Abby's distress at the separation from the mother were carefully considered.

ABBY AT 9 MONTHS

At the time treatment was brought to a close, Abby was a thriving 9-month-old. Her predominant mood was one of intense interest in her social and physical surroundings. In a familiar environment she used her parents as a secure base from which to explore, and readily crawled toward the toys prepared for her on the floor. When she was at a distance of a few feet from her parents, she divided her attention among her toys, her parents, and the therapist, and maintained contact with the adults by looking, smiling, and vocalizing. She regularly crawled back to the parents, particularly her mother, and signaled her desire to be picked up. She had a wide range of affect and expressed displeasure in no uncertain terms. She sobered appropriately to strangers, and although she was friendly and responsive to the therapist, she clearly responded differentially to the therapist and to her parents. Her cognitive and motor development were excellent, as tested by the Bayley Scales of Infant Development.

Discussion

For all parents, pregnancy evokes profound feelings in which dreams of the fulfillment of the deepest longings exist side by side with the stirrings of old memories. Anxiety and self-doubt are a normal part of experience of pregnancy. Mrs. Harris might easily have dismissed her own fears, but some wisdom about herself brought her to seek help in the month before her baby was born. She thought her fears were excessive, and she was afraid that her feelings might affect her capacity to be a good mother. It was love for the baby not yet born and the wish that all things should go well for her baby that brought her to seek help. There was something from the past that was intruding, and she could not name it. In the course of the therapeutic work she discovered the source of her anxiety and found resolution for old conflicts which were disturbing her joy in her baby.

During the last month of pregnancy and first months of Abby's life we saw the story unfold in treatment. There had been another baby in this mother's life, a baby brother to whom, as a 10-year-old child, she had been "mother" under most painful circumstances. The memories of that period were vivid. What was *not* remembered were the attendant feelings—helplessness, anger, a certainty that she was, as a child, an incompetent mother. And there were her own parents who had served as harsh models for a woman seeking a new role for herself as mother. What was not remembered was anger, helplessness in the face of the demands of her parents, and fears of loss of love for not meeting expectations.

As the story emerged in treatment we saw how early memories and feelings were revived, in the context of the relationship between mother and baby, and examined in a treatment which focused upon the baby and her parents. The baby was very much present in the interviews. Wherever old conflicts intruded into the relationship of love they were examined in the treatment, and Abby was freed of the impediments of her mother's painful childhood.

The mother's recall of the past was closely united with events in her pregnancy and events in the first nine months of her baby's life. We can retrace the steps in this process of recall:

1. The discovery during pregnancy of negative feelings that did not belong to a baby who was wanted and already loved.
2. The fear "I can't be a good mother."
3. Following the baby's birth, a comparison between the quiet Abby and the fretful brother who had been her "first baby."
4. The reproach she felt when the baby cried and she could not comfort

her; the feeling that Abby was disappointed in her and would not love her.

5. Memories of her own parents who demanded perfection in her; fears that she would lose their love unless she was perfect—Abby representing, strangely, Mrs. Harris's own demanding mother who could never be satisfied and representing also Mrs. Harris herself as someone in danger of losing love.

6. The emergence of feelings toward her own mother—anger, reproach.

7. The discovery of urges within herself to "push" Abby toward precocious accomplishment.

8. Emergence of a feeding problem in Abby in which Mrs. Harris found herself wanting to force her baby to eat.

9. The themes of "forcing" and "being forced" leading back to the struggle between Mrs. Harris and her own mother and the recollection of the feelings of helplessness and fear in herself as a small child. The painful recognition "I am like my mother!" The discovery with the help of the therapist that anger and fear had played a part in that first "identification with her mother as 'aggressor.' "

10. Helplessness, as a theme, moving toward another vital connection: the birth of her baby brother and her own helplessness and fears of her own competence as a 10-year-old "mother." This time the memories and the feelings came together in a profound insight.

As each of the links between past and present was discovered in the course of treatment, as the therapist gave meaning to these events through interpretation, Mrs. Harris was freed from the intrusive memories and feelings that disturbed her joy in her child. At the close of treatment, Abby and her parents were free in their love of each other. Where residues of the past still remained for Mrs. Harris, she could now recognize them as "belonging to the past" and not to Abby. This is the aim of infant-parent psychotherapy. Mrs. Harris, who had profited largely from this treatment, now wanted treatment for herself, no longer because she feared she could not be a good mother but because she wanted fulfillment in other areas of her life which were still affected by memories of the past.

XI

Martha: A Focused Clinical Use of the Bayley in Consultation

JEREE PAWL

JOHN W. BENNETT, JR.*

THIS CASE illustrates the way in which a request for a circumscribed developmental assessment of an infant (the Bayley Scales of Infant Development) can develop into a fruitful diagnostic and therapeutic consultation.

The Child Development Project received a phone call on behalf of a 9-month-old baby girl, Martha. A social worker at a private psychiatric hospital was in the process of making discharge plans for a young woman, Mrs. Jenner, who had been hospitalized for two months following serious decompensation and was now about to return home to her husband and daughter. She had been hospitalized once previously for psychiatric care, late in her pregnancy with Martha.

A public health nurse had visited the home after the baby had been born, up to the point of Mrs. Jenner's hospitalization, and these visits would continue after discharge. During her mother's hospitalization, Martha was cared for every day by the same person and at night by her father. The parents would be receiving outpatient treatment, and Mrs. Jenner would continue to spend some part of the day at the hospital in

---

*John W. Bennett, Jr. was the consultant; Jeree Pawl was the supervisor.

a controlled therapeutic environment. The agency specifically requested that a Bayley test be administered to the baby. The request was neither for an assessment, nor an evaluation, but was limited solely to a
Bayley testing.

The social worker appeared to have in mind getting the Bayley assessment of Martha so that there would be some reference point to
which the child could later be compared. We felt it was pertinent to explore exactly what was to be compared, and by whom. That there
might be a reasonable consultative role for the Child Development
Project seemed evident, but it was not specifically requested and would
need to be carefully articulated. What we could do, and for whom,
would have to be made very clear. It was necessary from the very beginning to work with the hospital social worker in order to clarify with
him exactly what his request was. It was necessary, not because we
knew and he didn't, but because neither of us knew. Experience had
taught us that a Bayley testing, in and of itself, can give some useful information about how a child is functioning in terms of cognitive motor
performance at a particular time in comparison with other infants his
own age. But it is not predictive, nor can variations in performance at a
later administration explain the complicated processes underlying the
variations. We knew from experience that a Bayley testing embedded
in a series of contacts with the parents could yield additional, different,
and more useful information. We needed to discover whether anything
in that realm of information was what was being asked for. We needed
to know what kinds of things the social worker hoped to learn as a result of this "testing."

Direct questioning might be helpful, but it is more likely to produce
answers that are either confused or of little more use than the initial request. What *is* useful is to ask permission to pose questions about the
baby to the person making the request. This can lead to a gradual eluci-
dation of the kinds of things there are to know about the baby and his
parents.

In this instance the consultant asked for the social worker's general
impressions of the baby, knowing he had seen her. The social worker
said he was not particularly knowledgeable about babies, but he had
noticed some things about Martha: "She smiles quite a bit when she
visits the hospital"; "She is active, but not overly active"; and "She
seems to be quite content a good deal of the time." He had other observations. While it seemed to the social worker that Mrs. Jenner couldn't
really notice or care about the baby at all when she was first hospitalized, he felt this was no longer the case, although it was difficult for
him to say exactly where that impression came from. Somewhere in
this conversation the Child Development Project consultant commented that if the baby were 8 to 9 months old, one would begin to expect

to see some sorts of reactions around separation and asked if the social worker had noted any. The social worker responded with a good deal of very important and pertinent information regarding the important people in Martha's life. He described how her days were typically structured, and he began to wonder how that sort of thing might affect the process of Martha's dealing with separation. As the discussion continued, it provided increasingly more meaningful detail about Martha's and her mother's experiences of separation and their reactions to them. The social worker went on to talk about Mrs. Jenner's recent inability to experience much pleasure in Martha and about Mrs. Jenner's sadness about this.

Gradually, in this way, by the mutual exploration of the child and her surround, important areas about which one might wish information were identified. It became clear that the social worker was not solely interested in Martha's cognitive motor performance on the Bayley. Rather, he was also interested in our assessment of the child's dominant mood and affect, in the child's social functioning, and in the indicators of attachment to the parents. Our view of Martha's general adaptive functioning would be useful to him. And he would welcome our observations not only of Martha herself but of interactions between Martha and her parents.

It was agreed that in order for observations to take place so that such information could be supplied, the cooperation and understanding of both parents would be necessary. The project consultant would meet with the parents and explain the purpose of the testing to them. The testing would also be followed by meetings with the parents in order to talk about the results.

Thus, this request for a "Bayley testing" expanded in the course of the phone call into an agreement to an evaluation which, though very focused and narrow, would take three or four sessions and provide some information about a child's general functioning and her relationship with her parents. This kind of brief engagement by us with various families has occurred in many slightly different forms, often from just such small beginning requests.

In this instance, the conversation had begun to clarify what would comprise the focus and content of the evaluation. There still remained the very important issue of designating clearly the consultee(s) for whom the evaluation was being done.

The hospital social worker responsible for coordinating after-care, the person requesting the evaluation, needed to remain a central person in the evaluation. Still, his role would end, except for the possibility of readmission, when Mrs. Jenner was discharged. It also became obvious from the conversation with the social worker that the public health nurse was extremely important in a variety of ways. She had provided the social worker with very useful information regarding Martha's early developmental history. Also, she was not someone, like the psychiatrist, who would only begin seeing the family after the mother's discharge and who at this point had no knowledge of or relationship with the family. The public health nurse had had a relationship with the family for nine months, and this would continue. When the social worker and consultant had clarified this, it became evident that the evaluation was being done primarily for the psychiatrist and the public health nurse, both of whom would have ongoing responsibility for the family. In effect, the "consultee" was not only the social worker who had called but also the psychiatrist and the public health nurse. It was agreed between the social worker and the consultant that the latter would convey the agreed-upon focus and use of the consultation to the psychiatrist. Because of the public health nurse's relationship with the family and her greater ongoing involvement, the consultant chose to include her in the process in a special way. He offered her the possibility of a brief consultation at the end of the assessment, if that should appear useful to her. It was understood that written reports would be sent to the social worker, the psychiatrist, and the public health nurse. As the social worker at the hospital was currently seeing the parents, he became the logical person to introduce the consultant to the family. The consultant made it clear that he wished the initial introduction to include the entire family. This would provide an opportunity to get to know them in a situation less formally structured than the Bayley provides.

The parents and Martha were introduced to the consultant by the social worker in his hospital office. Martha sat on her father's lap. She was chubby, shiny-haired, apple-cheeked, and bright of eye. As the consultant greeted Martha from a distance in a friendly way, Martha studied him intently. She frequently glanced at both of her parents and then back to the consultant. Her demeanor was sober. The consultant commented on how pretty the child was. He also said to Martha, "You know I'm new and different, don't you? It makes you feel better when you check and make sure your mother and dad are still there." A brief conversation between the consultant and the father regarding some of the skills Martha had recently acquired was interrupted by the social worker, who inquired if the consultant were going to tell the parents about the Bayley. The consultant apologized for not informing them he would take a little time to get acquainted with Mr. and Mrs. Jenner and Martha. It would give Martha a chance to look him over and hear his voice before they played together next week. The consultant then inquired as to time available. They all agreed to an additional half-hour.

Mrs. Jenner spoke up and said she was afraid Martha didn't remember her because of her being in the hospital so much and the visits being so few. The consultant acknowledged this as a natural concern and asked how the visits between them had been. Mrs. Jenner said that at first Martha had smiled at her during these visits, but now she didn't smile at her any more. The consultant acknowledged the disappointment a person would feel at that and said, "Martha looks to you a lot when she is confronted with a new person. I think that would mean she remembers you and that you are very important to her." As Mrs. Jenner and the consultant talked, Martha, from her father's lap, made an invitational gesture toward her mother, which the consultant pointed out to Mrs. Jenner. After a few more interchanges, the consultant began to talk about the process they would be undertaking. He began by inviting questions and concerns. He also utilized this time to inform the parents very concretely that he would be giving certain people information from these meetings with them and Martha. He specifically mentioned the social worker, the public health nurse, and the psychiatrist. The consultant made a point of telling the parents that time would be provided after the formal testing so that they could ask questions and so that he could talk with them about what he had learned about Martha and about exactly what information he would be giving out. This assurance served to reduce the anxiety of the parents regarding what might be said about them and their child.

Once this was discussed, the consultant focused on the Bayley itself. He said, "I will be giving Martha a number of things to do with simple toys. With these toys, I will be providing Martha with some simple problem-solving situations so that I can get an idea of how she approaches them and reacts to them. There will be a range of difficulty from ones I am sure Martha can easily handle, to ones I think she probably can't do." The consultant pulled the Bayley red ring from his pocket and dangled it in front of Martha, asking her to look at it. She immediately dropped a toy she was holding, looked up at both the ring and the consultant with great interest, and reached for the ring. She grasped it, examined it with her hands and eyes, and then passed it from hand to hand. The consultant explained to the parents that the ring was an actual Bayley item, but not one that he would be giving Martha during the evaluation. He pointed out to the parents how Martha passed the ring from hand to hand and he said, "Some children will do that at 4 months and others won't begin to do it until 8. Half the children will be doing it by around 5 months. If Martha were 5 months old and doing that, I would say she was doing something that was expected developmentally exactly at her age level." The consultant then used the string of the Bayley ring as another example. Again he described Martha's responses and compared her manipulations of the string to expectations at various age levels. He used a ball to further illustrate the simple kinds of items that would be employed. He emphasized that these tests were not to be merely passed or failed but to indicate where a child was functioning developmentally.

This introduction to the Bayley testing was followed by a request for permission to videotape the testing. The parents were told there were two main ways in which taping the testing could be helpful. First, it allows for the most useful consultation with colleagues at the Project if there are any questions. Second, and more important, it provides the best way for the consultant and the parents to review the testing and its results and to discuss them. The consultant also said that it was possible to do all of these things without a taping and that some people preferred not to have it used. Both parents readily agreed to the use of it.

Martha began babbling, and Mrs. Jenner mentioned that she does that a lot. Mr. Jenner added that she particularly does a lot of it in her crib. He said that she often says "momma" and "dadda." Mrs. Jenner said she wasn't sure that she knew *she* was momma, even though she said the word. The consultant replied that if she doesn't yet, she certainly has all the pieces, doesn't she? She has the word and she recognizes and knows that her mother is an important person, now all she needs to do is to link all of that together.

The consultant continued by outlining for the parents the number of times he wished to meet with them. They then discussed the schedule and set a time for an appointment.

After appropriate good-byes were said, the consultant spent some time with the social worker, who commented that he was beginning to get the idea that the Bayley might be something therapeutic for the family to experience. He also thought it was useful to point out the times when Mrs. Jenner and Martha were aware of one another and that it spoke to Mrs. Jenner's concerns in a very nice way. The consultant responded that he hoped it would be a useful experience and a benign one. He added that he felt the way the baby was functioning meant that both Mr. and Mrs. Jenner had been able to give sufficient time and energy to her, despite what must have been an extremely difficult period. He said he hoped they could take some pride in this. He commented that Martha's continual checking-in with her mother had been a most reassuring thing to see. The social worker then asked if the consultant had made any other observations. The consultant made a few comments about Martha's affect, which was somewhat subdued. He said that in new situations most babies will be somewhat sobered; it would be interesting to see whether that changed. There was then some mutual discussion of the stressful and difficult situation for every member of the family.

It seemed evident to the consultant that the social worker was very comfortable and even enthusiastic about the wider focus of the evaluation with the inclusion of a clinical assessment.

Both parents, as arranged, were present for the Bayley. By agreement, it took place at the Child Development Project. A brief time was set aside at the beginning so that the parents and Martha could get somewhat used to the setting and the presence of the camera and cameraperson. After some sense of comfort was established, the consultant began the administration of the Bayley. Throughout the administration the consultant made comments to the parents regarding Martha's performance. He complimented Martha on her good skills and on her enthusiastic involvement. He informed the parents of his expectations of Martha's performance on various items, in order to help them avoid making erroneous assumptions about what was really expected in response to an item.

At the end of the testing, time was allowed in order to answer the most pressing questions that it had raised in the parents' minds. In this instance, since Martha had done so uniformly well, the consultant's task of answering questions was a relatively easy one. After these initial questions were addressed, he arranged with the parents for a further session to discuss the meaning of the testing in which they had participated.

At that meeting the videotape was used to concretize the comments the consultant wished to make and to address the questions that the parents had raised. It was understood that the tape could be stopped at any point, reversed, replayed—anything that would aid in understanding. The consultant began by repeating again that Martha had done extremely well, and he used the tape to demonstrate her many successes. He described these successes in a way which allowed the parents to appreciate the many skills that coalesced in a successful engagement with even very simple tasks. He pointed out to the parents how important their interactions with Martha had been in her doing so well. Both parents had been very sensitive and supportive of Martha's efforts, encouraging her on difficult items and responding to her pleasure in her own success. The consultant related this to the parents' general efforts in staying invested and involved with Martha at a time when things were so very difficult for them both. Mr. and Mrs. Jenner responded very positively to this.

They all discussed Martha's persistence on difficult tasks and her ability to invest without becoming frustrated. The consultant focused on the importance of Martha's confidence that she could find objects that disappeared. He suggested that if the parents had not taken the time or had the energy to arrange and carry out visits for Martha, the resulting anxiety and upset at so sustained a loss of her mother could very well have been reflected in an inability to cope with such items. Instead, it was possible to see that the ability was developing sturdily. Her opportunities to intermittently renew her relationship with her mother were reflected in her confidence in the existence of objects that were not within her sight. At this time the consultant complimented the parents again on their ability during the difficult months to consider Martha and to provide so well for her development.

The parents then seemed comfortable enough to voice their concerns regarding Martha's mood—somewhat subdued, sometimes seeming even sad. The filmed session appeared to be a close match to what the parents saw at home, and it concerned them both. The consultant accepted the naturalness of their concern, but then he addressed the positive aspect of it. First, he talked about how the sadness reflected a loss, but a loss of something good. If what was lost had not been good, there would not be the sadness. Also, he said the sadness was really appropriate, healthy, and realistic. An infant who showed no signs of sadness over a loss, temporary but so important, would be an infant about whom one would need to worry. It made it harder for the parents, but it was actually a very healthy, appropriate response and spoke, as well, to the early good things that had been part of the baby's experience. This allowed Mrs. Jenner to address her sadness at the loss of Martha for those two months and particularly at the loss of closeness she felt they were experiencing. Mrs. Jenner was encouraged to expand in some slight way on what this meant. She said that one of the things it meant was that she felt Martha no longer really cared about her in the same way or wanted to be close to her in the same way. She had begun to feel that this closeness was simply something she was going to have to do without, though she missed it very much; perhaps Martha had outgrown her need for such closeness.

After some discussion, the consultant, by using the tape, was able to point out to Mrs. Jenner that something rather different was going on. He was able to show her very graphically that she and Martha were missing one another's cues. The evidence was incontrovertible on the tape that Martha would at times reach out to her mother and indicate a wish for more closeness to her, but that her mother would be oblivious to it. It was also clear that there were moments when the mother indicated that she wished to involve herself in a closer way with Martha, and Martha failed to notice it. The consultant suggested that, rather than having outgrown the need for closeness, they were instead out of the habit of being so quickly sensitive to one another. It would take a while for that to return. The important thing was that the wish was there, and that seemed to him undeniable. He went so far as to make suggestions to Mrs. Jenner about those occasions in which it would be most likely for this closeness to return: times when Martha was sleepy, when she was being read to or put to bed. It would be impossible to say how long-lasting Mrs. Jenner's grasp of the truth of this would prove to be, but there was no question that she understood it at the time. When it seemed to the consultant that they had exhausted what there was for them to discuss, he said as much. The parents agreed and indicated that the experience had been a very useful one to them. They suggested, in fact, that they could imagine finding it useful to have a similar assessment at a later time. The consultant said that if at any time they felt this would be useful, he was sure that all they needed to do was mention it to the psychiatrist or public health nurse, and it could then be arranged. There was general agreement that they had truly enjoyed, all of them, meeting one another.

This meeting with the family concluded the Child Development Project's contacts with them. What followed was the writing, by the consultant, of an extremely full and detailed report that was intended for the three consultees. In this instance, the same report was appropriate for all three, although in many other circumstances this would not be true. The report covered what had been agreed upon. In addition to presenting a review of the infant's recent history and current situation, it included clinical observations and, in a separate section, clinical inferences that might be drawn from those. It included a description of the dominant mood and affect of the child and of the child's general social and adaptive functioning. It also included a description of cognitive motor functioning as well as the formal Bayley scores. The more inferential section was labeled as just that, with warnings as to how it must be viewed in order for it to be useful. Nonetheless, is was possible on the basis of this analysis to make very useful recommendations as to what could be both looked for and worked with in the parents' treatment that would have to do with the harmony or disharmony in the infant-parent interactions. A strong case was made for following up on the observed instances in which Martha and her mother were missing one another's invitations and therefore missing one another.

The consultant also communicated very carefully in this report the degree to which and the level at which information had been discussed with the parents.

From the responses of the consultees, it seemed that they had all found the consultant's evaluation and report extremely useful. The response of the parents suggested that they too had found it interesting, helpful, and relatively benign in terms of the degree of anxiety it had provoked.

The consultant had the satisfaction of knowing that there was in writing a description of Martha and of her parents against which someone could usefully assess change at some future point, should it seem relevant. Perhaps most important at the moment, everyone could take pleasure in the fact that Martha was developing beautifully, that she was attached to her parents in a good and meaningful way, and that the potential was there for both mother and child to overcome the reactions to their separation. That this development needed careful watching was true, but the potential was there.

All of this seemed absolute justification for the time and energy it had taken to work out a meaningful interaction with the family, based on what was initially a very limited request.

XII

Beginning at the Beginning: The Introduction of Infant Mental Health Services to Community Mental Health Clinics

VIVIAN SHAPIRO
EDNA ADELSON
BETTY TABLEMAN

IN THIS CHAPTER we will describe a training program for infant mental health specialists which developed through the collaboration of the Michigan Department of Mental Health and the Child Development Project.

As we have described elsewhere in this book, our concept of infant mental health embraced services, professional training, and community organization on behalf of infants and their families. We did not conceive of the Child Development Project as a "model" but could imagine, even in the early stages of our work, that the underlying principles of this form of intervention could be applied in many settings other than our own and should in every instance be responsive to the needs of a community.

The Michigan Department of Mental Health had learned of our program and responded with considerable interest. In 1972 Betty Table-man (subsequently an administrator of prevention programming for the Michigan Department of Mental Health) met with Selma Fraiberg to discuss the possibility of developing a training program in infant mental health for professionals already working in community agencies in the state mental health system. In a series of meetings among senior staff members of the Child Development Project and Mrs. Tableman, we began to examine our own experience in training at the Child Development Project, to ask ourselves new questions which arose in extending a training program to a diverse group of experienced clinicians practicing in widespread geographic areas in the state. The program that evolved, which is described herein, represented the joint thinking of the Child Development Project staff and Mrs. Tableman. Edna Adelson served as director of the training program in 1973–74, and Vivian Shapiro was director during 1974–75.

Our own experience at the Child Development Project in both graduate and residency training provided a useful model, but one that would have to be modified in many respects for a group of trainees who had already received basic clinical training in their fields. They now needed from us an education specifically concerned with parent/infant relations in the first three years of life and the application of clinical skill to a population not yet served in mental health clinics, the at-risk baby and his parents. As in our own program at the Child Development Project, we did not conceive of infant mental health as a new discipline but rather an extension of professional education in the several mental health disciplines serving infants. This concept proved as congenial to the State Department of Mental Health as it was to us.

The main components of our intensive graduate training program at the Child Development Project were supervised casework and seminars. We saw these as the indispensable parts of the state program as well, but again, some additions and modifications would have to be made for this special group of trainees.

The training program called for a contract between the state, the Child Development Project, and twelve clinics. The budget, of necessity, would be a modest one. The trainees would be selected from community mental health clinics throughout the state of Michigan, representing diverse economic and geographic communities. Participation in the training program would be voluntary on the part of any clinic in the state network. Clinic administrators would not only offer support for the new program but would also have to participate, through workshops and special meetings, in the program's development. They would need to be facilitators of the program, within both their clinics and their communities.

The training program that was developed for the state consisted of the following major parts: one, the collaborative working agreement among the clinics, the state, and the Child Development Project; two, the development of the training program itself; and three, the initiation of new programs by the trainees which would lead to the extension of mental health services to infants.

The Collaborative Working Agreement

A collaborative working model among the state, the Child Development Project, and the twelve clinics was developed and modified over the two-year period 1973–75. The clinics were widely scattered but within a three-hundred-mile radius of Ann Arbor. They were located in rural, sparsely settled areas with minimal services and in urban areas densely populated and served by a full range of medical and social institutions. Some of the designated clinics were child guidance clinics, and others were general mental health clinics. The seminar members were equally diverse, ranging in age from the late twenties to the late fifties. Four participants were experienced clinicians and supervisors, while the others were at the staff level with varying amounts of experience. Their backgrounds were in social work, psychology, nursing, and counseling.

The diversity of the trainees and their clinics made it necessary to think of teaching methods that would satisfy individual and group needs. A combination of workshops, seminars, and individual supervisions was developed to address individual circumstances as well as to allow broad dissemination of knowledge and to foster clinic involvement. The trainees came to the Child Development Project for a year of biweekly seminars and case supervision. Workshops were distributed throughout the year and were used to introduce broad issues in infant mental health to clinic staff and community colleagues, thus building a background of support and understanding for the trainees from within their own work environments.

The state awarded the Child Development Project a contract which enabled it to undertake the training program. Individual clinics were asked to assume the cost of transportation, released time, and any additional clerical help needed for their trainees. In addition the clinics agreed to develop a program of infant mental health services as a condition to their participation. Mrs. Tableman, as state representative and organizer of the training program, kept in close touch with the clinics, the trainees, and the Child Development Project.

The Training Program: Goals and Format

It was hoped that each of these experienced clinicians could become the infant specialist in his clinic, someone who had knowledge about babies and their parents, who could evaluate the status of the infant's mental health and who could take the responsibility for getting appropriate help to the family at the critical time. The basis for the new skills was, of course, an intensive education in infant and early childhood development. The Child Development Project's own emphasis was on the centrality of infant-parent attachment for the emotional development of the infant. Thus the focus was not only on the baby but on the dyadic relationship between infant and parent.

Our experience at the Child Development Project had shown us that clinical assessment of the infant and the infant/parent relationship was central to every phase of our work. Our methods of assessment (see Chapter II) move from extended observation to clinical inference and formulation of treatment plans. Our training plan for graduate students and residents had shown us that a trainee from any clinical discipline could acquire competence in clinical assessment of the infant and his family in the course of one year of training. We could reasonably expect, therefore, that the trainees in the state program who were experienced child clinicians could attain competence in assessment through a one-year training program, even though the supervision and teaching were less intensive than in our in-house training programs. The trainees' clinical experience would greatly aid them. The clinician who already possessed a professional background and diverse experience in child and family work would, after all, come to an infant program with a body of knowledge and technical competence, and this could be translated to infant work with augmentation of new knowledge and specialized skills.

The methods of treatment which we had developed in our own program included developmental guidance on behalf of the infant, supportive treatment, and a form of infant-parent psychotherapy, all of which have been described in this volume. Each is a special adaptation for infant work of a body of professional skills which every experienced child clinician has developed for older children and their families. Of these methods only infant-parent psychotherapy is an invention of our own program which is not usually part of the professional experience of the child clinician. An experienced clinician, we felt, could be educated through the training program to translate his professional skills in developmental guidance and supportive treatment to infant work in one year. However our experience has shown us that infant-parent psychotherapy, which requires the most intensive supervi-

273

sion in our Child Development Project training program (and typically was the method of choice for the most severely disturbed infants and parents). We were less confident that these methods could be transmitted, even to experienced clinicians, with biweekly supervision.

Finally, we saw as one other very important outcome of the projected training program the development of a core of trained infant specialists who could bring to their communities new knowledge about the needs of infants and their parents and who could affect child service programs and community planning at many crucial points in the network that identifies children in need. Our trainees, we hoped, might bring the previously "invisible" infant into the center of community concern and service. They could be the spokesmen for the infant, the interpreters for the infant and his parents in consultation with community clinics and other agencies, and they would become themselves, in the broadest terms, the educators in infant mental health. As infant mental health specialists they could serve Protective Services, foster care agencies, social services, newborn nurseries, and primary medical care centers, bringing new ideas to those programs whose decisions so critically affect infants and young children. In this way, for the first time in many communities, plans for the prevention of mental health disorders would include the infants and could be conceived as the responsibility of every professional group concerned with the health and welfare of children.

As has been mentioned, the format for the training program was a combination of biweekly seminars, case supervision, and workshops. The seminars included a review of significant research findings in infant development in the fields of medicine, developmental and clinical psychology, and psychoanalytic studies. An important part of the seminars was the use of the Child Development Project's own library of videotapes and clinical research material which illustrated assessment and clinical case issues.

In our Child Development Project training program at the university, individual supervision was a primary method of clinical teaching. Students were able to begin their work by following study cases where they might learn about infant development in a relaxed mode by following the development of a normal baby over the course of a year. The state trainees brought in cases from their own clinics for supervision. For them, a slow-paced start was not possible. As soon as the trainee clinics opened their doors to infants, the most severely at-risk cases were referred, probably because these cases were the most visible and disturbing to the referring agencies. The trainees were thus quickly involved in serious cases, and much was expected of them by their clinics and their communities in a short period of time. The new responsibilities were often stressful, and the trainees were helped in this new clinical work by their case supervisors at the project and by their seminar colleagues, who offered support in framing diagnostic questions, if not in having ready answers.

The initial clinical training focused primarily on assessment. Most times these assessments led to the development of services and a therapeutic intervention for the infant and parents within the trainees' clinics, and resulted in good outcome. In exceptional cases the assessment led to recommendations for separation of the infant from the parent because no therapeutic help was available to reach the parent in time to save the child. The gaps in services for children became painfully apparent to the trainees. This experience led the trainees to become active consultants to their clinics and communities.

It was evident within the first year of training that through development of expertise in the new area of infant mental health, each trainee was becoming his clinic's infant specialist and community consultant. The demand for services was burgeoning, and the trainees moved to new roles as infant mental health consultants.

Pathway from Trainee to Infant Mental Health Consultant

A useful way to illustrate the nature and effectiveness of the training model is to consider in some detail the way two trainees used their experiences to expand their clinical work and then to move from direct casework in their own clinics to the role of agency and community infant mental health consultants. These examples are representative of the path that most trainees followed in becoming infant mental health specialists.

The first example is that of a clinician (Michael Trout) at North Central Michigan Mental Health Center, a four-county rural clinic. The first cases referred to Mr. Trout were severely endangered babies: a baby beaten by his 16-year-old mother, an infant who had been vomiting since birth, a baby with leukemia. He soon recognized that one mental health staff person alone could not make much of an impact on the high-risk infant family problems in his area. He realized too that there were some very competent and dedicated people in his community already dealing with infants. However, existing practice often reflected a lack of understanding of the needs of infants and parents. As a first step the trainee organized a multidiscipline team to discuss infant mental health needs. He visited eighteen people in public health, social services, the probate courts, the cooperative extension service, and the hospital, all of whom agreed to participate in a working group. The Infant Development Team began by reviewing what the trainee had learned about the identification of high-risk babies and modes of intervention. After working through the need for administrative sanction, the group coalesced into twelve to fifteen members meeting monthly for mutual learning and program discussion. That monthly meeting was augmented by a case coordinating committee which met weekly to review cases.

The trainee also provided consultation to public health nurses, the probate court, and others who were carrying the bulk of the infant caseload.

In the course of many weeks of discussion the group began to reexamine many types of problems in patients labeled "hard to reach." With new appreciation for the psychology of human attachment and the meaning of separation and loss for the mothers and fathers as well as the babies, new approaches were developed. The practitioner's ability to engage families, as well as the parents' responsiveness to the guidance and care being offered, was enhanced.

In a review of his first year of work Mr. Trout described the way in which one nurse used her new understanding of the parental need for mothering as a way of making contact with a previously unavailable mother. The nurse had been visiting a mother who chronically ignored and neglected her child. She had been unable to develop a working alliance with this mother, and was trying to understand the problems within the framework of her training. She wrote of the following turning point in her work with this mother:

> I was anxious to leave the W home. I had lots of visits to make that day and, besides, Mrs. W seemed far too manipulative and anxious for my attention for me to allow myself to stay. When I finally decided to sit down with her for a few moments, she kept talking about how her mother kept badgering her to come for a visit. What she was trying to tell me finally sank in and I said, "You seem to be telling me that you're lonely for your mother. I wonder if you would really like to spend some time with her?" Mrs. W became very quiet, reached over and picked up the child she had always ignored (on today's and previous visits), and with her child on her lap began telling me how lost she sometimes feels as a mother.

In this case, the nurse, with new understanding regarding bonding and human attachment, had used a psychological insight (into the mother's feelings of loss and her need for mothering) as a way to reach the mother. The mother, once having expressed her feelings and having these feelings acknowledged, had reached out for her child, something we have also seen in our work at the Child Development Project.

Mr. Trout's program continues to be recognized by his community and by the state for its contributions to the development of comprehensive mental health services to infants.

Another trainee (Mary K. Peterson), a skilled nurse from Marquette Community Mental Health Center, expanded children's services to include children under age three. While participating in our program, infants in families she had been seeing became more differentiated and visible to her. In this context, she became concerned about Karen, a 5-month-old twin baby girl. Her healthy twin, Sandra, was developing normally in all areas. This was not the case for Karen, who spent most of her days lying neglected in bed. The reciprocity that existed between mother and Sandra did not occur between mother and Karen, and the expected responsiveness of smile, recognition, and gaze were absent between them. Further, the Bayley criteria showed that she was behind the norms both cognitively and motorically. It became clear that mother avoided this baby.

The trainee undertook the case for assessment under supervision at the Child Development Project. The assessment raised the following questions: "What was the basis for Karen's poor development, and what accounted for the neglect of this baby by her mother?" The carefully supervised assessment revealed that there were complex diagnostic issues. Although both babies were premature, only Karen experienced poor health, which led to prolonged and repeated hospitalizations. There was now evidence of a severe impairment in the bonding process between Karen and her mother. Further, a psychiatric assessment revealed that mother was clinically severely depressed.

The assessment was not an easy one. Nor was the outcome a comfortable reunion of infant and mother. As a result of the crisis situation and the unavailability of intensive therapeutic care for the mother, the baby was temporarily placed in a foster home.

The trainee and her colleagues now realized that there had been critical points along the way where appropriate intervention could have promoted bonding between Karen and her mother. Karen's mother had needed early guidance about the developmental problems of premature babies. She had distanced herself from her baby whom she feared she might lose. She needed supportive therapy to respond to her own feelings of anticipated loss and to the difficulty in ministering at home to a baby who seemed indifferent and unresponsive after repeated separations.

In this case, the trainee, in the process of reaching a resolution, shared her new understanding of disorders of early attachment with the nurses and physicians in the hospital and the public health program. This led to the development of a multidiscipline, ongoing case review and discussion group. The work of this group led to the modification of practices in the newborn nursery of the pediatric unit, making possible preventive intervention in future cases. As a result, the trainee also became involved in consultation to Protective Services and child welfare workers. In her community there are now strong linkages between the public health program, the hospital, the child welfare agency, and the community mental health clinic. These linkages are also developing in the other communities where services are being offered by other trainees.

Impact of the Training Program

Since 1973 there have been major changes in the clinical roles of the trainees, the priorities within their clinics, and the provision of infant mental health services in the state of Michigan. In briefest summary, all of the trainees were able to acquire sufficient assessment skills so that they were able to coordinate the appropriate medical, psychological, and developmental understanding necessary for a complete assessment. Most of the trainees were able to provide guidance and supportive therapy to families using their new observational skills of the infant and the infant-parent pair and working on an outreach basis. Many of the trainees also began to undertake intensive infant-parent psychotherapy in cases where the infant was gravely at risk and there was significant parental pathology. This treatment depended primarily on the clinician's experience, confidence, agency sanction, and access to supervision and support. The year of biweekly training could only be a beginning of new infant-centered psychotherapeutic skills; continued growth would, of course, require continuing experience and supervision. In all, however, the effect of the clinical training on the development of infant mental health programming has been outstanding.

Some trainees have also used their training to become consultants to their clinics and communities. The consultations have been in the form of seminars and workshops, individual case consultations, the organizing of infant development teams and multidiscipline case review groups, and the guidance of new community programming for infants.

This work has resulted in changes in community agencies serving infants—changes in staff attitudes and practice in hospitals and medical practices, in public health programs, in the courts, and in Protective Services.

In almost half of the clinics the training resulted in the reallocation of staff resources so that trainees could spend all or half their time on infant work. In the remainder of clinics, it became apparent that new resources would have to be found to free the trainees to spend any substantial amount of time on infant work. In all clinics, however, there has been an extension of services to types of problems that previously would have been overlooked, turned away, or misdiagnosed.

On the state level, infant mental health programming is now moving into a new phase. The trainees have successfully developed a Michigan Association for Infant Mental Health with an interdisciplinary membership, a newsletter, and annual conferences which are widely recognized for their merit and are well attended. The Department of Mental Health has obtained funding for prevention programming, and development of infant services has been given a high priority. Beginning in 1976–77, for example, three of the clinics in the training program received special pilot demonstration grants, and one trainee has been involved at the state level in extending various types of infant programming to other areas. Considerable effort is going into the definition and evaluation of a community service model. Although infant mental health services have not yet become a part of mandated services in Michigan, widespread interest has been expressed by community mental health clinics, and there has been support from legislative study committees and the executive office. Recently, the state has agreed to collaborate with the Child Development Project in another training program for nine additional clinicians to staff existing and newly developing infant programs.

In summary, through our training program we learned that it is possible to train clinicians in community mental health centers to become their clinics' infant mental health specialists. We learned that an important new area of their work would be consultation to their own clinics and other community agencies. The trainees, therefore, need to be capable of both clinical and community organization/consultative skills. The most successful trainees are those who are able to develop relationships of trust and professional acceptance within both their clinics and their communities. As a group, they also need to offer each other support in order that individually they might carry the burden of the new knowledge and new responsibilities. In all, the program seems to have successfully expanded the treatment capacity to infants within the state's community mental health system. There is evidence of change in clinic practices and priorities and community programming, change which reflects an acceptance of infant mental health as an important area of concern. A major step has been taken toward the development of a comprehensive infant mental health program.